This book is explosive in the way that fireworks are explosive; it dazzles with its fire, it illuminates dark places in psychology, it celebrates the light towards which we can all go. At a time when our discipline is teetering on the precipice where we can choose to go backwards towards the Eurocentric frameworks that have defined and restrained psychology since its inception, or allow ourselves to have the courage to join in the liberatory project of decolonizing our understanding of humans in every setting, through all possible intersectional lenses, this volume is our guidebook to the territory of this emerging, powerful paradigm. Essential reading for all of us; for those, like myself, decades in the field; for those who teach and train and do research; for those offering healing. Brava/o to editors and authors alike.

–LAURA S. BROWN, PhD, ABPP, INDEPENDENT PRACTICE; DEPARTMENT OF PSYCHIATRY AND BEHAVIORAL SCIENCES, UNIVERSITY OF WASHINGTON, SEATTLE; AND PAST PRESIDENT OF APA DIVISIONS 35, 44, 56 AND WASHINGTON STATE PSYCHOLOGICAL ASSOCIATION

Comas-Díaz, Adames, and Chavez-Dueñas have aptly responded to an urgent call to examine past and current impacts of colonization on the discipline of psychology. The authors, in this significant volume, provide compelling information that is the basis for a sea change in how we approach theory, research, teaching, and practice. The authors' rich examples bring to life the profound problems of colonization as well as the profound potential for decolonial psychology.

–PRATYUSHA (USHA) TUMMALA-NARRA, PhD, BOSTON UNIVERSITY, BOSTON, MA

Few disciplines have taken the recent challenges of decolonization and the decolonial turn more seriously than the branches of psychology in the Global South that explore the linkages between subjectivity, community, and social life. Yet, the task is barely starting. Building on the work of figures like the famed psychiatrist and revolutionary fighter, Frantz Fanon, among others, the editors and authors in this book seek to further illuminate the path of decolonization, anticolonialism, and decoloniality in the contemporary world. The anthology provides invaluable resources in the effort to infuse psychology with decolonial transdisciplinary approaches, thereby taking psychology beyond its modern-colonial horizons. An essential reference for anyone heeding the call to consider decolonization as an unfinished project and as an imperative today.

–NELSON MALDONADO-TORRES, PhD, UNIVERSITY OF CONNECTICUT, STORRS

DECOLONIAL

PSYCHOLOGY

Cultural, Racial, and Ethnic Psychology Book Series

The Cost of Racism for People of Color: Contextualizing Experiences of Discrimination
  Edited by Alvin N. Alvarez, Christopher T. H. Liang, and Helen A. Neville

Decolonial Psychology: Toward Anticolonial Theories, Research, Training, and Practice
  Edited by Lillian Comas-Díaz, Hector Y. Adames, and
  Nayeli Y. Chavez-Dueñas

Evidence-Based Psychological Practice With Ethnic Minorities: Culturally Informed Research and Clinical Strategies
  Edited by Nolan Zane, Guillermo Bernal, and Frederick T. L. Leong

Liberation Psychology: Theory, Method, Practice, and Social Justice
  Edited by Lillian Comas-Díaz and Edil Torres Rivera

Positive Psychology in Racial and Ethnic Groups: Theory, Research, and Practice
  Edited by Edward C. Chang, Christina A. Downey, Jameson K. Hirsch, and Natalie J. Lin

Qualitative Strategies for Ethnocultural Research
  Edited by Donna K. Nagata, Laura Kohn-Wood, and Lisa A. Suzuki

Trauma and Racial Minority Immigrants: Turmoil, Uncertainty, and Resistance
  Edited by Pratyusha Tummala-Narra

Treating Depression, Anxiety, and Stress in Ethnic and Racial Groups: Cognitive Behavioral Approaches
  Edited by Edward C. Chang, Christina A. Downey, Jameson K. Hirsch, and Elizabeth A. Yu

DECOLONIAL

PSYCHOLOGY

TOWARD ANTICOLONIAL THEORIES, RESEARCH, TRAINING, *and* PRACTICE

LILLIAN COMAS-DÍAZ
HECTOR Y. ADAMES
NAYELI Y. CHAVEZ-DUEÑAS
editors

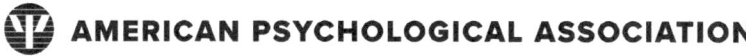 AMERICAN PSYCHOLOGICAL ASSOCIATION

Published by
American Psychological Association
750 First Street, NE
Washington, DC 20002
https://www.apa.org

Order Department
https://www.apa.org/pubs/books
order@apa.org

Typeset in Charter and Interstate by Circle Graphics, Inc., Reisterstown, MD

Printer: Sheridan Books, Chelsea, MI
Cover Designer: Mark Karis

Library of Congress Cataloging-in-Publication Data

Names: Comas-Díaz, Lillian, editor. | Adames, Hector Y., editor. |
  Chavez-Dueñas, Nayeli Y., editor.
Title: Decolonial psychology : toward anticolonial theories, research, training,
  and practice / edited by Lillian Comas-Díaz, Hector Y. Adames,
  and Nayeli Y. Chavez-Dueñas.
Description: Washington, DC : American Psychological Association, [2024] |
  Series: Cultural, racial, and ethnic psychology book series | Includes
  bibliographical references and index.
Identifiers: LCCN 2023036832 (print) | LCCN 2023036833 (ebook) |
  ISBN 9781433838521 (paperback) | ISBN 9781433838538 (ebook)
Subjects: LCSH: Social psychiatry. | Community psychology. | Cross-cultural
  counseling. | Decolonization--Psychological aspects. | Imperialism and science.
Classification: LCC RC455 .D393 2024 (print) | LCC RC455 (ebook) |
  DDC 616.89--dc23/eng/20231010
LC record available at https://lccn.loc.gov/2023036832
LC ebook record available at https://lccn.loc.gov/2023036833

https://doi.org/10.1037/0000376-000

Printed in the United States of America

10 9 8 7 6 5 4 3 2 1

*We dedicate this volume both in memory of Dr. Jean Lau Chin and of
Dr. Joseph L. White and to all who follow the path of decolonization.*

*To Communities of Color everywhere, may your decolonial
path transform oppression into liberation.*
—LILLIAN COMAS-DÍAZ

*To my community, familia, and chosen family above and beneath the sea.
Thank you for the gentle reminders that we are worthy of healing
and softness—the most precious gifts.*
—HECTOR Y. ADAMES

*To Indigenous and Black children all over the world, may you no
longer need to fight for your right to exist and walk on this earth
with dignity and respect. To Indigenous and Black parents,
may you be able and nourish your children's roots so they
can withstand the winds and storms of life's seasons.*
—NAYELI Y. CHAVEZ-DUEÑAS

Contents

Contributors   *xi*

Series Foreword—Frederick T. L. Leong   *xv*

Foreword—Gayle Skawen:nio Morse and Marie C. Weil   *xix*

Acknowledgments   *xxiii*

Introduction: Decoloniality as a Transformative Force in Psychology: An Orientation to This Book   **3**
Hector Y. Adames, Nayeli Y. Chavez-Dueñas, and Lillian Comas-Díaz

I. HISTORY AND KNOWLEDGE   **13**

1. **Colonial Mentality: Manifestations, Operations, and Psychological Implications**   **15**
   Hannah L. Rebadulla, Jonathan U. Guerrero, and E. J. R. David

2. **Naming and Unlearning Psychological Coloniality**   **41**
   Cristalís Capielo Rosario, Eduardo Lugo-Hernández, and Loíza A. DeJesús Sullivan

3. **Engaging With Decoloniality, Decolonization, and Histories of Psychology Otherwise**   **61**
   Sunil Bhatia, Wahbie Long, Wade Pickren, and Alexandra Rutherford

II. SCIENCE, METHODS, AND EPISTEMIC JUSTICE 87

4. Decolonizing and Building Liberatory Psychological Sciences 89
Helen A. Neville, B. Andi Lee, and Amir H. Maghsoodi

5. Beyond Decolonization: Anticolonial Methodologies for
Indigenous Futurity in Psychological Research 119
Jillian Fish and Joseph P. Gone

6. Disciplinary Disruptions: Strategies Toward a Decolonial
Community Psychology Praxis 143
Jesica Siham Fernández

7. Decolonizing in a Transnational Feminist Commons Perched
Precariously Between the Academy and Movements
for Justice 169
Adreanne Ormond, Puleng Segalo, María Elena Torre, and Michelle Fine

III. EDUCATION, PROFESSIONAL TRAINING, AND MENTORING 203

8. Decolonizing the High School and Undergraduate Curriculum 205
Edil Torres Rivera and Ivelisse Torres Fernández

9. Unlearning Colonial Practices and (Re)envisioning Graduate
Education in Psychology 219
Carrie L. Castañeda-Sound, Miguel Gallardo, and Susana O. Salgado

10. The Decolonial Mentoring Framework: Advancing an
Anticolonial Future in Psychology and Beyond 247
Mackenzie T. Goertz, Hector Y. Adames, Chelsea Parker, Nayeli Y.
Chavez-Dueñas, Radia DeLuna, and Jessica G. Perez-Chavez

11. Wise Face, Firm Heart: Ethics and Decolonial Psychology 271
Melinda A. García

IV. PSYCHOTHERAPIES 293

12. Decolonial Psychotherapy: Joining the Circle, Healing
the Wound 295
Lillian Comas-Díaz and Frederick M. Jacobsen

13. Decolonizing Psychoanalysis: Anti-Blackness, Coloniality,
and a New Premise for Psychoanalytic Treatment 321
Daniel Jose Gaztambide, Fabián E. Feliciano-Graniela,
José Luiggi-Hernández, and Edlyane Veronica Medina Escobar

14. Decolonizing Feminist Therapy 345
Thema Bryant, Carolyn Zerbe Enns, and Yuying Tsong

V. QUEER FUTURES, SELF-CARE, AND COMMUNITY CARE   367

15. Moving Psychology Toward Anticolonial Queer Futures   369
Della V. Mosley, Pearis L. Jean, Brittany Bridges, Maria Sobrino,
Jeannette Mejia, Sunshine Adam, Garrett Ross, and Roberto Abreu

**16. Your Self-Care Is Made of Capitalism: A Decolonial Approach
to Self and Community Care**   389
Arianne E. Miller and Nellie Tran

Index   *409*
About the Editors   *429*

Contributors

Roberto Abreu, PhD, Department of Psychology, University of Florida, Gainesville, FL, United States

Sunshine Adam, MA, Durham, NC, United States

Hector Y. Adames, PsyD, The Chicago School of Professional Psychology, Chicago, IL, United States, and the Immigration Critical Race and Cultural Equity Lab (IC-RACE)

Sunil Bhatia, PhD, Human Development, Connecticut College, New London, CT, United States

Brittany Bridges, MS, Department of Psychology, University of Florida, Gainesville, FL, United States

Thema Bryant, PhD, Graduate School of Education and Psychology, Pepperdine University, Los Angeles, CA, United States

Cristalís Capielo Rosario, PhD, Department of Counseling and Counseling and Psychology, Arizona State University, Tempe, AZ, United States

Carrie L. Castañeda-Sound, PhD, Graduate School of Education and Psychology, Pepperdine University, Los Angeles, CA, United States

Nayeli Y. Chavez-Dueñas, PhD, The Chicago School of Professional Psychology, Chicago, IL, United States, and the Immigration Critical Race and Cultural Equity Lab (IC-RACE)

Lillian Comas-Díaz, PhD, Transcultural Mental Health Institute and George Washington University, School of Medicine, Washington, DC, United States

E. J. R. David, PhD, Alaska Native Community Advancement in Psychology (ANCAP) Program, University of Alaska Anchorage, Anchorage, AK, United States

Loíza A. DeJesús Sullivan, MA, Department of Counseling and Counseling Psychology, Arizona State University, Tempe, AZ, United States

Radia DeLuna, MA, University of Illinois at Urbana Champaign, IL, United States, and the Immigration Critical Race and Cultural Equity Lab (IC-RACE)

Carolyn Zerbe Enns, PhD, Professor Emerita, Cornell College, Mount Vernon, IA, United States

Edlyane Veronica Medina Escobar, PhD, Department of Clinical Psychology, the New School for Social Research, New York, NY, United States

Fabián E. Feliciano-Graniela, BA, Departamento de Psicología, Universidad de Puerto Rico, Recinto de Río Piedras, San Juan, Puerto Rico, United States

Jesica Siham Fernández, PhD, Department of Ethnic Studies, Santa Clara University, Santa Clara, CA, United States

Michelle Fine, PhD, the Public Science Project and the Graduate Center, City University of New York, New York, NY, United States

Jillian Fish, PhD, Psychology Department, Macalester College, Saint Paul, MN, United States

Miguel Gallardo, PsyD, Graduate School of Education and Psychology, Pepperdine University, Irvine, CA, United States

Melinda A. García, PhD, Independent Practice, Albuquerque, NM, United States

Daniel Jose Gaztambide, PsyD, Department of Psychology, Queens College, Flushing, NY, United States

Mackenzie T. Goertz, PhD, Department of Psychiatry and Behavioral Medicine, Medical College of Wisconsin, Milwaukee, WI, United States, and the Immigration Critical Race and Cultural Equity Lab (IC-RACE)

Joseph P. Gone, PhD, Department of Anthropology, Harvard University, Cambridge, MA, and Department of Global Health and Social Medicine, Harvard Medical School, Boston, MA, United States

Jonathan U. Guerrero, MS, Clinical Community Psychology Program, University of Alaska Anchorage, Anchorage, AK, United States

Frederick M. Jacobsen, MD, MPH, Transcultural Mental Health Institute and George Washington University School of Medicine, Washington, DC, United States

Pearis L. Jean, PhD, Department of Psychology, Towson University, Towson, MD, United States

B. Andi Lee, MS, Department of Psychology, University of Illinois at Urbana-Champaign, Champaign, IL, United States

Frederick T. L. Leong, PhD, Retired, Department of Psychology, Michigan State University, East Lansing, MI, United States

Wahbie Long, PhD, Department of Psychology, University of Cape Town, Cape Town, South Africa

Eduardo Lugo-Hernández, PhD, Department of Psychology, University of Puerto Rico, Mayagüez, Puerto Rico, United States

José Luiggi-Hernández, PhD, MPH, Department of Psychology, Duquesne University, Pittsburgh, PA, and Department of General Internal Medicine, University of Pittsburgh, Pittsburgh, PA, United States

Amir H. Maghsoodi, MS, Department of Psychology, University of Illinois at Urbana-Champaign, Champaign, IL, United States

Jeannette Mejia, MS, Department of Psychology, University of Florida, Gainesville, FL, United States

Arianne E. Miller, PhD, Private Practice, Washington, DC, United States

Gayle Skawen:nio Morse, PhD, Department of Psychology, Russell Sage College, Albany and Troy, NY, United States

Della V. Mosley, PhD, The WELLS Healing Center, Durham, NC, United States

Helen A. Neville, PhD, College of Education, University of Illinois at Urbana-Champaign, Champaign, IL, United States

Adreanne Ormond, PhD, School of Government, Victoria University of Wellington, Wellington, New Zealand

Chelsea Parker, MA, LCPC, Love is Key Counseling LLC, Chicago, IL, United States, and the Immigration Critical Race and Cultural Equity Lab (IC-RACE)

Jessica G. Perez-Chavez, PhD, University of Wisconsin–Madison, Madison, WI; Cambridge Health Alliance, Harvard Medical School, Boston, MA,

United States; and the Immigration Critical Race and Cultural Equity Lab (IC-RACE)

Wade Pickren, PhD, Author, Editor, and Founder of Psychologies Otherwise/Earthwise, Ithaca, NY, United States

Hannah L. Rebadulla, MS, Institute of Social and Economic Research, University of Alaska Anchorage, Anchorage, AK, United States

Garrett Ross, MS, Department of Psychology, University of Florida, Gainesville, FL, United States

Alexandra Rutherford, PhD, Department of Psychology, York University, Toronto, Ontario, Canada

Susana O. Salgado, PhD, Mind Body Corazón, and Graduate School of Education and Psychology, Pepperdine University, Los Angeles, CA, United States

Puleng Segalo, PhD, Department of Psychology, University of South Africa, Pretoria, South Africa

Maria Sobrino, BS, Department of Basic and Applied Social Psychology, The Graduate Center of the City University of New York, New York, NY, United States

María Elena Torre, PhD, the Public Science Project and the Graduate Center, City University of New York, New York, NY, United States

Ivelisse Torres Fernández, PhD, Department of Counseling Psychology, Albizu University, San Juan, Puerto Rico, United States

Edil Torres Rivera, PhD, Interventions Service & Leadership in Education Department, Wichita State University, Wichita, KS, United States

Nellie Tran, PhD, Department of Counseling & School Psychology, San Diego State University, San Diego, CA, United States

Yuying Tsong, PhD, Division of Academic Affairs, California State University, Fullerton, CA, United States

Marie C. Weil, PsyD, ABPP, Independent Practice, Silver City, NM, United States

Series Foreword

As series editor of the American Psychological Association's (APA's) Division 45 (Society for the Psychological Study of Culture, Ethnicity and Race) book series on Cultural, Racial, and Ethnic Psychology, it is my pleasure to introduce another volume in the series: *Decolonial Psychology: Toward Anticolonial Theories, Research, Training, and Practice*, edited by Lillian Comas-Díaz, Hector Y. Adames, and Nayeli Y. Chavez-Dueñas.

The impetus for the series came from my presidential theme for Division 45: strengthening our science to improve our practice. Given the increasing attention to racial and ethnic minority issues within the discipline of psychology, I argued that we needed to both generate more research and make the existing research known. From the *Supplement to the Surgeon General's Report on Mental Health* (U.S. Department of Health and Human Services, 2001) to the *Unequal Treatment* report from the Institute of Medicine (Smedley et al., 2003)—both of which documented extensive racial and ethnic disparities in our health care system—the complex of culture, race, and ethnicity was becoming a major challenge in both research and practice within the field of psychology.

To meet that challenge, Division 45 acquired its own journal devoted to ethnic minority issues in psychology (*Cultural Diversity and Ethnic Minority Psychology*). At the same time, a series of handbooks on the topic were published, including the *Handbook of Racial and Ethnic Minority Psychology* (Bernal et al., 2003). Yet we felt that more coverage of this subdiscipline was imperative—coverage that would match the substantive direction of the handbooks, but would come from a variety of research and practice perspectives. Hence the Division 45 book series was launched.

The series—Cultural, Racial, and Ethnic Psychology—is designed to advance our theories, research, and practice regarding this increasingly crucial subdiscipline. It will focus on, but not be limited to, the major racial and ethnic groups in the United States (i.e., African Americans, Latinos, Asian Americans, and American Indians) and will include books that examine a single racial or ethnic group as well as books that undertake a comparative approach. The series will also address the full spectrum of related methodological, substantive, and theoretical issues, including topics in behavioral neuroscience, cognitive and developmental psychology, and personality and social psychology. Other volumes in the series will be devoted to cross-disciplinary explorations in the applied realms of clinical psychology and counseling, as well as educational, community, and industrial–organizational psychology. Our goal is to commission state-of-the art volumes in cultural, racial, and ethnic psychology that will be of interest to both practitioners and researchers.

As I end my tenure as the founding editor of this book series, I am very pleased to introduce this volume, *Decolonial Psychology*. Comas-Díaz, Adames, and Chavez-Dueñas have provided a pioneering volume on a critical issue facing contemporary psychology, namely the antecedents, nature, and consequences of colonialism in the science and practice of psychology. It courageously unpacks the underlying assumptions and biases of Eurocentric psychology with the aim of making the field more inclusive and relevant. The contributors to the volume do an excellent job of providing an in-depth discussion of the historical contexts, epistemology, models, and methods for decolonizing psychology. Psychology as it currently exists in the United States tend to be highly individualistic, decontextualized, and atemporal. The current volume counters these tendencies by examining the larger communities that can benefit from psychology as well as the historical context of why psychology is the way it is. It outlines the boundary conditions and limitations of a Eurocentric science based in part on a colonial mentality. Resistance to this volume is only to be expected; but a critical self-examination of our field will only improve it—if we are strong enough to endure it. I believe that the current volume, when viewed retrospectively, will represent a tipping point in the scientific development of our field.

Let me end by thanking the members of the editorial board who do the work of recruiting and reviewing proposals for the series: Guillermo Bernal, University of Puerto Rico; Beth Boyd, University of South Dakota; Lillian

Comas-Díaz, private practice; Sandra Graham, University of California Los Angeles; Gordon Nagayama Hall, University of Oregon; Helen Neville, University of Illinois Urbana-Champaign; Teresa LaFromboise, Stanford University; Richard Lee, University of Minnesota; Robert M. Sellers, University of Michigan; Stanley Sue, Palo Alto University; Joseph Trimble, Western Washington University; and Michael Zarate, University of Texas at El Paso. They represent leading scholars in psychology who have graciously donated their time to help advance the field. Finally, I am pleased to pass the baton to Dr. Chris Liang of Lehigh University, who will succeed me as the editor for this book series.

—Frederick T. L. Leong
Series Editor

REFERENCES

Bernal, G., Trimble, J. E., Burlew, A. K., & Leong, F. T. L. (2003). *Handbook of racial and ethnic minority psychology.* Sage.

Smedley, B. D., Stith, A. Y., & Nelson, A. R. (Eds.). (2003). *Unequal treatment: Confronting racial and ethnic disparities in health care.* National Academies Press.

U.S. Department of Health and Human Services. (2001). *Mental health: Culture, race, and ethnicity—A supplement to mental health: A report of the Surgeon General.* U.S. Department of Health and Human Services, Substance Abuse and Mental Health Services Administration, Center for Mental Health Services.

Foreword

All of us gather our minds together as one. We give thanks to our creator.
We always want it this way, peaceful, it's always this way. And now our
minds are one.

–Haudenosaunee Opening Address
Protecting and Defending our People:
Nakni Tushka Anowa (The Warrior's Path)

We are delighted to describe the Warrior's Path Report (WPR) journey with you all. At the height of the COVID-19 pandemic in 2020, a diverse group of graduate students, early, mid-, and late-career psychologists, and elders in the cultural and Indigenous psychology fields gathered together in community. This group of psychologists and psychologists-in-training were members of the Society for the Psychological Study of Culture, Ethnicity and Race, a Division (45) of the American Psychological Association (APA). They volunteered their time to work on a project in response to a call for service on the Warrior's Path Presidential Task Force (WPTF) from Dr. Art Blume, then president of Division 45. The task force, cochaired by Dr. Gayle Skawen:nio Morse, Dr. Jean Lau Chin, and Dr. Marie C. Weil, was trusted to produce a *Paper of Color Report* (rather than a white paper). The authors of the WPR were entrusted to serve as psychological "warriors in defense of our people inside and outside of psychology"

In the Warrior's Path Report (WPR), Dr. Art Blume stated, "The warrior's path is to oppose colonial and neocolonial forces that contribute to the psychological damage we address daily" (Aiello et al., 2021, p. 12). This volume—*Decolonial Psychology: Toward Anticolonial Theories, Research, Training, and Practice,* edited by Dr. Lillian Comas-Díaz (WPR coauthor), Dr. Hector Y. Adames, and Dr. Nayeli Y. Chavez-Dueñas—is a child of the WPR.

(Aiello et al., 2021, p. 13). The authors were asked to create a report that honored our elders and protected and respected the cultural history of Division 45. They also identified barriers within the APA that prevent the protection of our people and to truth and reconciliation processes. The report advocated for the decolonization of psychology with consideration of environmental and social justice in those processes. These goals align with the chapters *in Decolonial Psychology: Toward Anticolonial Theories, Research, Training, and Practice.* To expand their reach, the WPTF invited a discussion on the Division 45 listserv, administered a voluntary survey, collected stories from division members about how APA embodied colonialism in training, ethics, research, and publications, as well as how the structure of APA perpetuated colonial attitudes and discouraged representation of Black, Indigenous, and People of Color (BIPOC) leaders and employees in its ranks. The report delineated critical areas that required immediate attention and provided examples for decolonizing and dismantling APA's Eurocentric structure and practice. The report closed by exacting a call to action for healing and committed and sustained action. This outlined demands for change and the included an expectation that demands will be met. The WPR was downloaded more than 3,000 times in the first year of its publication. By the second year, the report was accessed worldwide. The impact of this transformational document has been widely felt in the world of psychology. The WPR was cited as a pivotal influence in three resolutions passed by the APA Council of Representatives in 2021:

- Apology to People of Color for APA's Role in Promoting, Perpetuating, and Failing to Challenge Racism, Racial Discrimination, and Human Hierarchy in U.S. (APA, 2021b)

- Role of Psychology and APA in Dismantling Systemic Racism Against People of Color in U.S. (APA, 2021c)

- Advancing Health Equity in Psychology (APA, 2021a)

These developments culminated in the Racial Equity Action Plan with a $1.1-million grant to fund equity, diversity, and inclusion work in psychology, education, training, and the workforce.

Recently, the WPR was cited in the APA Report and Apology to the First Peoples of the United States (2023) and has already been cited in numerous books, including *Applying Multiculturalism: An Ecological Approach to the APA Guidelines* (Clauss-Ehlers et al., 2023) and, most important, in this volume, *Decolonial Psychology: Toward Anticolonial Theories, Research, Training, and Practice* both published by APA. We thank all the chapter authors of this timely and critical book for their solidarity and hard work, which helps our various communities thrive. Also, we thank the editors for their invitation and opportunity to comment on this new and exciting volume. Let us continue to put our minds together to oppose colonial and neocolonial forces that harm humanity—together, let us uplift decoloniality in and outside psychology.

—Gayle Skawen:nio Morse, PhD
Marie C. Weil, PsyD, ABPP

REFERENCES

Aiello, M., Bismar, D., Casanova, S., Casas, J. M., Chang, D., Chin, J. L., Comas-Diaz, L., Salvo Crane, L., Demir, Z., Garcia, M. A., Hita, L., Leverett, P., Mendez, K., Morse, G. S., shodiya-zeumault, s., O'Leary Sloan, M., Weil, M. C., & Blume, A. W. (2021). Protecting and defending our people: Nakni tushka anowa (The Warrior's Path) final report. APA Division 45 Warrior's Path Presidential Task Force (2020). *Journal of Indigenous Research, 9*(2021), Article 8. https://doi.org/10.26077/2en0-6610

American Psychological Association, APA Indigenous Apology Work Group (APA). (2023). Report on an offer of apology, on behalf of the American Psychological Association, to First Peoples in the United States. https://www.apa.org/pubs/reports/indigenous-apology.pdf

American Psychological Association, Council Policy Manual (APA). (2021a). Advancing health equity in psychology. Resolution adopted by the APA Council of Representatives on October 29, 2021. https://www.apa.org/about/policy/resolution-advancing-health-equity.pdf

American Psychological Association, Council Policy Manual (APA). (2021b). Apology to People of Color for APA's role in promoting, perpetuating, and failing to challenge racism, racial discrimination, and human hierarchy in U.S. Resolution adopted by the APA Council of Representatives on October 29, 2021. https://www.apa.org/about/policy/resolution-racism-apology.pdf

American Psychological Association, Council Policy Manual (APA). (2021c). Role of psychology and APA in dismantling systemic racism against People of Color in the United States. Resolution adopted by the APA Council of Representatives on October 29, 2021. https://www.apa.org/about/policy/resolution-dismantling-racism.pdf

Clauss-Ehlers, C. S., Hunter, S. J., Morse, G. S., & Tummala-Narra, P. (2023). *Applying multiculturalism: An ecological approach to the APA Guidelines.* American Psychological Association.

Acknowledgments

Decolonial Psychology: Toward Anticolonial Theories, Research, Training, and Practice is possible because of our ancestors' echoes, reminding us that the past is the pathway to the future. Thank you for the continuous lessons on resisting oppression and creating a future where many worlds can fit—thank you for believing that we deserve better.

No edited volume comes to life without a community of outstanding and thoughtful scholars who generously share their minds, wisdom, and expertise. We are indebted to the chapter authors, who invite us to move toward anticolonial ways of creating psychological knowledge and practice. Your work and passion are helping shift the field.

We express our appreciation to the brilliant scholars Jessica G. Perez-Chavez, PhD, Frederick M. Jacobsen, MD, MPH, Ronald V. Hall, MD, Maryam M. Jernigan-Noesi, PhD, Helen A. Neville, PhD, Arianne E. Miller, PhD, Swati Sharma, and Shweta Sharma, PsyD, who provided feedback on the title and book cover, which powerfully captures the essence of the volume. We are also so thankful to Chris Kelaher, Kristen Knight, and Frederick T. L. Leong, PhD—our incredible editorial team at the American Psychological Association—for their guidance and belief in the promise of this decolonial project. Last thank you to the anonymous reviewers who generously took the time to read our manuscript and share their wisdom, judgment, and expertise.

DECOLONIAL

P S Y C H O L O G Y

INTRODUCTION

Decoloniality as a Transformative Force in Psychology:
An Orientation to This Book

HECTOR Y. ADAMES, NAYELI Y. CHAVEZ-DUEÑAS, AND LILLIAN COMAS-DÍAZ

The past is key to the future. Our past has the wisdom that can help us build
a future . . . by looking toward the past, toward those who were the first
inhabitants, to those who first had wisdom, who first made us.

−Marcos, 2002, p. 84

History carries the whispers of our ancestors layered in pain, hopes, and dreams. Whispers that remind us of a past that is still with us. Examining and understanding history is one way to recognize oppressive ideologies and practices that shape the day-to-day existence of Communities of Color. History also contains wisdom that can guide us toward detaching from and resisting the power structures designed to dehumanize, control, and exploit. In many ways, knowing history and its many lessons liberates. This notion of history mirrors the view and description provided by Chavez-Dueñas and Adames (2021), who state that

> History allows individuals to learn about themselves and their group's past
> while contextualizing and understanding their present day-to-day strengths,
> struggles, and realities. . . . However, when aspects of history are suppressed,
> ignored, or presented in biased ways, they can bind us to an existence that is

https://doi.org/10.1037/0000376-001
Decolonial Psychology: Toward Anticolonial Theories, Research, Training, and Practice,
L. Comas-Díaz, H. Y. Adames, and N. Y. Chavez-Dueñas (Editors)

3

stifling and defeating. This systematic suppression of history and knowledge is not an academic lapse; instead, it is used to manipulate minoritized groups into collaborating and participating in their own oppression. (p. 83)

A critical part of history that is often suppressed and ignored is the period of colonization. This historical era was steeped in destruction, exploitation, and genocide (Adames & Chavez-Dueñas, 2017; Kellogg, 2005; Livi-Bacci, 2008). Although colonization has ended in many countries, its ideologies and practices grounded in European colonialism, described as *coloniality*, are alive and thriving in contemporary society across the globe. Coloniality is responsible for policies and political systems that aim to control and erase Indigenous ways of knowing and being[1] in the world.

As a field, psychology in the United States and other Western, industrialized, wealthy countries is not immune to perpetuating coloniality. Recently, the American Psychological Association (APA; 2021) acknowledged U.S. psychology's collusion with coloniality by issuing a public apology that

Since its origins as a scientific discipline in the mid-19th century, psychology has, through acts of commission and omission, contributed to the dispossession, displacement, and exploitation of Communities of Color. This early history of psychology, rooted in oppressive psychological science to protect Whiteness, White people, and White epistemologies, reflected the social and political landscape of the U.S. at that time. Psychology developed under these conditions, helped to create, express, and sustain them, continues to bear their indelible imprint, and often continues to publish research that conforms with White racial hierarchy. (para. 8)

APA's apology is critical. It recognizes the harm of engaging in practices that promote a colonial enterprise that supports those in power while failing to uphold the ethical values of integrity, justice, and respect for people's rights and dignity (see Pope et al., 2021).

THE ABSENCE OF EPISTEMIC EQUITY IN PSYCHOLOGY KEEPS COLONIALITY ALIVE

Coloniality thrives by silencing those it seeks to control. In psychology, global Eurocentric voices, experiences, and methodologies are often centered and uplifted, and the narratives, realities, and practices from the Global South are

---

[1] Although the term *Indigenous* has often been used to describe people born in a specific place, the concept also represents the beliefs and experiences of a group of people who originally inhabited a country (Cunningham & Stanley, 2003). In this book, the authors use the latter usage.

devalued and suppressed. When the wisdom of the Global South is considered, their Indigenous knowledge, traditions, and methods are appropriated and exoticized (Gergen et al., 1996). For instance, Helms (2016) posited that for most of its history, psychology has used the perspectives of White, heterosexual men with power and privilege (WHMP) as "scientific" justification for dehumanizing Black, Indigenous, and other People of Color (BIPOC). This practice is a form of epistemic violence (Spivak, 1988; see also Brunner, 2021; Dotson, 2011) and is a dominant way of how coloniality operates in psychology. In other words, epistemic violence fails to reflect the lives of BIPOC and people from the Global South—it is the heartbeat that keeps coloniality alive in psychology today. Psychological science grounded in WHMP promotes a decontextualized perspective of people despite people's living in complex and constantly evolving and diverse environments (Gergen et al., 1996; Helms, 2016; see also Adames & Chavez-Dueñas, 2017; Comas-Díaz & Torres Rivera, 2020). Furthermore, it assumes an individualistic and Eurocentric hegemony and dismisses or minimizes the relevance of how sociopolitical contexts impact individuals and groups (Aiello et al., 2021; Comas-Díaz, 2007). As a result, the knowledge generated from a psychology not inclusive of BIPOC communities is incomplete, inadequate, and maintains the global order of coloniality; we need a paradigm shift.

DECOLONIAL PSYCHOLOGY AS A PARADIGM SHIFT TO LIBERATION

Decoloniality is a praxis—it is the process of constantly disrupting the legacies of inequities, dehumanization, domination, and WHMP (e.g., racism, sexism, gendered racism, heterosexism, cissexism, nativism, ethnocentrism, ableism) that maintains the global hierarchy of power. This notion of decoloniality reflects Walter Mignolo's (2011) description of decoloniality as "delinking from the colonial matrix of power" (p. 9). It also mirrors the Readsura Decolonial Editorial Collective (2022a), which states that decoloniality

> is an ongoing orientation toward being and knowing that seeks to unsettle the present, an open-ended mode of de-linking from Eurocentric modernity/coloniality in an attempt to imagine and give birth to another future. (p. 258)

In the field of psychology, the concept of decoloniality is gaining momentum (Barnes, 2018). Over the last decade, psychological work on decoloniality has appeared in professional conferences (see The New School, 2020; Teachers College, 2021), and has been the subject of books (see Beshara, 2019; Boonzaier & van Niekerk, 2019; Ciofalo, 2019) and special journal issues (see Readsura Decolonial Editorial Collective, 2022b). Additionally, the 2023 president of the American Psychological Association, Dr. Thema Bryant, has commissioned a presidential task force on decolonizing psychology. Building on this body of work, the current volume, *Decolonial Psychology: Toward Anticolonial Theories, Research, Training, and Practice*, seeks to contribute to helping address and remove the stubborn ways coloniality is practiced in psychology. Without paradigm shifts like these, coloniality in psychology will not fade away.

Decolonial Psychology: Toward Anticolonial Theories, Research, Training, and Practice presents a collective vision for the next steps in decoloniality in psychology, which aim to create spaces and methods for oppressed and impoverished communities to radically imagine their existence outside of the superimposed borders of coloniality, neoliberalism, racism, and other systems of oppression. It also emphasizes how people's subjectivity and connections to diverse social groups are influenced by history, context, and oppression; how these populations actively resist and survive attacks on their humanity; and how knowledge production is shaped not only by how data is interpreted but also by the nature of the questions asked and the individuals or entities posing those questions.

Together, we build on the emerging scholarship on decoloniality in and outside of psychology by convening a group of scholars, researchers, practitioners, and educators who have been thinking and writing about delinking psychology from its colonial legacy. A collective vision that unites the authors and editors in the book is the goal of developing an anticolonial[2] psychology that places "the power to challenge psychological research norms, assumptions, and outcomes squarely in the hands of Indigenous peoples" (p. 120, Chapter 5, this volume).

COLONIALITY POSITIONALITY-DECOLONIALITY PRAXIS

This coedited book offers you a path to embark on a decolonial–anticolonial journey and to contribute to psychology's paradigmatic transformation. On this journey, we recognize that how we interpret and experience the world and each other is shaped by many oppressive forces, including coloniality, and how we create joy, make connections, and build community with others. Among populations affected by oppressive and dehumanizing processes, some work to resist and delink their ideologies and actions from the hierarchy of power maintained by coloniality, whereas others support

---

[2]*Anticolonial* refers to Indigenous resistance and opposition to colonialism (see Chapter 5, this volume; Hartmann et al., 2019).

the status quo. In editing this book, we recognize the need for each of us to describe what we are coining and defining as a coloniality positionality–decoloniality praxis that openly names the social group identities affected by coloniality; describes how, if at all, scholars are working to disrupt and defy systems of power that keep the heartbeat of coloniality alive; and illustrates how lived experiences influence the production of knowledge. To demonstrate, we briefly apply the coloniality positionality–decoloniality praxis to ourselves as editors. We believe that beyond simply recognizing our social identities, we must engage in critical reflexibility about how those identities and experiences confer power and privilege which can influence our scholarship (see Grzanka & Moradi, 2021; Helms, 1993; Morrow, 2005). In other words, coloniality positionality–decoloniality praxis is not passive, it is not an odd form of exhibitionism or simply about naming our identities for the sake of sharing, but it is an intentional cycle of action–reflection–action that aims to disrupt coloniality and inform the knowledge making process while sharing our hearts and minds with the reader (see Grzanka & Moradi, 2021; Helms, 1993).

Lillian Comas-Díaz

I, Lillian, am a cisgender heterosexual Puerto Rican mixed-race woman with Taíno, African, and Iberian roots. I was born in Chicago and raised in Puerto Rico, the oldest colony in history. My journey and experiences led me to participate in the decolonization and liberation movements of the Global South. Such a path assisted me in connecting with ancestral spirituality and in recovering my historical memory. Several cultural translocations taught me to embrace Otherness and work toward antiracism in my work. I coined the term "LatiNegra" (see Comas-Díaz, 1994) and self-identify as one. As a scholar, psychotherapist, healer, and social justice warrior, I strive to infuse my life and work with decoloniality, liberation, and antioppression.

Hector Y. Adames

I am a cisgender, queer Afro Latino immigrant from Quisqueya, the island divided by superimposed borders now called Haiti and the Dominican Republic. I was born on the island of Quisqueya, the first space in the Americas where Black, White, and Indigenous people met. I come from a land and people who are intimately wrapped by a history of destruction and survival. As a queer man of African descent living in the 21st century of U.S. American imperialism, my experiences of oppression, survival, and resistance reverberate in and outside the academy. These historical and contemporary realities influence my work as a scholar, practitioner, and educator. It shapes all of who I am. I have devoted my career and talents to speaking the unspoken by naming and studying systemic forces that brutalize people through words, policies, and practices while developing methods that humanize and celebrate the strengths of who coloniality aims to vanish. To echo Junot Diaz, also from Quisqueya, "all of us must be free, all of us must be free, all of us must be free or none" (2016, 4:22). These experiences shape the questions I seek to explore and how I make sense of human behavior and mental processes.

Nayeli Y. Chavez-Dueñas

I am a cisgender, heterosexual, genderqueer Mexican immigrant who grew up in Michoacan, Mexico, the land of the Purepecha people, where remnants of colonization remain alive today. The exploitation of the land and its resources caused by colonization led to the decimation of my homeland and contributed to the forced migration of people to the north. Like millions of Mexicans before me, I crossed the imaginary border and entered the United States looking for the ever-evasive American dream. As a newly arrived teen immigrant, I worked as a day laborer and was affected by laws, policies, and practices anchored in the pillars of coloniality designed to control, dehumanize, and criminalize people for simply being a non-White and non-American. Simply put, people like me pay a heavy price for nurturing and exercising the audacity to cross the human-made borders established by imperial powers to maintain power. It is these experiences and realities that have shaped my scholarship and fueled my determination to continue using my privilege to speak truth to power in and outside of academia.

****

Recognizing and constantly reflecting on our coloniality positionality–decoloniality praxis influenced this volume's conceptualization, development, and editing process. We invite readers to engage in the process of action–reflection–action as they go through the various chapters so we can collectively continue to disrupt coloniality in psychological science, practice, and training.

CENTERING DECOLONIALITY IN PSYCHOLOGY: THE ORGANIZATION OF THIS BOOK

The current volume presents our collective effort to describe how Western psychology has contributed to coloniality and generate ideas and actions to center decoloniality in psychological research and practice. The volume comprises 16 chapters organized into five parts. Each chapter ends with a list of resources to further stimulate ideas to decolonize psychology and work toward creating anticolonial theories, research, and practice; examples include TED Talks, documentaries, podcasts, and additional readings.

Part I orients readers to the relevant history and foundational knowledge. Chapter 1 serves as a primer that introduces and describes colonial mentality and how it continues to be widespread and experienced by various minoritized racial and ethnic groups providing evidence for the urgent need to embrace and exercise decoloniality in psychology. Chapter 2 invites us to name and unlearn psychological coloniality. Chapter 3 assists us in interrogating and reimagining psychology's histories by examining the roots of postcolonial thought, that is, it focuses on how power relations maintain conditions of oppression beyond the binary of colonizer and colonized (Moore-Gilbert, 1997).

Part II centers on ways to decolonize knowledge production in psychology. Chapters in this part introduce novel frameworks for decolonizing psychological sciences (Chapter 4) and illustrate how an anticolonial stance can help challenge epistemic violence in psychology (Chapter 5). The last two of these chapters provide real case examples of the use of decolonial methods in community psychology (Chapter 6) and participatory action research (Chapter 7).

Part III centers on education and mentoring. Chapters 8 and 9 focus on decolonizing psychology's high school, undergraduate, and graduate curricula. Chapter 10 invites readers to reimagine professional mentorship in psychology through a novel decolonial mentoring framework. The section concludes with a chapter on the ethics of decoloniality in psychology for professionals and trainees (Chapter 11).

Part IV discusses psychotherapies. Chapters in this part focus on decoloniality in psychotherapy (Chapter 12), psychoanalysis (Chapter 13), and feminist therapy (Chapter 14).

Part V, the last section, takes us into two critical topics. Chapter 15 provides a rich discussion on ways to help move psychology toward anticolonial queer futures. Last, Chapter 16 presents a decolonial critique of traditional public and evidence-based notions of self-care and proposes how we might approach building decolonial community care.

We envision this volume as a guide for scholars, educators, practitioners, and students to disrupt coloniality in psychology and its epistemic violence and inequities. We hope the book serves as a road map to decoloniality in psychology and anticolonial futures. As Frantz Fanon argued, we need to build a decolonial society that represents all of us. Together we can advance decoloniality in psychology and strengthen the development of an equitable, inclusive, humane, and just society that benefits all.

REFERENCES

Adames, H. Y., & Chavez-Dueñas, N. Y. (2017). *Cultural foundations and interventions in Latino/a mental health: History, theory, and within group differences.* Routledge. https://doi.org/10.4324/9781315724058

Aiello, M., Bismar, D., Casanova, S., Casas, J. M., Chang, D., Chin, J. L., Comas-Díaz, L., Salvo Crane, L., Demir, Z., Garcia, M. A., Hita, L., Leverett, P., Mendez, K., Morse, G. S., shodiya-zeumault, s., O'Leary Sloane, M., Weil, M.C., & Blume, A. W. (2021). Protecting and defending our people: Nakni tushka anowa. *Journal of Indigenous Research, 9*(2021), 8. https://doi.org/10.26077/2en0-6610

American Psychological Association. (2021). *Apology to people of color for APA's role in promoting, perpetuating, and failing to challenge racism, racial discrimination, and human hierarchy in U.S. resolution adopted by the APA Council of Representatives* [Resolution]. https://www.apa.org/about/policy/racism-apology

Barnes, B. R. (2018). Decolonising research methodologies: Opportunity and caution. *South African Journal of Psychology, 48*(3), 379–387. https://doi.org/10.1177/0081246318798294

Beshara, R. (2019). *Decolonial psychoanalysis: Towards critical Islamophobia studies.* Routledge. https://doi.org/10.4324/9780429056611

Boonzaier, F., & van Niekerk, T. (Eds.). (2019). *Decolonial feminist community psychology.* Springer. https://doi.org/10.1007/978-3-030-20001-5

Brunner, C. (2021). Conceptualizing epistemic violence: An interdisciplinary assemblage for IR. *International Politics Reviews, 9*(1), 193–212. https://doi.org/10.1057/s41312-021-00086-1

Chavez-Dueñas, N. Y., & Adames, H. Y. (2021). Intersectionality awakening model of womanista: A transnational treatment approach for Latinx women. *Women & Therapy, 44*(1–2), 83–100. https://doi.org/10.1080/02703149.2020.1775022

Ciofalo, N. (Ed.). (2019). *Indigenous psychologies in an era of decolonization.* Springer. https://doi.org/10.1007/978-3-030-04822-8

Comas-Díaz, L. (1994). LatiNegra: Mental health issues of African Latinas. *Journal of Feminist Family Therapy, 5*(3–4), 35–74. https://doi.org/10.1300/J086v05n03_03

Comas-Díaz, L. (2007). Ethnopolitical psychology: Healing and transformation. In E. Aldarondo (Ed.), *Promoting social justice in mental health practice* (pp. 91–118). Lawrence Erlbaum.

Comas-Díaz, L., & Torres Rivera, E. (Eds.). (2020). *Liberation psychology: Theory, method, practice, and social justice.* American Psychological Association. https://doi.org/10.1037/0000198-000

Cunningham, C., & Stanley, F. (2003). Indigenous by definition, experience, or world view. *BMJ, 327*(7412), 403–404. https://doi.org/10.1136/bmj.327.7412.403

Dotson, K. (2011). Tracking epistemic violence, tracking practices of silencing. *Hypatia: A Journal of Feminist Philosophy, 26*(2), 236–257.

Fanon, F. (1967). *Black skin, white masks.* Grove Press.

Gergen, K. J., Gulerce, A., Lock, A., & Misra, G. (1996). Psychological science in cultural context. *American Psychologist, 51*(5), 496–503. https://doi.org/10.1037/0003-066X.51.5.496

Grzanka, P. R., & Moradi, B. (2021). The qualitative imagination in counseling psychology: Enhancing methodological rigor across methods. *Journal of Counseling Psychology, 68*(3), 247–258. https://doi.org/10.1037/cou0000560

Hartmann, W. E., Wendt, D. C., Burrage, R. L., Pomerville, A., & Gone, J. P. (2019). American Indian historical trauma: Anticolonial prescriptions for healing, resilience, and survivance. *American Psychologist, 74*(1), 6–19. https://doi.org/10.1037/amp0000326

Helms, J. E. (1993). I also said, "White racial identity influences White researchers." *The Counseling Psychologist, 21*(2), 240–243. https://doi.org/10.1177/0011000093212007

Helms, J. E. (2016, Fall). An election to save White heterosexual male privilege. *Latina/o Psychology Today, 3*(2), 6–7. https://www.nlpa.ws/assets/docs/newsletters/final%20lpt%20volume_3_no_2_2016.pdf

Kellogg, S. (2005). *Weaving the past: A history of Latin America's Indigenous women from the Prehispanic period to the present*. Oxford University Press.

Livi-Bacci, M. (2008). *Conquest: The destruction of the American Indios*. Polity.

Marcos, S. (2002). *Our word is our weapon: Selected writings*. Seven Stories.

Mignolo, W. D. (2011). *The darker side of Western modernity: Global futures, decolonial options*. Duke University Press.

Moore-Gilbert, B. (1997). *Postcolonial theory: Contexts, practices, politics*. Verso.

Morrow, S. L. (2005). Quality and trustworthiness in qualitative research in counseling psychology. *Journal of Counseling Psychology, 52*(2), 250–260. https://doi.org/10.1037/0022-0167.52.2.250

The New School. (2020). *Decolonizing psychology: Applications in research and clinical practice*. Retrieved from https://event.newschool.edu/decolonizngpsychologyconf

Pope, K. S., Vasquez, M. J. T., Chavez-Dueñas, N. Y., & Adames, H. Y. (2021). *Ethics in psychotherapy and counseling: A practical guide*. Wiley.

Readsura Decolonial Editorial Collective. (2022a). Psychology as a site for decolonial analysis. *Journal of Social Issues, 78*(2), 255–277. https://doi.org/10.1111/josi.12524

Readsura Decolonial Editorial Collective. (2022b). Special issue: Decolonial approaches to the psychological study of social issues, Installment 2: Psychology as a site for decolonial analysis. *Journal of Social Issues, 78*(2), 249–482.

Spivak, G. C. (1988). Can the subaltern speak? In C. Nelson & L. Grossber (Eds.), *Marxism and the interpretation of culture* (pp. 24–28). Macmillan.

Teachers College. (2021). *Decolonizing psychology training: Strategies for addressing curriculum, research, practices, clinical supervision, and mentorship*. https://www.tc.columbia.edu/decolonizing-psychology-conference/

PART I HISTORY AND KNOWLEDGE

1

COLONIAL MENTALITY

Manifestations, Operations, and Psychological Implications

HANNAH L. REBADULLA, JONATHAN U. GUERRERO, AND
E. J. R. DAVID

For many years to come we shall be bandaging the countless and sometimes indelible wounds inflicted on our people by the colonialist onslaught. Imperialism . . . sows seeds of decay (or germs of rot) . . . that must be mercilessly rooted out from our land and from our minds.

—Frantz Fanon, *Wretched of the Earth* (1965, p. 249)

As postcolonial scholar Frantz Fanon (1965) stated, colonialism is violent and pervasive and has long-lasting consequences. Colonialism's systematic use of violence in economic and political ways unavoidably also fragment peoples' cultures and ways of being (Fanon, 1965; Freire, 1970; Memmi, 1965). Thus colonialism's impact and legacy exist and persist not just in the political, material, and economic realms, but also in the psychological experiences of the colonized (Okazaki et al., 2008). Indeed, consistent with what Fanon called "seeds of decay" or "germs of rot," theoretical and empirical literature suggest that communities resisting their colonial status or dealing with the residual effects of colonization experience a psychological

https://doi.org/10.1037/0000376-002
Decolonial Psychology: Toward Anticolonial Theories, Research, Training, and Practice,
L. Comas-Díaz, H. Y. Adames, and N. Y. Chavez-Dueñas (Editors)

phenomenon commonly termed *colonial mentality* (CM), a specific type of internalized oppression wherein colonized individuals find themselves suffering from internalized negative views, a loss of dignity, and an overall sense of inferiority toward their colonizer.

Despite the fact that scholars and community leaders have long recognized the psychological damages of colonialism, and whereas other fields such as postcolonial studies, ethnic studies, and sociology have discussed it for decades, the field of psychology seems to have lagged behind in terms of how much attention it has paid to colonial mentality. For instance, a search on PsycInfo—the largest database of psychology and psychology-related literature abstracts in the world, with more than 5 million records from the 1800s and earlier up to the present—revealed only 95 results using the terms "colonial mentality" or "internalized colonialism" (as of September 29, 2021). This is particularly surprising given that psychology, with its focus on better understanding peoples' "mentalities," seems to be the field most naturally equipped to lead the study of colonial mentality. Nevertheless, there seems to be some spark of hope given that 88 of the results were published during the last 15 years, suggesting that psychology may finally be paying increased attention to colonial mentality. To this end, this chapter will highlight some studies in this growing body of literature and provide some research, clinical, and community recommendations to better understand and address CM as different communities experienced it.

THE PERVASIVENESS OF COLONIAL MENTALITY

Colonialism was pervasive; thus it follows that its psychological consequences are equally ubiquitous. Fanon's (1965) observations of the damages wrought by French colonization of Algeria are arguably among the most well-known works on colonialism and colonial mentality. Synthesizing Fanon's writings on colonialism and applying the colonial model to the experiences of African Americans, criminal justice scholar Becky Tatum (1994) argued that there seem to be four typical phases of colonialism. The first is the forced entry of a foreign group into a geographic territory with the intention of exploiting the native peoples' natural resources, including the peoples themselves. The second involves cultural imposition of the colonizers' worldviews and ways of doing onto the native peoples, cultural disintegration of the native peoples' ways, and cultural recreation of the native peoples' ways as inferior to those of the colonizers. Once a clear contrast is established between the supposedly superior colonizer and the supposedly inferior colonized—wherein the colonized are portrayed as wild, savage peoples whom the colonizer has to police, educate, civilize, and tame—a rationale is essentially created to put oppression and domination into practice, which is the third phase. The fourth and final phase is the development and institutionalization of policies and systems (political, social, economic) that carry out the colonizer's supposedly noble intention of civilizing, educating, or enlightening the colonized, creating a society wherein those who adhere or assimilate to the colonizer's ways reap some benefits whereas those who do not are punished.

What happens to the people who live in such an oppressive colonial climate? According to Fanon and other noted postcolonial studies scholars, such as Tunisian essayist Albert Memmi (1965) and Brazilian educator Paolo Freire (1970), colonized people may eventually succumb to the inferiorizing messages about their heritage that permeate—and are reinforced by— the colonial society. Colonized people may feel ashamed and embarrassed because of their heritage and develop a desire to distance themselves from the stigma that has been attached to their ethnicity and culture. Consequently, because the colonial society portrays as better, more civilized, and more beneficial the ways of the colonizers, the colonized may begin to emulate the colonizer in various ways such as adopting their language, values, mannerisms, worldviews, standards, and ways of doing things. Furthermore, colonized people might develop a sense of gratitude or indebtedness to the colonizers for civilizing them, enlightening them, teaching them, or saving them. This may manifest as tolerating, minimizing, or even justifying the oppression and injustices they face—historically and contemporarily—because such injustices have come to be seen as the natural cost for "progress" or "civilization."

These influential works are consistent with how Jose Rizal, a Filipino national hero who was executed by Spanish colonizers in 1896, described Filipinos' experiences under Spanish rule. In 1889, Rizal wrote,

> little by little they lost their old traditions, the mementos of their past; they gave up their writing, their songs, their poems, their laws in order to learn by rote other doctrines which they did not understand, another morality, another aesthetics different from those inspired by their climate and their manner of thinking . . . degrading themselves in their own eyes; they became ashamed of what was their own; they began to admire and praise whatever was foreign and incomprehensible; their spirit was dismayed and it surrendered . . . to this disgust of themselves. (Rizal, 1912, p. 33)

This powerful passage suggests that CM has been a salient issue among Filipinos as far back as the 1800s. It is not surprising, therefore, that the majority of the scant literature on CM has included Filipinos. For instance, of the 95 PsycInfo results on "colonial mentality" or "internalized colonialism," 74 either referred to "Filipinos" or had "Filipinos" as a keyword.

One of the more explicit calls for increased psychological attention on CM was when David and Okazaki (2006a) argued that the construct is a critical factor to consider when conceptualizing Filipino Americans' psychological experiences and mental health. They followed this up with the development of the Colonial Mentality Scale (CMS) for Filipino Americans (David & Okazaki, 2006b), which they hoped would spark more psychological research on CM not just among Filipinos but also among other communities with similar experiences of colonialism or oppression. Since then, the CMS has been adapted and used successfully among Ghanaians (Utsey et al., 2014), Puerto Ricans (Capielo Rosario et al., 2019), and Asian Indians (Nikalje & Çiftçi, 2021), making available psychometrically developed measures of CM for different social groups that, in turn, can stimulate even more research on this topic. Beyond the CMS, other literature on CM addresses it as experienced by Samoans (Faaleava, 2020), Mexicans (Miranda, 2011), and Peoples of Color in general (Hal, 2011). Relatedly, work has increased on internalized racism—a more general term often used interchangeably with CM—among other communities with similar histories of colonialism and oppression such as Latinx people (Hipolito-Delgado et al., 2014), Indigenous peoples of North America (Gonzalez et al., 2014), African Americans (Bailey et al., 2011), Vietnamese Americans (Huynh, 2022), Pacific Island Peoples (Salzman & Laenui, 2014), and Peoples of Color in general (Campón & Carter, 2015). Indeed, from the classic literature on colonialism to the more contemporary body of research on its psychological consequences, it is clear that CM is a worldwide phenomenon.

Manifestations of Colonial Mentality

Many of the CM-focused research over the past 15 years has explored how different groups express CM. In their validation of the CMS, David and Okazaki (2006b) found through exploratory and confirmatory factor analyses that Filipino Americans typically express CM in five ways: feelings of inferiority for being of one's ethnicity and culture; feelings of shame and embarrassment related to one's ethnicity and culture; discriminating against less-Westernized members of one's group because such people are seen as backward or inferior; regarding European physical characteristics such as having lighter skin tones and more bridged noses as more desirable and attractive; and feeling thankful and indebted to colonizers for civilizing, educating, and enlightening one's community. Utsey et al. (2014) investigated the factor structure of the CMS on a sample of Ghanaians and obtained results that map on quite well with David and Okazaki's findings. Specifically, Utsey et al. found that Ghanaians tend to typically express CM in four ways: feelings of shame and inferiority, within-group discrimination, physical characteristics, and colonial debt. Similarly, Nikalje and Çiftçi (2021) found that Asian Indians tend to manifest CM as feeling ashamed and inferior for one's culture, preferring lighter skin color, discriminating against less-Americanized Indians (e.g., speaking with an Indian accent), and feeling indebted for colonization. Among Puerto Ricans, whose colonial experience is quite similar to that of Filipinos (Spanish and American colonialism), Capielo Rosario et al. (2019) found that CM is commonly expressed through feelings of inferiority, shame, and embarrassment for being Puerto Rican, discriminating against less-Americanized Puerto Ricans, regarding European physical features as more desirable, and colonial debt.

Studies with other communities that explore the manifestations of the more general construct of internalized racism found similar results as the studies on colonial mentality. For example, Bailey and colleagues (2011) found that African Americans typically express internalized racism by devaluing African worldview and motifs, altering their physical appearance, internalizing negative stereotypes about Black people, and changing their hair. Another example is a study by Campón and Carter (2015) who—using data from almost 700 participants who identified as Black, Asian, Latinx, Native American, or multiracial—found that the common manifestations of internalized racism among Peoples of Color are feelings of shame, embarrassment, or inferiority for one's racial group; subscribing to the White American standard or definition of beauty; and minimizing or justifying racism or injustices. Thus, despite some slight differences in how racial groups may specifically express it (e.g., changing one's hair for Black people), overlap is clear and strong in how CM—or more generally internalized racism—is experienced by historically colonized or oppressed groups. That is, CM or internalized racism seems to be commonly manifested by the denigration of one's self, body, and cultural heritage, discrimination against others who are less assimilated to a colonizer's culture, and toleration or justification of historical and contemporary experiences of oppression.

With regard to their prevalence, studies with different communities (Filipino Americans, Ghanaians, Puerto Ricans, and Asian Indians) consistently find that approximately one-third endorse at least one CM manifestation (Capielo Rosario et al., 2019; David & Okazaki, 2006b; Nikalje & Çiftçi, 2021; Utsey et al., 2014). As prevalent as CM seems to be, however, indications are that CM manifestations are experienced or witnessed even more frequently. For example, although only around 30% of their Filipino American sample endorsed at least one of the five common CM manifestations, David and Okazaki (2006b) found that 85% of their sample have witnessed a family member express CM attitudes and behaviors, 88% have witnessed a friend display CM, and 90% have seen CM manifestations in their larger community. The same study also found that exposure to CM manifestations was positively correlated with CMS scores. Even further, studies with Filipino Americans (David & Okazaki, 2006a, 2006b, 2010) and Asian Indians (Nikalje & Çiftçi, 2021) found that more frequent experiences of racism were also positively correlated with the feelings of inferiority and/or cultural shame/embarrassment subscales of the CMS, which are theorized to be the initial stages of CM development. The combination of these findings suggest that CM may develop and be passed down intergenerationally through socialization and continued oppression. Interestingly, the CMS subscale of Colonial Debt (i.e., feeling indebted to previous colonizers) was negatively correlated with experiences of racial discrimination in both Filipino American and Asian Indian samples. This CM dimension can be expressed as the toleration, minimization, and even justification of historical and contemporary oppression. Thus this finding highlights how CM—particularly the Colonial Debt manifestation—may be perpetuating and even justifying an oppressive status quo, which in turn can lead to the development of colonial mentality.

Automaticity of Colonial Mentality

Although the increasing availability of self-report scales to capture CM has helped facilitate the growth of CM-focused research, that CM is a sensitive and undesirable construct many people may not be as forthcoming to admit having is undeniable. Additionally, even the studies using self-report measures of CM consistently find that components of CM that are more covert and focused on internal mechanisms (e.g., attitudes, feelings, beliefs) might be less easily identifiable and reportable than more overt and behavior-oriented manifestations (e.g., discriminating against less-Westernized people, changing one's physical traits). Further, CM has been defined as an automatic and uncritical rejection of anything from one's heritage and an automatic and uncritical preference for anything American or Western (David & Okazaki, 2006a), suggesting that some components of CM may be more covert, less obvious, and even automatic. Thus a need seems apparent for tools or methods that are less susceptible to potential response biases and that can capture the less blatant and possibly automatic component of colonial mentality.

To fill this gap, the application of tools and methods commonly used in social cognition research to the study of CM seems to be promising. For example, David and Okazaki (2010) applied a simple word-completion task to test whether a CM-consistent cognitive schema—wherein Filipino-related stimuli activate inferior thoughts and American-related stimuli activate superior thoughts—exist among Filipino Americans. They found that participants who completed Filipino word fragments first (e.g., Phil_p_ines, Taga_o_, Bro_n) were more likely to complete the word fragment "_ _ _ erior" as "Inferior" than participants who completed American word fragments first (e.g., Uni_ed S_ates, Engl_s_, Whit_). In contrast, they also found that participants who completed American word fragments first were more likely to complete the word fragment "_ _ _ erior" as "Superior" than participants who completed Filipino word fragments first. Furthermore, they replicated this study with a sample of Filipino Americans who outwardly express their pride and interest in their identity (i.e., attendees of a Filipino American conference), suggesting that even people who may seem satisfied and secure with their heritage may still harbor automatic thoughts of inferiority toward such heritage.

To further investigate the automaticity of CM, David and Okazaki (2010) used the lexical decision-priming task and found that Filipino American participants reacted more quickly and committed fewer mistakes when pleasant target words (e.g., beautiful) followed a subliminal "American" prime, than when pleasant target words followed a subliminal neutral prime. Participants were not faster and not more accurate when unpleasant words followed an American prime than when unpleasant words followed a neutral prime. This suggests that Filipino Americans have automatically associated American culture with positivity, but not with negativity. However, participants reacted more quickly and more accurately when unpleasant target words (e.g., ugly) followed a subliminal "Filipino" prime, than when unpleasant target words followed a subliminal neutral prime. Participants were not faster and not more accurate when pleasant words followed a Filipino prime than when pleasant words followed a neutral prime, suggesting that Filipino Americans have automatically associated Filipino culture with negativity, but not with positivity. These findings demonstrate that CM may be activated automatically and influence colonized peoples' cognitions by mere exposure to colonized or colonizer-related stimuli.

Another commonly used social cognition method that has been applied to the study of CM is the Implicit Association Test (IAT). Following typical IAT paradigms, David and Okazaki (2010) and David (2010) developed the CM-IAT, in which in the first block participants distinguished between an American word or a Filipino word. Block 2 was similar in that participants distinguished between a pleasant word and an unpleasant word. In block 3, participants were asked to press one computer key if they saw either an American or pleasant word, or to press another if they saw either a Filipino or unpleasant word. Block 4 simply switched the keys, and block 5 asked participants to press one key if they saw either a Filipino or pleasant word, or to press another if they saw either an American or unpleasant word.

The hypothesis was that if Filipino Americans have automatically associated anything pleasant with American and anything unpleasant with Filipino, then they would find block 3 easier than block 5. To put it another way, if CM operates automatically, then participants would have faster reaction times and commit fewer mistakes in block 3 than in block 5, because block 3 is consistent with a cognitive system that reflects colonial mentality. Consistent with the hypothesis, their results showed that participants committed more errors and were slower when American words were paired with unpleasant words or when Filipino words were paired with pleasant words. In contrast, they were faster and committed fewer errors when American words were paired with pleasant words or when Filipino words were paired with unpleasant words. Altogether, the results of these social cognition studies suggest that CM can be covertly and overtly expressed and may exist and operate automatically outside of one's awareness, intention, or control.

PSYCHOLOGICAL IMPLICATIONS OF COLONIAL MENTALITY

As evidenced by the literature discussed in the previous section, the effects of colonialism extend beyond political and physical means of violence and oppression. Those who have experienced historical and contemporary forms of colonialism are also affected psychologically. CM influences the way individuals from colonized groups perceive themselves, other members of their group, as well as how they regard and behave toward dominant groups in society. Indeed, as Fanon (1965) stated, "Because it is a systematic negation of the other person and a furious determination to deny the other person all attributes of humanity, colonialism forces the people it dominates to ask themselves the question constantly: 'In reality, who am I?'" (p. 250), suggesting that one of colonialism's many damages is that it leaves the colonized in a perpetual identity crisis—a highly distressing psychological condition that can lead to other mental health concerns. Thus, in this section, we review some studies on the influences of CM on acculturation, ethnic and racial identity formation, and mental health.

Colonial Mentality, Acculturation, and Ethnic or Racial Identity

Research shows that acculturation is an important factor in understanding the psychological experiences of different racial or ethnic groups (for a review, see Balls Organista, Organista, & Kurasaki, 2003). Briefly, *acculturation* is the adjustment process among all involved that occurs when groups from different cultures interact with one another (Berry, 2003). Acculturation does not occur in a vacuum, however, and larger sociopolitical factors affect how people acculturate and which people are more pressured to adjust. Power imbalances between groups inevitably force groups with less power to adjust or change more than groups with more power. Given the pervasiveness of colonialism and continued oppression—important historical and contemporary sociopolitical factors—CM is therefore a vital factor to consider in how various groups acculturate. Indeed, in their studies with Filipino Americans, David (2008) and David and Okazaki (2006b) found that all factors of CM related with lower levels of enculturation (i.e., the extent to which one adheres to one's heritage culture). Further, participants who endorsed more overt expressions of CM (i.e., within-group discrimination, physical characteristics) also tended to have stronger assimilation attitudes. Similarly, colonial debt positively correlated with mainstream acculturation and negatively correlated with enculturation. These findings suggest that CM may lead to either marginalization or assimilation, two acculturation strategies that literature suggests are not as psychologically beneficial as when individuals are connected with their heritage culture (i.e., enculturation) or both their heritage and the mainstream cultures. Consistent with these findings, Capielo Rosario and colleagues (2019) also found that CM among Puerto Ricans is related to higher levels of acculturative stress.

Furthermore, although most studies on acculturation tend to focus on the experiences of immigrants as they adjust to their adopted country, it is important to recognize that the process of acculturation for historically colonized peoples have been happening in their heritage lands for a much longer time. That is, because of colonialism and its legacies, historically and contemporarily colonized peoples have been dealing with the process of acculturation and acculturative stress in their own countries for generations. For example, David and Nadal (2013) found that Filipino American immigrants commonly experienced ethnic and cultural denigration as they were growing up in the Philippines—often from their own family, friends, and community—before they even emigrated to the United States. These experiences were also found to be associated with the development of CM within Filipino American immigrants, and their CM was further reinforced by racism experiences after they arrived in the United States.

Another important psychological construct that is theoretically related to acculturation and CM is ethnic or racial identity (ERI). Briefly, *ERI* is defined as the connotation, significance, and interpretation that individuals use to construct their perspective of being a member of their ethnic or racial group (Sellers et al., 1998). Enculturation is theorized to lead toward the development of a positive ERI (i.e., positive regard of their ethnic or racial group), which is associated with better self-esteem, psychological well-being, and mental health (e.g., Gong et al., 2003; Phinney, 1992; Phinney et al., 1992; Wilson et al., 2017). Similar to acculturation, ERI development does not happen in a vacuum and is also influenced by larger sociopolitical factors (e.g., Berry, 2003; Phinney, 1992; Yeh & Huang, 1996). Thus CM may also impact the extent to which historically colonized or oppressed peoples develop positive or negative regard of their ethnic or racial group, consistent with Helms' (1995) argument that the primary goal of ethnic or racial identity development among Peoples of Color is to overcome internalized racism. Indeed, studies with Filipino Americans suggest that CM is related to lower levels of ERI (David, 2008; V. E. Tuazon et al., 2019). On a more general level, studies on internalized racism with various ethnic or racial groups have also found internalized racism to be related to lower levels of ERI (e.g., Choi et al., 2017; Hipolito-Delgado, 2016; Lee, 2005; Maxwell, et al., 2015; Willis et al., 2021; see also Cokley, 2002).

Colonial Mentality and Mental Health

Given the emerging evidence that CM is related to other constructs (i.e., acculturation, acculturative stress, ethnic and racial identity) that are known to influence the mental health and well-being of historically colonized or oppressed groups, many CM-focused studies have also investigated the potential relationship between CM and various indicators of mental health and well-being. In recent years, studies with various ethnic groups with colonized histories have demonstrated that CM is consistently associated with poorer well-being and mental health such as lower levels of personal self-esteem and collective self-esteem (e.g., David & Okazaki, 2006b; Utsey et al., 2014), lower life satisfaction (e.g., David, 2008), and higher levels of body dissatisfaction (Cajucom, 2016). Some studies with Filipino American (Clement, 2014) and Ghanaian (Utsey et al., 2014) participants have also found a positive relationship between CM and anxiety symptoms. Much of the literature investigating the mental health implications of CM, however, has focused on its relationship with depression symptoms (e.g., Capielo Rosario et al., 2019; David, 2008, 2010; David & Okazaki, 2006b; Nikalje & Çiftçi, 2021; Utsey et al., 2014).

With the goal of creating a model that better captures the etiology of depression among Filipino Americans, David (2008) found that even though a conceptual model that incorporated other related variables such as personal and collective self-esteem, acculturation, ethnic identity, and life satisfaction had good fit with the data and captured a substantial proportion of the variance in depression (32.5%), a model that also included CM still had better fit statistics and accounted for a significantly higher proportion of the variance in depression (62.4%). Similarly, due to Ghana's long history of being colonized and oppressed, Utsey and colleagues (2014) postulated that Ghanaians would also exhibit parallel patterns of relationships between CM and mental health variables. Indeed, they found that CM was related to lower personal and collective self-esteem, and higher levels of depression. Likewise, positing that centuries of colonialism and its psychological consequences may better explain the high rates of depression among Puerto Ricans than the typical acculturative stress paradigm, Capielo Rosario and colleagues (2019) tested a conceptual model that included CM and found that it explains 76% of the variance in depression. Furthermore, they also found that acculturative stress fully mediates the positive relationship between CM and depression symptoms. Altogether, these studies suggest that CM is an important factor to consider when conceptualizing the mental health and well-being of historically colonized groups.

Given CM's negative impact on mental health and well-being, some studies have also investigated CM's potential influence on another important mental health–related variable: help-seeking. Overall, the findings from these studies consistently suggest that CM is related to lower likelihood of seeking help for mental health concerns (Bartlett, 2010; A. C. A. Tuazon, 2013; V. E. Tuazon et al., 2019). For example, a recent study found that CM among Filipino Americans significantly predicted negative mental health help-seeking attitudes above and beyond ethnic identity, acculturation, social support, and demographic variables (V. E. Tuazon et al., 2019). The authors also found that CM is related to lower levels of social support, and that social support significantly predicted positive help-seeking attitudes for participants with mental health problems. The researchers theorized that CM acts as an isolating mechanism where Filipino Americans with high CM are less interested in building relationships with those in their culture. This disconnection or lack of enculturation eventually leads to a reduced social support network and ultimately a lower probability of help-seeking for mental health problems. Thus combining the body of research suggesting that CM is related to mental health concerns with the findings that CM is also related to lower likelihood of mental health help-seeking, it is probable that many people with histories of colonialism may not be receiving the services they might need. This compounding impact on mental health and help-seeking represents yet another troubling psychological consequence of colonial mentality.

FROM COLONIAL TO DECOLONIAL MENTALITY: CLINICAL AND COMMUNITY EFFORTS

The growing body of empirical evidence suggesting that CM has many negative mental health consequences is consistent with Fanon's (1965) statement that colonialism has inflicted "countless wounds" on colonized peoples. Fanon, who was also a psychiatrist in addition to being a leader of Algeria's liberation efforts against French colonialism, further stated that "bandaging" or "rooting out" these colonial wounds "from our land and from our minds" will require plenty of work, signifying that both individual- and systemic-level changes are necessary to eradicate CM and its many associated damages. To this, we now highlight some efforts to address CM in both clinical and community settings (see David, 2014, for a review).

Addressing Colonial Mentality in the Clinical Context

Several traditional clinical approaches (e.g., humanistic, psychoanalytic, and so on) can be used to conceptualize and address colonial mentality. One modality that seems to have more potential than others, however, is cognitive-behavioral therapy because of its practicality, familiarity, and wide-scale use in health care settings (David, 2009). Using cognitive-behavioral theories, CM, or internalized racism more generally, may be understood as a set of self-defeating cognitions, attitudes, and behaviors that have been shaped by an oppressive environment. Furthermore, CM may be conceptualized as a distorted view of oneself and others (i.e., one's group, other oppressed peoples, dominant group) because of the messages propagated by an oppressive environment. Colonized people consistently receive the message that they are inferior to the dominant group. Eventually, members of colonized groups may no longer need the oppressive society to perpetuate such inferiorizing messages; they begin telling themselves. As supported by the findings of social cognition studies on CM (David, 2010; David & Okazaki, 2010), colonized peoples may eventually internalize the oppression they experience in such a deep way that it creates within them a distorted cognitive system characterized by automatic negative perceptions of their heritage. Consistent with cognitive-behavioral theories on psychopathology (e.g., Beck et al., 1979), underlying such automatic thoughts, attitudes (e.g., "lighter skin is more attractive or desirable") or behaviors (e.g., discriminating against less-Westernized members of the same ethnic group) are maladaptive general beliefs (e.g., "being White is better") that have been developed from oppressive experiences (e.g., colonialism, boarding schools, contemporary oppression). Such thoughts and beliefs contribute to the creation of dysfunctional self-schemas (e.g., "I am not White, therefore I am not attractive") that may lead to distress and various psychopathology.

As potentially useful as traditional clinical frameworks are in conceptualizing and addressing CM, however, all of them are still reductionist (David & Derthick, 2018). In other words, they all conceptualize pathology and change at the individual level. The cognitive behavior therapy (CBT) approach described previously, for example, is still focused on changing individuals' thoughts, attitudes, and behaviors. Thus traditional clinical approaches neglect to address the contexts beyond the individual, such as oppression or colonialism, which are the roots of colonial mentality. To treat the psychological impacts of oppression or colonialism, clinical efforts must look beyond the individual level and also acknowledge their sociopolitical context. Indeed, liberation psychologists have argued that the role of psychologists is to help clients understand their psychological experiences in the context of the broader sociopolitical structures that exist (Martín-Baró, 1994; Torres Rivera, 2019). When psychologists consider clients' historical, political, and cultural contexts in their conceptualizations, they can better understand the experiences of their clients, improve their therapeutic relationship, reduce cultural mistrust, and form effective interventions (David, 2013). Furthermore, clients' experiences of oppression are legitimized. As a result, clients can learn how to externalize and name the ways in which they have been or continue to be oppressed and find ways to change those oppressive systems.

Decolonial Clinical Approaches

Decolonial clinical approaches that incorporate clients' sociopolitical context include liberation psychotherapy and the social justice counseling model (Comas-Díaz, 2020; Ratts, 2009). Liberation psychotherapy is rooted in liberation theory (Comas-Díaz, 2020). The practice is grounded in a deep understanding of the sociopolitical, historical, and cultural contexts of oppressed people. Liberation psychotherapy considers each context and the ways they affect a client's psychological experience. Liberation psychotherapists, therefore, acknowledge the insidious psychological effects of colonization. Liberation psychotherapists examine how the structures of power and privilege that were established by colonizers continue to impose the colonizer's values and ideals on colonized people (Comas-Díaz, 2020; Quijano & Ennis, 2000). They address CM by helping clients to "deconstruct (neo)colonizing stories, reformulate personal and collective identities, develop a sociopolitical consciousness, and foster transformative changes" (Comas-Díaz, 2020, p. 170). Liberation psychotherapists validate and encourage the cultural and spiritual practices of clients, help clients recover historical memory, raise clients' critical consciousness, and nurture clients' healing, growth, and desire for social justice action. Unlike many Western clinical approaches, liberation psychotherapists incorporate psychospiritual, Indigenous healing, and holistic approaches into their practice (Comas-Díaz, 2020).

Inspired by liberation psychology and conscientization, or critical consciousness (Freire, 1970; Martín-Baró, 1994), Ratts's (2009) Social Justice Counseling Model is another decolonial clinical approach that addresses the limitations of traditional therapy modalities (David & Derthick, 2018). Like liberation psychotherapy, social justice counseling looks beyond the individual level and recognizes that clients' sociopolitical, historical, and cultural contexts affect their mental health. Because the model is based on raising critical consciousness, social justice therapists help clients address internalized oppression by helping them identify oppressive structures in their environment. In doing so, clients begin to feel empowered to act against the systems that perpetuate coloniality, thereby breaking the cycle of CM in their lives (David & Derthick, 2018; Ratts, 2009). Furthermore, social justice therapists believe that clinical work and interventions extend beyond the therapy room. Ratts (2009) states that social justice counselors engage in community-based work and advocacy to change systems that negatively affect the well-being of marginalized clients and communities.

To embody decoloniality when working with clients, the therapist's identity and role beyond the therapeutic relationship must be addressed. Liberation psychotherapy and the social justice counseling model both emphasize the importance of reflecting on the therapist's positionality. In both approaches, therapists must examine the ways in which they hold and represent power and privilege and how that may affect their clients (Comas-Díaz, 2020; David & Derthick, 2018; Ratts, 2009). Liberation psychotherapy and the social justice counseling model recommends that therapists use power differential analyses (Worrell & Remer, 2003), the ADDRESSING (age, developmental disability, disability acquired later in life, religion and spiritual orientation, ethnic or racial identity, socioeconomic status, sexual orientation, Indigenous heritage, national origin, and gender) framework (Hays, 2001), and other methods to identify their areas of power, privilege, and oppression. For example, a young White heterosexual woman therapist seeing a client who is an older gay Asian man should be mindful of her power and privileges as a White heterosexual person while keeping an eye on how age and gender dynamics may play a role in the therapeutic relationship. These types of models recommend that therapists contrast their areas of power, privilege, and oppression with that of their clients and, when appropriate, disclose their findings with their clients when such power dynamics may be influencing therapeutic processes and outcomes (Comas-Díaz, 2020; David & Derthick, 2018).

Decolonial Community Efforts to Address Colonial Mentality

Although useful and necessary, however, clinical efforts to address CM are not enough. To end the insidious cycle of CM or internalized racism, it is imperative that we also take decolonial community-based approaches to address systems that maintain and perpetuate oppression. Community efforts to address CM may include raising a community's awareness of an issue, developing community programs, educating the community, and psychological decolonization.

One way that psychologists can address CM or internalized racism is to prevent people from being exposed to oppression. David and Derthick (2018) state that this can be done by directly changing or eliminating systems and institutions that perpetuate injustice and oppression (e.g., criminal justice system, police departments, schools, and so on). Psychologists can collaborate with communities to raise awareness of the oppressive institutions or systems in place by suggesting tactics such as townhall discussions, media campaigns, and other outreach efforts. Once a community becomes aware and identifies the oppressive system they want to change, psychologists can collaborate with communities in organizing social change movements, lobbying, collaborating with community and organizational leaders, partnering with nonprofit organizations, and more.

Communities can also be key stakeholders in the development of community programs. They can identify the strengths and needs of their community and what an intervention program would need to enhance protective factors in the community that may prevent the internalization of the oppressive messages that permeate society. Although community intervention programs may not directly address oppression at the source, they can be designed and implemented to prevent or buffer the development and effects of CM by enhancing ethnic identity, increasing cultural connectedness, and teaching about colonial history (David & Derthick, 2018; Halagao, 2004; Lin & Israel, 2012; Neblett et al., 2012; Strobel, 2015).

Psychologists can also address CM by making information about history, colonialism, and oppression more open and accessible to the public. Many marginalized and oppressed people do not have the privilege to access resources and safe spaces where they can talk about oppression and internalized oppression. Psychologists can hold spaces in communities, in online video-conferencing platforms, or on social media for people to share their stories and have ongoing conversations about CM and decoloniality. They can also teach communities by sharing psychological concepts and findings related to CM and oppression in a jargon-free, readable way (David & Derthick, 2018). Psychologists have used social media platforms, online blogs, YouTube, magazines and newspapers, and podcasts and radio stations to make psychological theories and concepts more accessible and relatable to the public.

Psychological decolonization efforts within communities can also address colonial mentality. Briefly, psychological decolonization efforts attempt to reduce CM by examining the cognitive, emotional, and behavioral manifestations of CM and linking it back to people's historical and contemporary experiences of oppression (David, 2013). Although remembering that decolonization is not metaphor, in that decolonization for historically and contemporarily colonized peoples literally means liberation from settler colonizers and repatriation of lands and resources (Tuck & Yang, 2012), psychological decolonization efforts seem to help people from various colonized groups develop a critical consciousness in which they have a more accurate and realistic understanding of their experiences of oppression (Freire, 1970). From there, colonized peoples can presumably begin to address oppressive systems.

Various psychological decolonization frameworks have been developed by colonized peoples for colonized peoples (David, 2013; Halagao, 2004; Laenui, 2000; Strobel, 2015). One psychological decolonization framework was created for the Kanaka Maoli, that is, Native Hawaiian (Laenui, 2000). Laenui defined five stages of psychological decolonization: rediscovery or recovery, mourning, dreaming, commitment, and action. Rediscovery or recovery requires individuals to learn and acknowledge that their people have been colonized. In the mourning stage, people grieve for what they have lost due to colonization. The dreaming stage, perhaps the most crucial, is when people begin to imagine what all aspect of decolonization and self-determination may look like. It is when they can begin to express their hopes of new sociopolitical and cultural structures. In the commitment stage, people can commit to changing the oppressive systems and commit to a direction in which they want their society to move. The action stage is when people take proactive measures to promote decolonization on a larger level.

Another psychological decolonization framework was developed for Filipino Americans (Strobel, 2015). Strobel notes three stages of psychological decolonization: naming, reflecting, and acting. The naming stage occurs when people can name and understand the impact of CM on their identity. The reflection stage is when people critically reflect on the impact of colonial narratives on their personal experiences and the experiences of their family members and their community. In the acting stage, people give back to their communities by helping others in their psychological decolonization process and empowering their community to eliminate systems of coloniality. Similarly, Halagao (2004) also led a psychological decolonization effort that involved six Filipino Americans in a semester-long curriculum on Filipino history and culture during which the students engaged in extensive discussions and wrote journal reflections. Their experiences revealed valuable implications for decolonizing education. The curriculum encouraged the students to think critically about the historical and cultural knowledge that they had about themselves. It helped the students to become aware of how CM manifests within them and others. The curriculum enhanced the students' ethnic identification and inspired them to engage in social action.

Inspired by Strobel's (2015) and Halagao's (2004) work, David (2013) also implemented a psychological decolonization effort with Filipino Americans and found that four types of connections are necessary to address CM and facilitate systems-level changes. The first is making historical–contemporary connections: realizing how the violent, oppressive, and traumatic systems established in colonialism are still operating in today's modern structures and systems and ways of doing things. The second is connecting oppressive environmental social factors with individual and community issues: going beyond individual thoughts, feelings, and behaviors to explain individual and community struggles toward a focus on oppressive systems. The third is making connections between one's individual experiences with those of others in their community: this type of connection helps people realize that they are not alone in their struggles and may help them realize that their confusions, difficulties, pain, anger, sadness, and sometimes feelings of desolation and despair are legitimate responses to an oppressive world. Finally, the fourth connection is seeing the links between the experiences of one's community with the experiences of other communities: making between-groups connections addresses horizontal violence and hostility, and allow various communities to more accurately diagnose the problem of oppression as a complex, multipronged, and multifaceted issue, and address it more accordingly and effectively. Indeed, as Assata Shakur (1987) wrote,

> Any community seriously concerned with its own freedom has to be concerned about other peoples' freedom as well. The victory of oppressed people anywhere in the world is a victory for (all oppressed) people. Each time one of imperialism's tentacles is cut off we are closer to liberation. . . . Imperialism is an international system of exploitation, and we, as revolutionaries, need to be internationalists to defeat it. (p. 267)

Altogether, the four psychological decolonization efforts highlighted here involve learning about one's historical and contemporary experiences of oppression, gaining cultural knowledge, and dismantling systems of oppression and coloniality through social action. Most important, psychological decolonization efforts are not only an individual process. They also need to be done in community with one's group as well as in coalition with other groups to help each other become aware of CM, decolonize their minds, and embody decoloniality.

WAYS TO DECOLONIZE RESEARCH AND INTERVENTIONS ON COLONIAL MENTALITY

Without a doubt, the significant growth of CM-focused work over the past 15 years has contributed to a better understanding of the construct. We now know that CM is pervasive, prevalent, and may exist and operate outside our awareness, intention, or control. We also know that CM may be learned and passed on to later generations through socialization and continued experiences of oppression, and that CM is related to various psychological constructs including well-being and mental health variables. Further, some clinical and community efforts intended to reduce, eliminate, and even prevent colonial mentality are promising. Despite such progress, however, many questions remain, as do many areas of improvement pertaining to CM-focused work. To this end, we now turn to some recommendations for how CM research and interventions can be improved.

In the research context, it is clear from this review that a majority of CM-focused literature is about Filipino Americans. Thus, more work is needed on CM as experienced by other historically and contemporarily colonized peoples (e.g., Chamorus). Relatedly, the development of scales or other methods (e.g., implicit association tests) to empirically explore how CM is manifested by other communities are needed to spark more CM-focused research on such groups. Further, as promising as the use of social cognition methods are in capturing CM, such studies have so far been exclusively conducted with Filipino Americans. Future CM research that applies social cognition methods with other groups may therefore yield better understanding of CM's automaticity. Much of the recent literature on CM has used quantitative methods. Qualitative methods may generate a more nuanced understanding of the effects of colonialism, such as with Faaleava's (2020) study that found colonial resilience—the ability to resist the colonial pressures to negatively regard and replace one's heritage—to be a more salient construct than CM among Samoans.

More studies are also needed to explore the mental health consequences of CM with various groups. Further, the mental health implications of CM have so far been focused on mood and affective outcomes, such as depression and anxiety and other closely related constructs (e.g., self-esteem, life satisfaction). Thus, future research may explore CM's implications on other variables (e.g., substance use, diet). Even further, despite growing empirical evidence supporting the notion that CM is an important factor to consider with regard to the mental health of colonized peoples, studies suggest that the relationship between CM and mental health may be more complex. For instance, among Filipino Americans, covert CM manifestations (feelings of inferiority, shame, and embarrassment) seem to be more strongly related to mental health issues than overt CM (discriminating against less-Americanized people, desiring White physical features; David, 2008, 2010; David & Okazaki, 2006b). Among Ghanaians (Utsey et al., 2014), only feelings of shame and embarrassment and colonial debt were correlated with more anxiety and depression symptoms. Discriminating against less-Westernized Ghanaians positively correlated with anxiety only, whereas desiring White physical features positively correlated with depression only. Similarly, among Asian Indians (Nikalje & Çiftçi, 2021), higher levels of within-group discrimination were related to fewer depressive symptoms, suggesting that discriminating against less-Americanized members of one's group may function as a protective factor against depression. Altogether, these findings suggest that facets of CM may be differentially related with various mental health outcomes, depending on the particular community one is working with and the mental health variable one is looking at.

Future research on CM should also use decolonial and Indigenous research methodologies because these can further our understanding of the psychological effects of colonialism across historically and contemporarily colonized peoples. According to Chilisa (2019),

> Indigenous research has four dimensions: (1) It targets a local phenomenon instead of using extant theory from the West to identify and define a research issue; (2) it is context-sensitive and creates locally relevant constructs, methods, and theories derived from local experiences and indigenous knowledge; (3) it can be integrative, that is, combining Western and indigenous theories; and (4) in its most advanced form, its assumptions about what counts as reality, knowledge, and values in research are informed by an indigenous paradigm. (p. 9)

Using Indigenous research methodologies, psychologists could collaborate with historically oppressed peoples to identify culturally appropriate methods to study the consequences of colonialism and develop a more accurate understanding of the impacts of colonialism. This type of method is community based and participatory wherein the participants from the community are coresearchers who identify the research questions and determine the appropriate research methods, data analysis and interpretation, and dissemination of the results. Other examples of Indigenous research methods include the pagtatanong-tanong interview method rooted in Filipino culture (Pe-Pua, 1989), the diviner-client interviewing strategy from southern Africa (Chilisa, 2019), the focused life-story method developed with Māori people (Edwards et al., 2005), and talking circles that are familiar with many Indigenous peoples of North America (Wilson & Wilson, 2000). Psychologists could use Indigenous research methods to investigate the relationship between CM and other behavioral and mental health concerns (i.e., suicide, substance use, domestic violence, high-risk behaviors), develop culturally appropriate measures of CM, and examine potential factors that may buffer against the development of colonial mentality.

With regard to decolonial interventions, psychologists need to incorporate liberation and social justice frameworks into their practice. Psychologists should be aware of and understand the inherent powers and privileges they hold and how they may perpetuate the oppression of others. They need to go beyond their Western training to expand their competencies and knowledge base when working with historically colonized groups to ensure that they are understanding clients' cultures, worldviews, and experiences. For instance, psychologists can attend trainings such as Blanket Exercises (a participatory workshop on the painful colonial history of Indigenous peoples intended to foster healing and reconciliation), traditional medicine workshops, and community events. More specifically, attending community events such as protests or townhalls provide therapists a unique opportunity to learn about important issues directly from community members in a nonclinical setting. This could increase psychologists' understanding of sociopolitical factors and oppressive policies that affect their clients. Additionally, psychologists should also incorporate liberation and social justice frameworks when working with clients from groups who benefit from oppression and colonization. Just as psychologists work to become aware of the ways that they may hold power and privilege, they can also help clients identify how they hold powerful and privileged positions. This may lead both psychologists and clients to recognize and accept responsibility in propagating oppression, whether it is intentional or unintentional, and healing the wounds of oppression by striving to promote equitable solutions and practices in their day-to-day lives.

Regarding systemic-level interventions, Martín-Baró (1994) believed that psychology holds the potential to encourage people to participate in social justice activism and work together to change existing oppressive social structures. He therefore stated that psychologists have a duty to change the world. Psychologists and psychology training programs need to reframe the roles and duties of a psychologist to include a liberation and social justice orientation. Psychologists' roles extend beyond that of being teachers, researchers, therapists, and administrators. By including a liberation and social justice orientation, psychologists and psychologists-in-training can begin to embody an epistemology and a praxis that transforms their roles and realities into one that includes working collaboratively with historically oppressed peoples as consultants, community organizers, and coalition builders (David & Derthick, 2018).

CONCLUSION

Circling back to Frantz Fanon's (1965) quote at the beginning of this chapter, did colonialism leave behind "germs of rot" or "seeds of decay"? Yes, it did. Did colonialism inflict these damages on "our lands" and also "in our minds"? Yes, Fanon was right. Do these germs of rot or seeds of decay inflict "countless wounds" on colonized peoples? Yes, Fanon was correct about that as well. Does "bandaging" or "rooting out" these wounds require generations of multilevel work? Yes, Fanon seems to be correct on this too. Although many of the things Fanon said seem to have been proven true, we hope he is wrong about the "indelible" part; we hope that these colonial wounds can be healed, reversed, or erased. We hope these damages are not permanent. We truly hope Fanon is wrong on that one.

RESOURCES

CBS News. (2020, February 7). *Shady business: The illegal sale of skin-whitening creams* [TV series segment]. YouTube. https://www.youtube.com/watch?v=SgO-4SzJVHE

Davis, K. (2007, May 4). *A girl like me: A brief documentary on colorism in the Black community* [Video]. YouTube. https://www.youtube.com/watch?v=YWyI77Yh1Gg

Doan, T. (2020, June 5). *A Vietnamese woman describes her identity development and her struggles with colonial mentality* [Video]. YouTube. BAVC Media. https://www.youtube.com/watch?v=qhhrSRIbsGY

Good Morning America. (2020, July 24). *The emotional effects of skin lightening* [TV series segment]. YouTube. https://www.youtube.com/watch?v=xm1pnslhqzl

Lim, S. B. (2017, December 2). *Influenced identities: How colonial mentality shapes one's cultural character* [Video]. YouTube. https://www.youtube.com/watch?v=3-pE5Vii8JO

Next Day Better. (2019, October 15). *How a Filipino raises his kids with his Native Alaskan wife* [Video]. YouTube. https://youtu.be/IN2S_grP2ZE

REFERENCES

Bailey, T.-K. M., Chung, Y. B., Williams, W. S., Singh, A. A., & Terrell, H. K. (2011). Development and validation of the Internalized Racial Oppression Scale for Black individuals. *Journal of Counseling Psychology, 58*(4), 481–493. https://doi.org/10.1037/a0023585

Bartlett, C. A. (2010). *Enculturation, colonial mentality and help-seeking attitudes among Filipino Americans* (Publication No. 3452386) [Doctoral dissertation, Ateneo de Manila University]. ProQuest Dissertations & Theses Global.

Beck, A. T., Rush, A., Shaw, B., & Emery, G. (1979). *Cognitive therapy of depression.* Guilford Press.

Berry, J. W. (2003). Conceptual approaches to acculturation. In K. M. Chun, P. Balls Organista, & G. Marín (Eds.), *Acculturation: Advances in theory, measurement, and applied research* (pp. 17–37). American Psychological Association. https://doi.org/10.1037/10472-004

Cajucom, K. M. R. (2016). *Body dissatisfaction as a mediator and a moderator of colonial mentality and depression in Filipino Americans* (Publication No. 10162501) [Doctoral dissertation, University of La Verne]. ProQuest Dissertations & Theses Global.

Campón, R. R., & Carter, R. T. (2015). The Appropriated Racial Oppression Scale: Development and preliminary validation. *Cultural Diversity & Ethnic Minority Psychology, 21*(4), 497–506. https://doi.org/10.1037/cdp0000037

Capielo Rosario, C., Schaefer, A., Ballesteros, J., Rentería, R., & David, E. J. R. (2019). A caballo regalao no se le mira el colmillo: Colonial mentality and Puerto Rican depression. *Journal of Counseling Psychology, 66*(4), 396–408. https://doi.org/10.1037/cou0000347

Chilisa, B. (2019). *Indigenous research methodologies* (2nd ed.). Sage Publications.

Choi, A. Y., Israel, T., & Maeda, H. (2017). Development and evaluation of the Internalized Racism in Asian Americans Scale (IRAAS). *Journal of Counseling Psychology, 64*(1), 52–64. https://doi.org/10.1037/cou0000183

Clement, L. F. (2014). *Is there a correlation between colonial mentality and anxiety in Filipino Americans?* (Publication No. 3619001) [Doctoral dissertation, School of Professional Psychology, Alliant International University]. ProQuest Dissertations & Theses Global. https://www.proquest.com/openview/928852b48a13001a12c1572a8fafbb88

Cokley, K. (2002). Testing Cross's revised racial identity model: An examination of the relationship between racial identity and internalized racism. *Journal of Counseling Psychology, 49*(4), 476–483. https://doi.org/10.1037/0022-0167.49.4.476

Comas-Díaz, L. (2020). Liberation psychotherapy. In L. Comas-Díaz & E. Torres Rivera (Eds.), *Liberation psychology: Theory, method, practice, and social justice* (pp. 169–185). American Psychological Association. https://doi.org/10.1037/0000198-010

David, E. J. R. (2008). A colonial mentality model of depression for Filipino Americans. *Cultural Diversity & Ethnic Minority Psychology, 14*(2), 118–127. https://doi.org/10.1037/1099-9809.14.2.118

David, E. J. R. (2009). Internalized oppression, psychopathology, and cognitive-behavioral therapy among historically oppressed groups. *Journal of Psychological Practice, 15*(1), 71–103.

David, E. J. R. (2010). Testing the validity of the colonial mentality implicit association test and the interactive effects of covert and overt colonial mentality on Filipino American mental health. *Asian American Journal of Psychology, 1*(1), 31–45. https://doi.org/10.1037/a0018820

David, E. J. R. (2013). *Brown skin, white minds: Filipino-/American postcolonial psychology (with commentaries)*. Information Age Publishing.

David, E. J. R. (Ed.). (2014). *Internalized oppression: The psychology of marginalized groups*. Springer.

David, E. J. R., & Derthick, A. O. (2018). *The psychology of oppression*. Springer Publishing Company.

David, E. J. R., & Nadal, K. L. (2013). The colonial context of Filipino American immigrants' psychological experiences. *Cultural Diversity & Ethnic Minority Psychology, 19*(3), 298–309. https://doi.org/10.1037/a0032903

David, E. J. R., & Okazaki, S. (2006a). Colonial mentality: A review and recommendation for Filipino American psychology. *Cultural Diversity & Ethnic Minority Psychology, 12*(1), 1–16. https://doi.org/10.1037/1099-9809.12.1.1

David, E. J. R., & Okazaki, S. (2006b). The colonial mentality scale (CMS) for Filipino Americans: Scale construction and psychological implications. *Journal of Counseling Psychology, 53*(2), 241–252. https://doi.org/10.1037/0022-0167.53.2.241

David, E. J. R., & Okazaki, S. (2010). Activation and automaticity of colonial mentality. *Journal of Applied Social Psychology, 40*(4), 850–887. https://doi.org/10.1111/j.1559-1816.2010.00601.x

Edwards, S., McManus, V., & McCreanor, T. (2005). Collaborative research with Māori on sensitive issues: The application of tikanga and kaupapa in research on Māori sudden infant death syndrome. *Social Policy Journal of New Zealand, 25*(July), 88–104.

Faaleava, F. (2020). *Identifying colonial mentality among Samoans in America* (Publication No. 28091164) [Doctoral dissertation, Alliant International University]. ProQuest Dissertations & Theses Global.

Fanon, F. (1965). *The wretched of the earth*. Grove Press.

Freire, P. (1970). *The pedagogy of the oppressed*. Continuum.

Gong, F., Takeuchi, D. T., Agbayani-Siewert, P., & Tacata, L. (2003). Acculturation, psychological distress, and alcohol use: Investigating the effects of ethnic identity and religiosity. In K. M. Chun, P. Balls Organista, & G. Marín (Eds.), *Acculturation: Advances in theory, measurement, and applied research* (pp. 189–206). American Psychological Association. https://doi.org/10.1037/10472-012

Gonzalez, J., Simard, E., Baker-Demaray, T., & Eyes, C. I. (2014). The internalized oppression of North American Indigenous peoples. In E. J. R. David (Ed.), *Internalized oppression: The psychology of marginalized groups* (pp. 31–56). Springer.

Hal, R. E. (2011). A psychogenesis of color-based racism: The implications of colonialism for people of color. *Psychology, 2*(3), 220–225. https://doi.org/10.4236/psych.2011.23034

Halagao, P. E. (2004). Holding up the mirror: The complexity of seeing your ethnic self in history. *Theory and Research in Social Education, 32*(4), 459–483. https://doi.org/10.1080/00933104.2004.10473265

Hays, P. A. (2001). *Addressing cultural complexities in practice: A framework for clinicians and counselors*. American Psychological Association.

Helms, J. E. (1995). An update of Helms's White and People of Color Racial Identity Models. In J. G. Ponterotto, J. M. Casas, L. A. Suzuki, & C. M. Alexander (Eds.), *Handbook of multicultural counseling* (pp. 181–198). Sage.

Hipolito-Delgado, C. P. (2016). Internalized racism, perceived racism, and ethnic identity: Exploring their relationship in Latina/o undergraduates. *Journal of College Counseling, 19*(2), 98–109. https://doi.org/10.1002/jocc.12034

Hipolito-Delgado, C. P., Payan, S. G., & Baca, T. I. (2014). Self-hatred, self-doubt, and assimilation in Latina/o communities: Las consecuencias de colonización y opresión. In E. J. R. David (Ed.), *Internalized oppression: The psychology of marginalized groups* (pp. 109–136). Springer.

Huynh, J. (2022). Understanding internalized racial oppression and second-generation Vietnamese Americans. *Asian American Journal of Psychology, 13*(2), 129–140. https://doi.org/10.1037/aap0000211

Laenui, P. (2000). Processes of decolonization. In M. Battiste (Ed.), *Reclaiming Indigenous voice and vision* (pp. 150–160). University of British Columbia Press. https://www.sjsu.edu/people/marcos.pizarro/maestros/Laenui.pdf

Lee, R. M. (2005). Resilience against discrimination: Ethnic identity and other-group orientation as protective factors for Korean Americans. *Journal of Counseling Psychology, 52*(1), 36–44. https://doi.org/10.1037/0022-0167.52.1.36

Lin, Y. J., & Israel, T. (2012). A computer-based intervention to reduce internalized heterosexism in men. *Journal of Counseling Psychology, 59*(3), 458–464. https://doi.org/10.1037/a0028282

Martín-Baró, I. (1994). *Writings for a liberation psychology*. Harvard University Press.

Maxwell, M., Brevard, J., Abrams, J., & Belgrave, F. (2015). What's color got to do with it? Skin color, skin color satisfaction, racial identity, and internalized racism among African American college students. *Journal of Black Psychology, 41*(5), 438–461. https://doi.org/10.1177/0095798414542299

Memmi, A. (1965). *The colonizer and the colonized*. Beacon Press.

Miranda, L. (2011). *Internalized colonization and decolonizing Mexican American youth* (Publication No. 3517214) [Doctoral dissertation, Alliant International University]. ProQuest Dissertations & Theses Global.

Neblett, E. W., Jr., Rivas-Drake, D., & Umaña-Taylor, A. J. (2012). The promise of racial and ethnic protective factors in promoting ethnic minority youth development. *Child Development Perspectives, 6*(3), 295–303. https://doi.org/10.1111/j.1750-8606.2012.00239.x

Nikalje, A., & Çiftçi, A. (2021). Colonial mentality, racism, and depressive symptoms: Asian Indians in the United States. *Asian American Journal of Psychology, 14*(1), 73–75. Advance online publication. https://doi.org/10.1037/aap0000262

Okazaki, S., David, E. J. R., & Abelmann, N. (2008). Colonialism and psychology of culture. *Social and Personality Psychology Compass, 2*(1), 90–106. https://doi.org/10.1111/j.1751-9004.2007.00046.x

Organista, P. B., Organista, K. C., & Kurasaki, K. (2003). The relationship between acculturation and ethnic minority health. In K. M. Chun, P. Balls Organista, & G. Marín (Eds.), *Acculturation: Advances in theory, measurement, and applied research* (pp. 139–161). American Psychological Association. https://doi.org/10.1037/10472-010

Pe-Pua, R. (1989). Pagtatanong-tanong: A cross-cultural research method. *International Journal of Intercultural Relations, 13*(2), 147–163. https://doi.org/10.1016/0147-1767(89)90003-5

Phinney, J. S. (1992). The Multigroup Ethnic Identity Measure: A new scale for use with diverse groups. *Journal of Adolescent Research, 7*(2), 156–176. https://doi.org/10.1177/074355489272003

Phinney, J. S., Chavira, V., & Williamson, L. (1992). Acculturation attitudes and self-esteem among high school and college students. *Youth & Society, 23*(3), 299–312. https://doi.org/10.1177/0044118X92023003002

Quijano, A., & Ennis, M. (2000). Coloniality of power, Eurocentrism, and Latin America. *International Sociology, 15*(2), 215–232. https://doi.org/10.1177/0268580900015002005

Ratts, M. J. (2009). Social justice counseling: Toward the development of a fifth force among counseling paradigms. *Journal of Humanistic Counseling, Education and Development, 48*(2), 160–172. https://doi.org/10.1002/j.2161-1939.2009.tb00076.x

Rizal, J. (1912). *The Philippines a century hence.* Philippine Education.

Salzman, M., & Laenui, P. (2014). Internalized oppression among Pacific Island peoples. In E. J. R. David (Ed.), *Internalized oppression: The psychology of marginalized groups* (pp. 83–107). Springer.

Sellers, R. M., Smith, M. A., Shelton, J. N., Rowley, S. A. J., & Chavous, T. M. (1998). Multidimensional model of racial identity: A reconceptualization of African American racial identity. *Personality and Social Psychology Review, 2*(1), 18–39. https://doi.org/10.1207/s15327957pspr0201_2

Shakur, A. (1987). *Assata: An autobiography.* Lawrence Hill.

Strobel, L. M. (2015). *Coming full circle: Narratives of decolonization among post-1965 Filipino Americans* (2nd ed.). Center for Babaylan Studies.

Tatum, B. (1994). The colonial model as a theoretical explanation of crime and delinquency. In A. T. Sulton (Ed.), *African American perspectives on crime causation, criminal justice administration, and crime prevention* (pp. 33–68). Sulton Books.

Torres Rivera, E. (2019). Is quality a culturally-based or universal construct? *Interamerican Journal of Psychology, 47*(1), 1–7. https://doi.org/10.30849/rip/ijp.v53i1.1175

Tuazon, A. C. A. (2013). *Colonial mentality and mental health help-seeking attitudes among Filipino Americans* (Publication No. 3581166) [Doctoral dissertation, The Wright Institute]. ProQuest Dissertations & Theses Global.

Tuazon, V. E., Gonzalez, E., Gutierrez, D., & Nelson, L. (2019). Colonial mentality and mental health help-seeking of Filipino Americans. *Journal of Counseling and Development, 97*(4), 352–363. https://doi.org/10.1002/jcad.12284

Tuck, E., & Yang, K. W. (2012). Decolonization is not a metaphor. *Decolonization, 1*(1), 1–40. https://jps.library.utoronto.ca/index.php/des/article/view/18630/15554

Utsey, S. O., Abrams, J. A., Opare-Henaku, A., Bolden, M. A., & Williams, O., III. (2014). Assessing the psychological consequences of internalized colonialism on the psychological well-being of young adults in Ghana. *Journal of Black Psychology, 41*(3), 195–220. https://doi.org/10.1177/0095798414537935

Willis, H. A., Sosoo, E. E., Bernard, D. L., Neal, A., & Neblett, E. W. (2021). The associations between internalized racism, racial identity, and psychological distress. *Emerging Adulthood, 9*(4), 384–400. https://doi.org/10.1177/21676968211005598

Wilson, P., & Wilson, S. (2000). Circles in the classroom: The cultural significance of structure. *Canadian Social Studies, 34*(2), 11–12.

Wilson, S. L., Sellers, S., Solomon, C., & Holsey-Hyman, M. (2017). Exploring the link between Black racial identity and mental health. *Journal of Depression & Anxiety, 6*(3), 272–276. https://doi.org/10.4172/2167-1044.1000272

Worrell, J., & Remer, P. (2003). *Feminist perspectives in therapy: Empowering diverse women* (2nd ed.). Wiley.

Yeh, C. J., & Huang, K. (1996). The collectivistic nature of ethnic identity development among Asian-American college students. *Adolescence, 31*(123), 645–661. https://pubmed.ncbi.nlm.nih.gov/8874610/

2 NAMING AND UNLEARNING PSYCHOLOGICAL COLONIALITY

CRISTALÍS CAPIELO ROSARIO, EDUARDO LUGO-HERNÁNDEZ,
AND LOÍZA A. DEJESÚS SULLIVAN

Even when psychologists have the best intentions to participate in efforts to advance social justice, the frameworks and actions we adopt and uphold often are the same oppressive structures, institutions, theories, and actions we are attempting to transform. This is most evident in our field's continued reliance on psychological models that essentialize culture, cultural differences, and cross-cultural interactions as the main determinants of psychological outcomes and primary targets of psychological interventions, research, training, and advocacy. In this way, we reproduce colonial power dynamics and logics by creating a cultural other on which we act. Moreover, we do this while disregarding the impact this coloniality of power has on the other and the long history of psychological theory and praxis anchored in postcolonialism and decoloniality. With this chapter, we hope to contribute to the continued coconstruction and reimagining of a psychology rooted in liberation and delinked from the domination of histories, knowledge, logics, and experiences. We start with a review of postcolonial and decolonial critique and how each provides a framework for understanding the rise of Western, mainstream

Correspondence about this chapter should be addressed to Cristalís Capielo Rosario, PhD, at cristalis.capielo@asu.edu.

https://doi.org/10.1037/0000376-003
Decolonial Psychology: Toward Anticolonial Theories, Research, Training, and Practice,
L. Comas-Díaz, H. Y. Adames, and N. Y. Chavez-Dueñas (Editors)

psychology as a method for colonial oppression. We then discuss how psychological knowledge production in the United States continues to function as an axis of colonial domination and the efforts of anticolonial and decolonial psychologists have put forward to unsettle psychological coloniality. We also reorient the readers to the postcolonial and decolonial theory and praxis developed by Black, Indigenous, and Latinx psychologists. We end the chapter by offering two examples of how we practice a postcolonial and decolonial psychology with our Puerto Rican communities in the United States and Puerto Rico. We support our discussion with two examples of community psychological interventions to help the reader better understand the application of postcolonial and decolonial critique in producing psychological knowledge.

BRIEF REVIEW OF TERMINOLOGY

The origins of postcolonial and decolonial thought and critique are broad and diverse (Bhambra, 2014); hence we begin the chapter with a brief review of the terms we will discuss. We could describe each through a historical and political lens to gain a helpful distinction between both terms. Emerging from the works of American, Caribbean, Middle Eastern, and South Asian scholars such as Aimé Césaire, Edward Said, Franz Fanon, Homi Bhabha, and Gayatri Spivak, postcolonial critique offers a framework for examining the consequences of Western colonialism, empire, and enslavement that were unleashed by the 18th-century European modernity campaign (Bhambra, 2014; Mignolo, 2007). In this effort, postcolonial study seeks to historicize, critique, and interrupt discourses that distort and sublimate Western European modernism (Bhabha, 1994). Decolonial thought, on the other hand, is primarily associated with the scholarship of African, American, South Asian, and South Pacific thinkers such as Oyèrónkẹ́ Oyěwùmí, Audre Lorde, María Lugones, Anibal Quijano, Enrique Dusel, Walter Mignolo, Upolu LumaVaai, and Unaisi Nabobo-Baba and their work on understanding the origins of European incursion and colonialism across the globe (Bhambra, 2014; Duong-Pedica, 2021). Although similar to postcolonialism in its intent to interrogate how Western European imperialism and colonialism invented and raced the colonized, decolonialism departs from postcolonialism by also calling us to unlearn "hegemonic ways of thinking and being, and a relearning of other ways of thinking and being" (Duong-Pedica, 2021, p. 147). In other words, when we unlearn the logics that created conditions of colonialism, we can set the stage for learning what existed before colonialism as well as create new ways of thinking and being delinked from the colonizer (Mignolo, 2002,

2007). Therefore, decolonial critique does not just try to change the content of the discussion (postcolonialism), but it also changes the terms and conditions of the discussion.

COLONIALITY AND DECOLONIALITY EFFORTS IN PSYCHOLOGY

For psychologists, transforming the content, terms, and conditions of our work needs to begin by acknowledging how the dominant sector of our discipline, White Western psychology, has had an enormous role in creating the infrastructure that supports colonialism (Okazaki et al., 2008). Psychology owes its recognition and prominence as part of the modern social sciences to its role in informing, promulgating, and popularizing logics based on the idea of colonial difference (the colonizer is superior to the colonized). The logic of colonial difference first racializes non-White Others and then establishes the rationale for disposing the ways of knowing and being of non-White Others. Thus colonial difference helped create scientific methods that rejected all epistemologies and ontologies not created by Western White Christian men's minds and lived experiences (Fanon, 1967; Memmi, 1965; Mignolo, 2002; Tomicic & Berardi, 2018). The information these methods yielded further entrenched colonial difference as an early foundation of White Western psychology when the psychological concepts, frameworks, and practices generated by these approaches presumed their universal application and validity across all peoples, locations, and times (Chávez et al., 2016; Goodman & Gorski, 2015; Mignolo, 2002). Within these conditions of epistemological coloniality and embargo, subalterns could not produce knowledge, development, economies, politics, social structures, or technologies (Dussel, 1995; Fals-Borda, 1987; Fanon, 1967; Maldonado-Torres, 2007; Mignolo, 2007; Moane, 2003; Okazaki et al., 2008; Quijano, 2002). The knowledge and methods created by White Western psychology and led by White men was also articulated into values and ethics that, in the name of helping, developing, and/or correcting the colonized, helped institutionalize scientific and intervention methods that led to the labor, economic, political, sexual, and cultural exploitation, exclusion, and control of the colonized. White Western psychology's role in post–Civil War segregation, eugenics and sterilization campaigns, and opposition to racial mixing, are just some examples of how White Western psychology helped establish or promote racial and colonial difference (see American Psychological Association, 2021; Gould, 1996; Yakushko, 2019).

Although mainstream White Western psychology has taken steps toward rectifying its racist past, the power dynamics of colonial difference are still evident within the practice of psychology in two significant and interconnected ways: (a) the expertization of psychological knowledge over community knowledge and (b) the promulgation of interventions that essentialize racial and cultural differences without critically historicizing the origins or attributes we assign to race and culture. In the first dynamic psychologists may operate under the premise that knowledge production and transformational change are top-down processes. Under this assumption, psychologists assume a position of acting on communities rather than colearning and coacting with communities to generate psychological knowledge and healing. From this position, psychologists also conceptualize the race and culture (e.g., language, values) of marginalized communities as their main assets and determinants of their thoughts, feelings, and behaviors. Accordingly, instead of learning a psychology that comes from the people, efforts focus on generalizing and translating psychological interventions and understanding racial and cultural differences. As Goodman and Gorski (2015) noted, by focusing only on race and culture, psychologists—even those who want to advance a multicultural psychology—end up recrafting and reproducing the lie that the sole contribution of oppressed communities is their race and culture. In Latinx psychology, for example, this dynamic is palpable in the centrality of cultural values in psychological research, interventions, and training curricula aimed to serve Latinxs. This practice should be considered epistemic violence for three reasons: first, because it negates a psychology that is born outside academic spaces; second, because it reduces the complexity of lived experiences into a set of monolithic values believed to be inherent to the community; and, third, because it fails to question how the mind and behaviors and even the values assigned to marginalized communities are influenced by oppressive power dynamics. This violence can happen even when we have the intention to decolonize psychology. For example, African and American decolonial philosophers argue that when social scientists make attempts to change the terms and location of knowledge production we often engage in a double bind (e.g., Bernasconi, 1997; Chimakonam, 2017). First, during times when we are willing to learn another psychology, we struggle to recognize its substantive contribution. In this condition, we say, "what they offer is not that different from what we offer." Therefore, our reflex is to again try to generalize theoretical and practical concepts across all populations and locations. In the second condition, when psychology is broadened and relocated in the community, psychological coloniality again flexes its muscle by gatekeeping and questioning the merits of what communities present as psychological knowledge or methods of psychological knowledge production. In this second bind we say, "that departs too much from what psychology is, so it is not psychology." Our continued participation in these power dynamics ends up undermining our intentions and efforts to disrupt colonial psychological narratives and ultimately decolonize psychology. In his essay discussing the need for social scientist to make way to other principles of knowledge and understandings, Walter Mignolo (2002) provided important insights about why social scientists continue to be ineffective in their efforts to decolonize social sciences:

> The belief that social scientists with goodwill toward social transformation will be endorsed by the "people," whose interest the social scientist claims to defend, would be difficult to sustain today. First, this is because the people (e.g., social movements of all kind) do not need intellectuals from outside to defend their interests. Second, the transformation of knowledge (and social transformation, of course), to which the social scientist could contribute, is located not so much in the domain of the people as in learned institutions and the mass media. (pp. 73–74)

In other words, decolonial efforts will fail as long as psychologists continue to herald their expertise over the expertise and experiences of the community and to only create knowledge outside the community. Therefore, a decolonized psychology can only emerge when we are willing to unlearn hegemonic ideas of what and where psychological knowledge and understandings are as well as the social, political, economic structures that came from hegemonic psychology.

In response to this continued psychological coloniality, an increasingly rich literature has sought to unlearn and unsettle the reproduction of colonial logics and power dynamics in the psychology profession (e.g., Cohen, 2022; Goodman & Gorski, 2015; Okazaki et al., 2008; Stevens & Sonn, 2021; Teo, 2015). Scholarly efforts have also focused on critiquing and understanding the psychology of colonial oppression on formerly and currently colonized populations (e.g., Capielo Rosario et al., 2022; Cokley, 2002; David, 2008; Gone & Trimble, 2012; Okazaki et al., 2008; Speight, 2007; Utsey et al., 2015). A review of the literature shows that part of the efforts to dismantle psychological coloniality has also centered on offering postcolonial and decolonial psychological methods, theories, and practices, including critical consciousness of anti-Black racism (Mosley et al., 2021), ethnopolitical psychology (Comas-Díaz, 2007), intersectionality in psychotherapy (Adames et al., 2018), healing ethno-racial trauma (Chavez-Dueñas et al., 2019), historical trauma (Hartmann et al., 2019), Indigenous culture as treatment (Pomerville & Gone, 2019), liberation psychology (Martín Baró, 1986; Montero, 2003), marginal methods (Trimble, 2021), social analysis (Moane, 2003), and the psychology of radical healing (Adames et al., 2022; French et al., 2020). Informed by the works of postcolonial and decolonial scholars from the Global North and South, these frameworks collectively focus on the urgency of changing the ethics and politics of psychological knowledge, seeking reparative justice, and creating a just society. To accomplish this, they call on psychologists in alliance with communities to

- reconnect to or create knowledge that affirms the experiences and lives of oppressed peoples;

- demand the end of settler-colonialism and call for the return of stolen land and resources;

- help build critical consciousness about the role of colonialism in the lives of oppressed communities; and

- envision new knowledge, economies, governments, and politics that can help create and sustain a pluriversal society.

We dedicate the rest of this chapter to describe how we try to meet these responsibilities in the work we do in collaboration with our Puerto Rican communities.

THE NECESSITY OF A PUERTO RICAN POSTCOLONIAL AND DECOLONIAL PSYCHOLOGY

Puerto Rico has been under U.S. rule since 1898 and is one of the world's last remaining colonies (Trías Monge, 1997). Its political status as unincorporated U.S. territory does not allow its residents the right to vote for the U.S. president or to have voting representation in the U.S. Congress despite being governed by U.S. law. This establishes a different category of U.S. citizenship for the residents of this colonial state. Lack of representation in the democratic process and the corruption and neglect of some of its public officials, has resulted in a financial crisis that led to bankruptcy proceedings and a federally mandated fiscal board imposing a series of austerity measures on the public. An estimated 39.8% of adults and 57% of children live below poverty levels relative to 16% of children living in the United States (Instituto de Desarrollo de la Juventud, n.d.; Instituto de Estadísticas de Puerto Rico, 2019). Furthermore, the Merchant Marine Act (Jones Act) of 1917, which establishes that any maritime commercial exchange between the United States and Puerto Rico must occur through the U.S. merchant marine (one of the most expensive in the world), hampers Puerto Rico's economic development and prevents foreign governments from supplying aid in times of crisis, such as natural disasters (Venator-Santiago & Meléndez, 2017).

Fiscal austerity measures and several catastrophes related to the climate crisis have also resulted in mass migration to the United States. Between 2006 and 2017, Puerto Rico lost about 14% of its population to migration to the mainland (Hinojosa & Meléndez, 2018). This migration is even larger than between the 1940s and the 1960s, a movement known as the Great Puerto Rican migration (Gonzalez et al., 2021). Migration has been especially high among professionals who leave the archipelago due to problems with the health care system and insurance agencies. This has resulted in increasing problems with accessibility of health services, particularly among those living in remote rural areas. Once Puerto Ricans are in the United States, colonial power dynamics continue to have profound health and economic consequences for them. After migration, Puerto Ricans who do not fit White European American racial and language standards continue to be racialized as non-White Others because of their linguistic, physiological, and cultural differences (Aranda, 2007; Godreau & Bonilla, 2021). This racialized post-migration context in turn helps explain the intergenerational socioeconomic and health disparities and injustices affecting Puerto Ricans in the United States (Burgos & Rivera, 2012; Vélez, 2017). It is clear that Puerto Rico's colonial situation is a human rights issue that increasingly affects Puerto Ricans' well-being in both Puerto Rico and the United States.

Puerto Rico's colonial relationship with the United States also has an influence on Puerto Rican psychology. Counseling and clinical psychology programs have to be accredited by the American Psychological Association and school psychology programs are accredited by the National Association for School Psychologists. Accreditation standards from these associations promote a coloniality of knowledge that has profound consequences for student training, theory development, and interventions. Deciding not to be accredited by these bodies, however, can severely hinder students from being able to apply to internships and later employment opportunities in Puerto Rico and the United States. Although relationships and connections with Latin American psychologists are present, these relationships have not translated into curricula that center decolonial efforts. Hence the influence of the Global South is scarce and traditionally limited to community psychology circles outside of Puerto Rico.

As Puerto Rican psychologists and psychologists-in-training, we experience firsthand the colonial violence against our communities in Puerto Rico and the United States. Our lived and shared experiences as citizens of a colonial state (those living in Puerto Rico) and colonial migrants (those living in the United States) guide why and how we are propelled to promote a postcolonial and decolonial Puerto Rican psychology. For Cristalís, these efforts focus on disrupting psychological discourses that ignore or deny the impact that past and ongoing U.S. colonialism has on the mental health and migration of Puerto Rican populations through research collaborations with Puerto Rican communities in the United States. Eduardo and Loíza, on the other hand, embody work that strives to create a Puerto Rican psychology that resists colonial narratives and delinks it from colonial frameworks. Eduardo and Loíza describe their collaborations with Puerto Rican communities in Puerto Rico and Chicago.

Eduardo Lugo-Hernández's Work With Impacto Juventud and Aula en La Montaña

Hurricanes Irma and Maria devastated the archipelago of Puerto Rico in 2017. The immediate aftermath of these hurricanes included the destruction of the power grid (some places had no electricity for more than 10 months), impassable roads (97% were affected), lack of drinking water, the destruction of basic service infrastructure (health and education) and death (more than 4,000 people perished; RAND Corporation, n.d.). Given the basic infrastructure damage, it took months for youth to return to school and universities. When they were finally able to do so, they faced many hardships associated with the slow rebuilding process and the trauma of these events. Research has shown that the direct impact of climate change in the form of extreme weather events has a deleterious effect on youth mental health (Fritze et al., 2008).

It is against this backdrop that Impacto Juventud [Youth Impact] was created. Students from a psychology of adolescence course at the University of Puerto Rico Mayaguez (UPRM) developed a documentary to expose child poverty in Puerto Rico and promote dialogue with experts and other youth about possible actions to eradicate child poverty. The documentary was shown at a movie theater close to the university with participants from the university, middle and high school students, professors, and community members. After the showing, students from the course expressed that for the first time after Maria that they felt a sense of empowerment and sociopolitical agency that should continue in a more sustainable manner—hence the birth of Impacto Juventud.

Impacto Juventud has the goal of providing a space for young people ages 15 to 25 to gain knowledge and skills related to civic and political engagement. It also places youth in community projects, advocacy initiatives, community organizations, citizen coalitions, and research projects to promote their voices. This is anchored on a firm belief that youth need to have a place at the table on issues that affect them, as stated in the Declaration of the Rights of the Child (United Nations, 1989). They are also experts of their own realities, positioning them in a place where they can inform others about their experiences, the development of interventions, and public policies. This approach tries to dismantle traditional oppressive adult-centric approaches, which are rooted in colonial power structures and modes of subordination (DeJong & Love, 2015).

After 4 years, Impacto Juventud has grown to include youth and young adults from municipalities across Puerto Rico, representing a diversity of gender, race, sexual orientation, educational, and economic backgrounds. From the beginning, Impacto Juventud was anchored on decolonial, feminist, and antiracist approaches. It sought to build coalitions of youth interested in promoting children's rights and youth's participation in policy development and advocacy. Inevitably, these conversations also allowed youth to discuss issues of coloniality and decoloniality, power dynamics, community action, and empowerment.

The project has a strong social media presence recognizing the influence of this platform on youth organizing and social action. On these platforms (e.g., Facebook, Instagram, Twitter, YouTube), the youth of Impacto Juventud share educational content and have dialogues with other youth, both locally and internationally. We also interview experts on various topics that affect youth and lead policy campaigns to promote antiracist, antipoverty, and antisexist actions. For example, youth from Impacto Juventud helped craft and advocate for antipoverty legislation recently signed by Puerto Rico's Senate after initiating and sustaining a long public awareness campaign about child poverty in Puerto Rico. Impacto Juventud has also designed and led interventions and workshops across public schools in Puerto Rico to increase children's participation in antigendered violence efforts. It has developed activities to reclaim historical events that have been omitted from our history books that exemplify our oppression and struggle for liberation. We believe that the reclaiming of history is part of identity development and a catalyst for sociopolitical action to transform our reality. To increase their reach across Puerto Rico, the youth of Impacto Juventud have created a podcast titled *Generación Cambio* (*Generation Change*), a radio program called *Salud y Justicia Social* (*Health and Social Justice*), and a social media platform on Facebook called *Chiqui Impacto* (*Kid Impact*) to serve younger children (0–12) in Puerto Rico and offer educational, health, and recreational support during the COVID-19 pandemic.

Impacto Juventud is a place of healing in the midst of colonial trauma. It has created a coalition of youth who question the roots of poverty in Puerto Rico, the meanings of colonial economic dependence, the importance of a culture-based education that recognizes cultural roots, historical oppressions and strengths, and alternative actions to promote decoloniality. It connects youth with each other recognizing the collective and intergenerational nature of our struggle. It helps them translate pain into actions based on solidarity and mutuality.

The COVID-19 pandemic was the catalyst for the development of another Impacto Juventud Initiative. Through our community work, we collaborated with the rural community of el Rucio, Quebradilla sector in Peñuelas (southwest region of Puerto Rico), with the goal of promoting energy and food sustainability, child development, and physical and mental health through community empowerment. This community faces many structural challenges that limits access to basic services and elevates their risk when faced with a natural disaster. When the COVID-19 pandemic started, community leaders quickly identified education access as a main priority. Children were at home with inadequate technology, many with no or poor internet connections and with need for specialized educational services. In this environment, Aula en la Montaña (School in the Mountain) was launched.

Aula en la Montaña is an educational and socioemotional support intervention for the school aged children of the community. The project is based on an awareness that the Puerto Rican educational system is predicated on inequality, colonialism, and lack of understanding and appreciation for diversity. Informed by a decolonial and antiracist pedagogy, Aula en la Montaña provides weekly educational support to students and remote homework support during the week. It emphasizes a historical-cultural component through systematic readings of children's books related to race, gender, and issues around Puerto Rico's colonial history. Bomba classes are also taught. Bomba is a traditional African dance that has been a symbol of resistance since slavery and has had a resurgence after Hurricane Maria. Aula en la Montaña also includes an agroecology project in which children connect with the land, learning about the importance of food security and sustainability as part of community development and self-determination. In collaboration with community leaders, we see these factors as essential for promoting psychological well-being. The cocreation of knowledge and the problematization of oppressive circumstances is part of a liberation psychology process necessary for emancipation in a colonial context. Working from a psychology of liberation, not only with adults, but also with children, allows for critical dialogues that are not present in children's traditional schooling. It also creates a space for unsettling dominant social messages that promote coloniality in Puerto Rico.

Our approach to working with children dismantles adult-centric relationships in the educational context. Central to our pedagogy is children's voice and participation. This is part of our relationships, program evaluation, and the activities children engage in. Some of the things children have done through the project were meeting with Puerto Rican senators to discuss child poverty and its manifestation in their communities, publishing newspaper columns about their experiences, and developing a children's guide in conjunction with the Puerto Rico Public Health Trust to teach other children COVID-19 prevention strategies in school.

Education and learning do not occur in a vacuum. Children's lives are complex and their life experiences influence their ability to engage in effective learning. This is the case with the impact that the climate crisis has had on these children. The impact of Hurricane Maria and the earthquakes, a few years later, has elevated children's anxiety and posttraumatic stress disorder symptoms. For example, Raquel (a pseudonym), who is 8 years old, experienced panic attacks every time it began to get cloudy and when it rained. She would shake and ask about when Aula en la Montaña was going to end that day so that she could go home. One rainy day when she arrived home, she knocked on the door and her mother was not there (was just two houses down the street). Raquel started screaming and crying desperately and one of our psychologists had to manage her crisis with skills she had been learning in Aula. Raquel had seen her roof blown off during Hurricane Maria, and rainy days were especially difficult for her.

Aula en la Montaña children have poor access to mental health services. Through our partnership, we offer mental health support for them and their families. Interventions break with traditional forms of therapy, they are not grounded in an office space, they rely on everyday observations and conversations, and provide psychosocial accompaniment (Watkins, 2015) and skills to help them effectively manage their situations. Mental health and physical activity are integrated in a wellness component to dismantle the conception that mind and body are separate. This approach has not only increased accessibility to services but also significantly reduced the stigma of mental health services in children and their parents. In the case of Raquel, after months of conversations and skill-practice with our wellness team, she has been able to speak about her experience and gain skills to manage her anxiety symptoms. Other children have started adopting these skills not only in relation to climate situations but also in other anxiety-provoking situations such as test taking.

The impact of this intervention is not only observed in children and families but also on the psychologists and graduate students involved in the Aula en la Montaña. It has provided them with a different framework for delivering services and a higher awareness of the structural factors that impinge on children's well-being and the ability of their parents to access services. The collaborative work with the communities served by Aula en la Montaña is also grounded on mutuality. For example, because we all share similar experiences of disaster and colonial trauma, an important component of our work is to build relationships based on shared feelings and experiences. This in turn allows us to cocreate a collaborative working relationship that facilitates mutual healing. We have also articulated egalitarian and horizontal relationships with our graduate and undergraduate students recognizing their knowledge and skills and prioritizing conversations when they are respected and listened to. We have also highlighted the importance of multisystemic interventions, including policy interventions, to address the oppressive circumstances that the community faces. Many students have stated that traditional training methods lacked depth (particularly referring to structural dimensions of mental health) and this type of approach seems more attuned to the needs of Puerto Ricans' colonial experience.

Engaging in liberation praxis through Aula en la Montaña has been a healing process for our team members, who also face the struggles of the colonial context and the climate crisis. As Comas-Díaz and Torres Rivera (2020) wrote, "one does not come to help; rather, one accompanies others in a mutual healing and liberation journey" (p. 293). We are wounded people with intergenerational traumas associated caused by brutal colonial processes. We come from diverse backgrounds and have decided to engage in a transdisciplinary journey to generate possibilities of healing with our community partners. Our praxis is *sentipensante* (sensing, thinking) in that we do not separate reason and knowledge from feeling. Experiences in this sense are discussed in our team and with the community to which we are grateful for this opportunity to join in liberating action and hope.

Loíza A. DeJesús Sullivan's Work With Youth Group at the Segundo Ruiz Belvis Cultural Center in Chicago

In the 1950s, Puerto Rican colonial migrants began to migrate to urban centers throughout the United States. Chicago became home to a large community of Puerto Ricans recruited to work in the city's factories. Puerto Ricans in Chicago find themselves subject to the colonial reality on the archipelago due to continued contact with family and circular migration, and the internal colonial reality in Chicago. Over the decades, these early migrants, their children, and the migrants who came after developed cultural institutions and created social support networks to mitigate the effects of their colonial reality. Organizations such as the Pedro Albizu Campos Puerto Rican High School, the Juan Antonio Corretjer Puerto Rican Cultural Center, Casa Central (Central House), and the Segundo Ruiz Belvis Cultural Center were created to provide services and support for Puerto Ricans in Chicago. Today, most of Chicago's Puerto Rican community resides in what is known as the Puerto Rican Influence Area (PRIA; Cintrón et al., 2012). According to Cintrón et al. (2012), the PRIA consists of census tracts with a Puerto Rican concentration of at least 10 percent. This includes the Chicago neighborhoods Humboldt Park, Logan Square, Hermosa, and Belmont Cragin, among others.

My family migrated to the PRIA from Puerto Rico in the 1960s. I was raised in the PRIA and spent my formative years participating in community and cultural events at the various institutions there. In January 2020, when the opportunity to apply for a Schweitzer Fellowship arose—a funding opportunity for aspiring health professionals interested in addressing health disparities—I immediately thought of working with one of the organizations that had been most influential in my upbringing, the Segundo Ruiz Belvis Cultural Center (SRBCC). The SRBCC is the oldest operating Latinx cultural center in Chicago and the only one dedicated to preserving and promoting Afro–Puerto Rican culture and history. Originally based in the now-gentrified Logan Square neighborhood, and now located in the increasingly Puerto Rican Hermosa community, the SRBCC provided Afro-Puerto Rican music and dance lessons primarily to high school youth. I began conversations with Omar Torres-Kortright, the executive director of the SRBCC, with the aim of collaborating on an art and culture-based youth empowerment program. Then COVID hit.

By the time I was awarded the Schweitzer Fellowship, the city was officially in lockdown. Omar and I decided to switch tactics. We were in a crisis and we needed to respond to the immediate needs of the youth of the community. The project needed to be redesigned and the youth needed to be at the center of the redesign. We had conversations with the youth already engaged in SRBCC programming and with various community stakeholders. In the beginning, the youth requested a space to socialize and support each other. They requested that we cut the time commitment from five hours to two hours per week. They requested financial assistance.

Omar and I created a budget and obtained funding to pay the youth a small stipend. We started preparing the SRBCC for the eventual end of lockdown. We met weekly to socialize and support each other. The youth needed a space to vent, to unburden, to be themselves, to be kids. My role shifted from teaching to *acompañamiento*. According to Watkins (2015), acompañamiento involves bearing witness and walking in solidarity with those who are suffering. It also involves recognizing the structural and systematic roots of the suffering and moving past individualistic notions of health to community well-being.

The first hour of each session was a check-in. We all took turns in updating the group on our week, how we felt, what we struggled with, and what we wanted to celebrate. We had structured problem-solving sessions. We also set weekly goals (e.g., practice communication and stress management skills) and provided an update on the status of the plan from the previous week. The second hour was structured as a youth-led space. During this hour, the group discussed issues of racism, homelessness, sexual and gender identity, police brutality, pandemic stress, and gang violence. My role was to witness and collaborate with the youth to problematize these experiences. Although this may sound like a typical support group, it was just by nature of its existence in that community with those youth at that period in time, a political act. It was also a space of collective healing. A compliment on one youth's new hairstyle turned into an hour-long discussion on the trauma of being lesbian, gay, bisexual, transgender, queer, or beyond in religious and misogynistic spaces. One youth's comment about wanting to continue online learning after lockdown evolved into a discussion on relative privilege and the differences in safety between different PRIA neighborhoods. As the youth discussed issues, they externalized what they had perceived as internal and individual problems. Instead, we could all name how our collective experiences were influenced by systemic erosion of power, resources, and rights. For example, struggling at school was no longer seen as caused by being lazy or unintelligent but instead as the result of attending schools with limited resources with policies that were designed to make them fail. They were doing the work of *concientización,* consciousness raising. What they needed from me was a safe space, and occasionally a little context and some resources.

The space was ever changing based on the needs and requests of the youth. It was truly a youth-led space. At the request of youth who could not participate in the weekly group sessions and those who needed additional support (e.g., college coaching), I also conducted college and career coaching in one-on-one sessions. My role was to be what the youth needed me to be. I was a mentor, a friend, a teacher, a counselor, a social worker, a coach, and a cheerleader. It was terrifying and so rewarding. It certainly was not what was taught in our ethics and counseling skills classes. That is, as clinicians we are taught to remain objective and avoid holding multiple roles with the communities we serve. As the weeks passed and I saw the youth engaging, I began to let go of colonial narratives that told me that *acompañamiento* was not ethical and that it was not appropriate work for a future psychologist. In fact, these boundary crossings and multiple roles set the stage for collective healing (Capielo Rosario et al., 2022).

Eventually, the project evaluation and later outcomes would speak for themselves. I conducted a brief anonymous online survey of the youth.

Sixteen youths were involved in at least one session, 12 attended at least half of the sessions, and eight attended three quarters of the sessions. Of the youth who participated in the survey ($N = 8$), the majority felt the project helped them recognize and understand their emotions ($n = 7$), communicate their emotions to others ($n = 7$), and meet academic demands during the pandemic ($n = 7$). All participants reported improved self-esteem and self-confidence, a clear understanding of their identity, better COVID-19 stress management, and better conflict resolution with family and peers.

The youth entered the project believing that therapy and mental health issues are for others, for White people, or the severely mentally ill. By the end of the project, the youth had requested more frequent sessions and additional workshops on coping skills and stress management, and six had requested referrals for individual therapy. One had even convinced a parent to give therapy a try. Breaking stigmas and barriers is how I measure the success of this project.

CONCLUSION

Whether working with youth in Chicago or in Puerto Rico, our collective work provides a wide range of engagement experiences and opportunities for unlearning and relearning. Our communities have taught us that our work has to be rooted in a complex array of mechanisms for change that considers innovative spaces and traditional spaces. We have also witnessed how this leads to practical experiences that

- provide opportunities to connect with historical, sociopolitical, and land resources that colonialism has attempted to deny or distort;

- provoke a reflexive process that allows us to become aware of and later question our colonial reality and how this reality impacts our lives;

- provide spaces that promote the community's agency to envision and demand change; and

- enhance solidarity between members of oppressed communities in a dynamic change process.

We hope our lived experiences serve as an example of a postcolonial and decolonial psychology centered on working toward a vision of a life free of oppression. To learn more about our ongoing community work in Puerto Rico and Chicago, we encourage readers to use the following resources.

RESOURCES

Aula en la Montaña. (n.d.). *Home* [Facebook page]. Facebook. Retrieved October 10, 2023 from https://www.facebook.com/profile.php?id= 100071696760571

Impacto Juventud. (n.d.). *Programa de radio Salud y Justicia Social* [Healing and Social Justice radio program] [Playlist]. YouTube. https://www. youtube.com/c/ImpactoJuventud

Impacto Juventud. (2018, January 24). *¡Conoce a Impacto Juventud!* [Meet Youth Impact!] [Video]. YouTube. https://www.youtube.com/watch?v= I62f13Bz3TA

Segundo Ruiz Belvis Cultural Center. https://www.segundoruizbelvis.org

Torres-Kortright, O. (Host). (2020, October 31). Interview about the youth performance and project at the Segundo Ruiz Belvis Cultural Center (No. 1) [Video podcast episode]. In *Abrazo virtual*. Segundo Ruiz Belvis Cultural Center, Chicago. https://fb.watch/eWiITb3-JV/

REFERENCES

Adames, H. Y., Chavez-Dueñas, N. Y., Lewis, J. A., Neville, H. A., French, B. H., Chen, G. A., & Mosley, D. V. (2022). Radical healing in psychotherapy: Addressing the wounds of racism-related stress and trauma. *Psychotherapy, 60*(1), 39–50. Advance online publication. https://doi.org/10.1037/pst0000435

Adames, H. Y., Chavez-Dueñas, N. Y., Sharma, S., & La Roche, M. J. (2018). Intersectionality in psychotherapy: The experiences of an AfroLatinx queer immigrant. *Psychotherapy, 55*(1), 73–79. https://doi.org/10.1037/pst0000152

American Psychological Association. (2021). Historical chronology: Examining psychology's contributions to the belief in racial hierarchy and perpetuation of inequality for People of Color in U.S. https://www.apa.org/about/apa/addressing-racism/historical-chronology

Aranda, E. M. (2007). Struggles of incorporation among the Puerto Rican middle class. *Sociological Quarterly, 48*(2), 199–228. https://doi.org/10.1111/j.1533-8525.2007.00076.x

Bernasconi, R. (1997). The violence of the face: Peace and language in the thought of Levinas. *Philosophy and Social Criticism, 23*(6), 81–93. https://doi.org/10.1177/019145379702300606

Bhabha, H. K. (1994). *The location of culture*. Routledge.,

Bhambra, G. K. (2014). Postcolonial and decolonial reconstructions. In G. K. Bhambra, *Connected sociologies* (pp. 117–140). Bloomsbury Publishing. https://doi.org/10.5040/9781472544377.ch-006

Burgos, G., & Rivera, F. I. (2012). Residential segregation, socio-economic status, and disability: A multi-level study of Puerto Ricans in the United States. *Centro Journal, 24*(2), 14–47.

Capielo Rosario, C., Schaefer, A., Ballesteros, J., Rentería, R., & David, E. J. R. (2019). A caballo regalao no se le mira el colmillo: Colonial mentality and Puerto Rican depression. *Journal of Counseling Psychology*, *66*(4), 396–408. https://doi.org/10.1037/cou0000347

Capielo Rosario, C., Torres Fernández, I. T., & Wejrowski, B. (2022). Puerto Rico se levanta: Advocacy service and research in the aftermath of Hurricane María. *Qualitative Psychology*, *9*(3), 312–320. https://doi.org/10.1037/qup0000199

Chávez, T. A., Fernández, I. T., Hipolito-Delgado, C. P., & Rivera, E. T. (2016). Unifying liberation psychology and humanistic values to promote social justice in counseling. *Journal of Humanistic Counseling*, *55*(3), 166–182. https://link.gale.com/apps/doc/A467681285/AONE

Chavez-Dueñas, N. Y., Adames, H. Y., Perez-Chavez, J. G., & Salas, S. P. (2019). Healing ethno-racial trauma in Latinx immigrant communities: Cultivating hope, resistance, and action. *American Psychologist*, *74*(1), 49–62. https://doi.org/10.1037/amp0000289

Chimakonam, J. O. (2017). Conversationalism as an emerging method of thinking in and beyond African philosophy. *Acta Academica*, *49*(2), 11–33.

Cintrón, R., Toro-Morn, M., García Zambrana, I., & Scott, E. (2012). *60 years of migration: Puerto Ricans in Chicagoland* [Puerto Rican Agenda Research Program final report]. https://static1.squarespace.com/static/5ada4708cc8fed32bd40cda6/t/5ae601bf8a922de4679df164/1525023200816/Full_report.compressed.pdf

Cohen, E. (2022). *The psychologisation of Eastern spiritual traditions: Colonisation, translation, and commodification.* Routledge.

Cokley, K. O. (2002). Testing Cross's revised racial identity model: An examination of the relationship between racial identity and internalized racialism. *Journal of Counseling Psychology*, *49*(4), 476–483. https://doi.org/10.1037/0022-0167.49.4.476

Comas-Díaz, L. (2007). Ethnopolitical psychology: Healing and transformation. In E. Aldarondo (Ed.), *Advancing social justice through clinical practice* (pp. 91–118). Lawrence Erlbaum.

Comas-Díaz, L., & Torres Rivera, E. (2020). Conclusion: Liberation psychology—Crossing borders into new frontiers. In L. Comas-Díaz & E. Torres Rivera (Eds.), *Liberation psychology: Theory, method, practice, and social justice* (pp. 283–295). American Psychological Association. https://doi.org/10.1037/0000198-016

David, E. J. R. (2008). A colonial mentality model of depression for Filipino Americans. *Cultural Diversity & Ethnic Minority Psychology*, *14*(2), 118–127. https://doi.org/10.1037/1099-9809.14.2.118

DeJong, K., & Love, B. J. (2015). Youth oppression as a technology of colonialism: Conceptual frameworks and possibilities for social justice education praxis. *Equity & Excellence in Education*, *48*(3), 489–508. https://doi.org/10.1080/10665684.2015.1057086

Duong-Pedica, A. (2021). Thinking Kanaky decolonially. *Artha Journal of the Social Sciences*, *20*(2), 141–164.

Dussel, E. (1995). *The invention of the Americas: Eclipse of "the other" and the myth of modernity.* Continuum.

Fals-Borda, O. (1987). The application of participatory action-research in Latin America. *International Sociology*, *2*(4), 329–347. https://doi.org/10.1177/026858098700200401

Fanon, F. (1967). *Black skin, white masks.* Grove Press.

French, B. H., Lewis, J. A., Mosley, D. V., Adames, H. Y., Chavez-Dueñas, N. Y., Chen, G. A., & Neville, H. A. (2020). Toward a psychological framework of radical healing in communities of color. *Counseling Psychologist, 48*(1), 14–46. https://doi.org/10.1177/0011000019843506

Fritze, J. G., Blashki, G. A., Burke, S., & Wiseman, J. (2008). Hope, despair and transformation: Climate change and the promotion of mental health and wellbeing. *International Journal of Mental Health Systems, 2*(1), 13. Advance online publication. https://doi.org/10.1186/1752-4458-2-13

Godreau, & Bonilla, Y. (2021). Nonsovereign racecraft: How colonialism, debt, and disaster are transforming Puerto Rican racial subjectivities. *American Anthropologist, 123*(3), 509–525.

Gone, J. P., & Trimble, J. E. (2012). American Indian and Alaska Native mental health: Diverse perspectives on enduring disparities. *Annual Review of Clinical Psychology, 8*(1), 131–160. https://doi.org/10.1146/annurev-clinpsy-032511-143127

Gonzalez, K. A., Capielo Rosario, C., Abreu, R. L., & Cardenas Bautista, E. (2021). "It hurts but it's the thing we have to do": Puerto Rican colonial migration. *Journal of Latina/o Psychology, 9*(2), 140–160. https://doi.org/10.1037/lat0000181

Goodman, R. D., & Gorski, P. C. (2015). *Decolonizing multicultural counseling through social justice.* Springer.

Gould, S. J. (1996). Space, time and the human being. *International Social Science Journal, 48*(150), 449–460. https://doi.org/10.1111/j.1468-2451.1996.tb00099.x

Hartmann, W. E., Wendt, D. C., Burrage, R. L., Pomerville, A., & Gone, J. P. (2019). American Indian historical trauma: Anticolonial prescriptions for healing, resilience, and survivance. *American Psychologist, 74*(1), 6–19. https://doi.org/10.1037/amp0000326

Hinojosa, J., & Meléndez, E. (2018). *Puerto Rican exodus: One year since Hurricane Maria.* https://centropr-archive.hunter.cuny.edu/sites/default/files/RB2018-05_SEPT2018%20%281%29.pdf

Instituto de Desarrollo de la Juventud. (n.d.). Child and youth well-being index. https://idj-testproject-1.webflow.io/datos-dimensiones-economia/puerto-rico

Instituto de Estadísticas de Puerto Rico. (2019). Perfil del migrante 2018–2019 [Profile of the immigrant]. https://estadisticas.pr/files/Publicaciones/PM_2018-2019_1.pdf

Instituto de Estadísticas de Puerto Rico. (2020). Baja levemente el porcentaje de familias en pobreza en Puerto Rico [Slight decrease in the percentage of families in poverty in Puerto Rico]. https://censo.estadisticas.pr/sites/default/files/Comunicados/CP_SDCPR_3_17_2022_PRCS_2011-145vs_2016-20%20%2817032022%29_1.pdf

Maldonado-Torres, N. (2007). On the coloniality of being: Contributions to the development of a concept. *Cultural Studies, 21*(2–3), 240–270. https://doi.org/10.1080/09502380601162548

Martín-Baró, I. (1986). Hacia una psicología social de la liberación [Toward a social psychology of liberation]. *Boletín de Psicología, 5*(22), 219–231.

Memmi, A. (1965). *The colonizer and the colonized.* Orion Press.

Mignolo, W. D. (2002). The geopolitics of knowledge and the colonial difference. *South Atlantic Quarterly, 101*(1), 57–96. https://doi.org/10.1215/00382876-101-1-57

Mignolo, W. D. (2007). Delinking. *Cultural Studies, 21*(2–3), 449–514. https://doi.org/10.1080/09502380601162647

Moane, G. (2003). Bridging the personal and the political: Practices for a liberation psychology. *American Journal of Community Psychology, 31*(1–2), 91–101. https://doi.org/10.1023/A:1023026704576

Montero, M. (2003). *Teoría y práctica de la Psicología Comunitaria. La tensión entre comunidad y sociedad* [Theory and practice of Community Psychology. The tension between community and society]. Paidós.

Mosley, D. V., Hargons, C. N., Meiller, C., Angyal, B., Wheeler, P., Davis, C., & Stevens-Watkins, D. (2021). Critical consciousness of anti-Black racism: A practical model to prevent and resist racial trauma. *Journal of Counseling Psychology, 68*(1), 1–16. https://doi.org/10.1037/cou0000430

Okazaki, S., David, E. J. R., & Abelmann, N. (2008). Colonialism and psychology of culture: Colonialism and psychology. *Social and Personality Psychology Compass, 2*(1), 90–106. https://doi.org/10.1111/j.1751-9004.2007.00046.x

Pomerville, A., & Gone, J. P. (2019). Indigenous culture-as-treatment in an era of evidence-based mental health practice. In C. Fleming & M. Manning (Eds.), *Routledge handbook of Indigenous well-being* (pp. 237–247). Routledge. https://doi.org/10.4324/9781351051262-20

Quijano, A. (2002). The return of the future and questions about knowledge. *Current Sociology, 50*(1), 75–87. https://doi.org/10.1177/0011392102050001006

RAND Corporation. (n.d.). Hurricanes Irma and Maria: Impact and aftermath. https://www.rand.org/hsrd/hsoac/projects/puerto-rico-recovery/hurricanes-irma-and-maria.html

Speight, S. L. (2007). Internalized racism: One more piece of the puzzle. *Counseling Psychologist, 35*(1), 126–134. https://doi.org/10.1177/0011000006295119

Stevens, G., & Sonn, S. S. (Eds.). (2021). *Decoloniality and epistemic justice in contemporary community psychology.* Springer. https://doi.org/10.1007/978-3-030-72220-3

Teo, T. (2015). Critical psychology: A geography of intellectual engagement and resistance. *American Psychologist, 70*(3), 243–254. https://doi.org/10.1037/a0038727

Tomicic, A., & Berardi, F. (2018). Between past and present: The sociopsychological constructs of colonialism, coloniality and postcolonialism. *Integrative Psychological & Behavioral Science, 52*(1), 152–175. https://doi.org/10.1007/s12124-017-9407-5

Trías Monge, J. (1997). *Puerto Rico: The trials of the oldest colony in the world.* Yale University Press.

Trimble, J. E. (2021). "The circling spirits call us home;" The shaman, marginal methods, and relational approaches to healing research. In D. F. Ragin & J. Keenan (Eds.), *Handbook of research methods in health psychology.* Routledge/Taylor & Francis Group.

United Nations. (1989). *Convention on the rights of the child.* https://www.ohchr.org/sites/default/files/crc.pdf

Utsey, S. O., Abrams, J. A., Opare-Henaku, A., Bolden, M. A., & Williams, O., III. (2015). Assessing the psychological consequences of internalized colonialism on the psychological well-being of young adults in Ghana. *The Journal of Black Psychology, 41*(3), 195–220. https://doi.org/10.1177/0095798414537935

Vélez, W. (2017). A new framework for understanding Puerto Ricans' migration patterns and incorporation. *Centro Journal, 29*(3), 126–153.

Venator-Santiago, C. R., & Meléndez, E. (2017). U.S. citzenship in Puerto Rico: One hundred years after the Jones Act. *Centro Journal, 29*(1), 14–37.

Watkins, M. (2015). Psychosocial accompaniment. *Journal of Social and Political Psychology, 3*(1), 324–341. https://doi.org/10.5964/jspp.v3i1.103

Yakushko, O. (2019). Eugenics and its evolution in the history of Western psychology: A critical archival review. *Psychotherapy and Politics International, 17*(2).

3 ENGAGING WITH DECOLONIALITY, DECOLONIZATION, AND HISTORIES OF PSYCHOLOGY OTHERWISE

SUNIL BHATIA, WAHBIE LONG, WADE PICKREN, AND
ALEXANDRA RUTHERFORD

Decolonizing history is an exercise that we must start by questioning the story that is told, who tells it, and which voices have been silenced and still live among us.

—Naknanuk, 2021, p. 12

This multivocal chapter explores how the decolonial turn can help us interrogate and reimagine psychology's history. The decolonial turn is a transdisciplinary movement that takes the coloniality of being and knowing as the central problem of (post)modernity (see Maldonado-Torres, 2011). Critical historians and decolonial scholars have shown how both individual psychologists and the psy-disciplines writ large have enforced European American political, cultural, and intellectual domination and continue to reproduce the coloniality of being and the coloniality of knowledge. These scholars have done so by surfacing psychology's direct involvement, both historically and in the present, in such colonial projects as modernization theory (see Pickren & Rutherford, 2010) to the shaping of neoliberal selves in India (Bhatia &

https://doi.org/10.1037/0000376-004
Decolonial Psychology: Toward Anticolonial Theories, Research, Training, and Practice,
L. Comas-Díaz, H. Y. Adames, and N. Y. Chavez-Dueñas (Editors)

Priya, 2018). Indigenous scholars have also powerfully expressed how the dominant idea of what history is needs to be radically disrupted if it is to be decolonized. For example, Linda Tuhiwai Smith (2012) outlined several Western, modernist beliefs about the nature of history that function to rule Indigenous peoples' knowledge out of the bounds of history. These include the belief that narratives should be rooted in linear chronologies that reveal progression over time; the idea that history can and should be told as a completely coherent and unmediated narrative that reflects what happened in the past; and the idea that history is innocent, that the facts tell an unmotivated story absent of interpretation or power interests.

In addition to reiterating this important critique, we imagine histories of psychology otherwise. What could histories of psychology that foreground other-than-Enlightenment—that is, based on Eurocentric White male, Cartesian dualist—rationality, for example, look like? What other actors, experiences, knowledges, feelings, and practices might become central, and how might historians need to engage in new praxes to think, write, and feel with—rather than about—their subjects? Given that each coauthor is undertaking their decolonial projects from specific places, geographies, histories, and ongoing conditions of coloniality, we make some initial steps toward undoing the assumed universality and "view from nowhere" valorized by modernity and coloniality by foregrounding our positionality. That is, we use both positionality and multivocality to intentionally and explicitly challenge the idea that knowledge—and history—exists in some rarified state uninfluenced by the social position of the knower. We reinforce that local, place-based, and situated knowledges are not only epistemologically valid but also consistent with, and demanded by, the decolonial turn. Through a decolonial analysis, we challenge the ontological and epistemological bases of the psy-disciplines that function as the way psychologies, knowledges, and histories otherwise have been, and continue to be, excluded from consideration.

Our first voice is that of Sunil Bhatia, who encountered a deeply colonial psychology throughout his undergraduate and graduate education in Pune, India, a psychology that openly enforced the superiority of Eurocentric psychological knowledge. After migrating to the United States, he experienced how the universal, colonial, and empirical designs of U.S. psychology were unreflectively accepted as providing the standards for the rest of the world, rather than as reflecting local norms. Sunil is followed by Wahbie Long, who provides a perspective from South Africa. Early on in his clinical psychology training, he became sensitized to the shortcomings of psychology's social relevance in a country beset by stark racial and material divisions. This inspired his critical work into the historical problem of relevance in South African psychology.

He reminds us, too, that decolonization does not and cannot mean only one thing, a point we wish to emphasize by highlighting our different vantage points. Long is followed by Alexandra Rutherford, a White, settler-colonial feminist scholar based in Canada, who draws inspiration for decolonizing historical practice from both Indigenous scholars on Turtle Island and Black feminist scholars grappling with the coloniality of the archive. We end our multi-vocal chorus with Wade Pickren, a historian of psychology whose history is marked by his working-class upbringing in the racially divided southern United States. This upbringing sensitized him to questions of oppression and liberation, questions that have guided and shaped his historical inquiry and practice.

THE DECOLONIAL TURN: SUNIL BHATIA

Theories of decoloniality and decolonization are now increasingly part of our academic discourse and have been described by Maldonado-Torres (2011) as a sign of the decolonial turn. The decolonial turn does not advance a particular position. Instead, it is made up of a family of diverse, contradictory, and scattered positions that share the view that coloniality poses one of the central challenges for a vast majority of the people in the world who are living in the age of unequal globalization and thus decolonization is a critical unfinished undertaking (Bhatia, 2018). Decolonial thinking and resistance are not new, but they have existed since modern colonization forms began in the early 16th century (W. D. Mignolo, 2007). Decolonial resistance projects, therefore, have come from many different scholars and activists, fields, localities, and geographies with radically different ideas about justice, freedom, and liberation (Tuck & Yang, 2018).

Decolonization within the framework of especially North American settler colonialism is primarily focused on land, sovereignty, and territory (Coulthard, 2014; Grande, 2015). In contrast, the decolonial turn, or decoloniality, emerged out of the conquest, exploitation, and exercise of the coloniality of power in the Americas (W. D. Mignolo, 2007). Coloniality does not merely refer to the colonization of Indigenous culture in the Americas; instead, it refers to a whole system of thought, a mentality, and a power structure that constructs "the hegemonic and Euro centered matrix of knowledge" (W. D. Mignolo, 2010, p. 11). Postcolonial scholars focus on understanding the social and cultural consequences of Euro-American colonization on the formation of Third World diasporas in First World communities and investigating the creation of cultural practices under imperialism (E. W. Said, 1979), transportation of indentured labor and slavery, and the formation of postcolonial identities (Spivak, 1988). Scholars using a postcolonial lens focus on under-standing the representation of the colonized subjects by the colonizer in terms of power, race, gender, ethnicity, creation of nations, and nationalism in relation and opposition to the influential discursive practices of Europe and the United States (Ashcroft et al., 1995). Epistemological differences in decolonial, postcolonial, and decolonization approaches are crucial, but they provide us with radical possibilities in unsettling and undoing the coloniality of psychological sciences (Bhatia, 2020; Macleod et al., 2020). Decolonizing psychology entails examining how European American scientific psychology becomes the standard-bearer of psychology worldwide and how specific local cultural flows and ideas play an important role in shaping social and personal identities and institutional structures, cultures, and practices across the globe.

Positionality and Decolonization

Positionality is key to understanding mutual struggles, incommensurability, and differing praxis and social justice ideas in decolonial projects. We often undertake decolonial projects from specific places, geographies, and histories of colonization. Acknowledging positionality does not mean that no room is left for developing solidarity across decolonial projects. Instead, articulating positionalities shows the spaces where coalitions are possible and where tensions exist, and collaborations may not be possible (Tuck & Yang, 2018). South African psychologists Peace Kiguwa and Puleng Segalo (2018) argued that

> Such positioning matters for how we choose what we teach, how it is pack-aged, and how it is presented. This is part of engaging the hidden curriculum. Engaging the socio-history of the discipline—its worldviews and philosophical underpinnings—is linked to our specific orientations and view of the self-in-the-world. (p. 13)

My decolonial consciousness began to take root when I first encountered colonial psychology in my undergraduate and graduate education at the University of Pune, India. That curriculum was not hidden or concealed, and it was pretty brazenly colonial in its orientation and paraded Eurocentric psychological knowledge as superior to Indigenous frameworks. Britain's colonial rule of India was racist and ruthless because it oppressed, imprisoned, and tortured Indians for more than 200 years. Its policies created famines that killed more than 35 million Indians. Another million died, and more than 13 million people became displaced during India's violent and tragic partition in 1947 (Tharoor, 2017). The British used psychological and social science knowledge to justify their descriptions of my ancestors as animals, primitives, rude, backward, lazy, and ignorant; Winston Churchill called them "beastly people." Yet in my seven years of undergraduate and graduate psychology, I was taught that British and European theories of people and culture were more correct, legitimate, and superior to Indian culture and history. All of the psychology books in my college and university curriculum were written by British and American authors (Bhatia, 2020).

Subsequently, when I migrated to the United States, the psychology I encountered in my graduate school was also primarily built on colonial knowledge, universalistic principles, and Eurocentric cultural assumptions about individuality and rationality. It was a psychology based on 5% of the human population, yet it had the power to speak on behalf of the other 95% of humanity (Arnett, 2008). The universal, colonial, and empirical designs of American psychology were local norms conceived as standards for the rest of the world. My introduction to postcolonial scholars allowed me to articulate the legacy of colonialism that lived inside me. The "Empire" was deeply intertwined with my evolving self. From my positionality both as a postcolonial subject in India and as a migrant occupying space on Indigenous land, I have made efforts to decolonize psychology.

Epistemological Decolonization

A critical dimension of decolonization is epistemological decolonizing (Quijano, 2000; Richards, 2014; Smith, 2012). This involves delinking from Eurocentric knowledge systems, theories, ideas, and practices anchored in colonialism and coloniality (W. D. Mignolo, 2007). Epistemological decolonizing means dismantling the colonial structure of the academy or university and asking questions of what counts as knowledge, who is an expert, what is healing, feeling, thinking, and doing research relationally, spiritually, ecologically, to whom are we accountable in our research, and for what purposes (Smith, 2012). Epistemic decolonization means naming the cultural values and assumptions embedded in European American colonial knowledge systems that have caused epistemic violence (Bhatia, 2020; Teo, 2011) and what Santos (2014) has called epistimicide (the killing of non-Western knowledge). Decolonization of knowledge means explaining how people experience alienation as a psychic and material reality and theories that connect social structures with individual experiences of trauma and violence (Long, 2021). Several critiques of psychology have shown how Eurocentric psychological knowledge is largely based on a racialized, ahistorical, apolitical, and decontextualized framework (e.g., Adams et al., 2018; Bhatia & Priya, 2018; Kessi, 2017; Pickren & Rutherford, 2010). The field of psychology has neglected to examine how colonialism and coloniality shape how people remember, form relationships, create connections with family, community, divinity, myth, place, stories, rituals, and culture (Bhatia & Priya, 2018; Bulhan, 1985; Gone, 2021; Seedat & Suffla, 2017; Watkins, 2019). Decolonizing psychology highlights the asymmetrical balance of power in the geography of knowledge production, and the Eurocentric assumptions embedded in mainstream psychology, and the need for contextualized epistemologies, methodologies, and practice (Macleod et al., 2020).

Decolonization and Imagining Generative Possibilities

Scholars in decolonial psychology have argued that we have to map out and investigate the colonial wounds, historical trauma (Gone, 2021), and the structural violence that was unleashed by the shackles of colonialism, slavery, and genocide and spell out what was psychology's role in advancing slavery and genocide (Bhatia, 2002, 2020). This project has barely been addressed in psychology.

Before we undo coloniality, we first need to understand what kind of violence colonialism has unleashed at the structural, personal, familial, and psychopolitical level to marginalized populations in North America and the masses of humanity in the Global South. The term Global South can be broadly used as a political project and refers to the populations of Latin America, Asia, Africa, and Oceania (Bhatia & Priya, 2018). Many of the people who live in these spaces are low income and marginalized and are often used as extractive labor by Europe and the United States. The phrase Global South signals a "shift from a central focus on development or cultural difference toward an emphasis on geopolitical relations of power" (Dados & Connell, 2012, p. 12).

Epistemic decolonization focuses on centering and retrieving knowledge from the Global South. Ndlovu-Gatsheni (2013), a development studies scholar, argued that understanding how the coloniality of knowledge operates in the current global system of knowledge production is central to the project of decolonizing psychology. Ndlovu-Gatsheni (2013) wrote,

> coloniality of knowledge speaks directly to the epistemological colonization whereby Euro-American techno-scientific knowledge managed to displace, discipline, destroy alternative knowledge that it found outside the Euro-American zones (colonies) while at the same time appropriating what is considered useful to global imperial designs. (p. 54)

Epistemological decolonization is not just about adding new theories to psychology but also about fundamentally rethinking psychology. It means examining what possibilities mean or what it means "to imagine possibility differently" (Escobar, 2020, p. x). One of the main assumptions of decolonial thinking is that modern knowledge systems are tied to capitalism, racism, gender violence, and genocidal violence. Thus modernity entails coloniality. Psychology is born of modernity or coloniality. We cannot set up a new school of decoloniality while keeping intact the more prominent Eurocentric modes of knowing, thinking, and feeling based on Western ontologies and epistemology (W. D. Mignolo & Walsh, 2018). Second, the decolonial turn is built on the assumption that to construct a decolonized world, we have to delink from the current system of thinking and create solidarities to build new knowledge systems that signify an "epistemic reconstitution" or new forms of epistemic freedom (W. D. Mignolo & Walsh, 2018, p. 246). The majority population residing in the Global South does so in conditions where access to basic material resources needed for livelihood are missing, and access to food, housing, education, work, and a clean environment is a recurrent challenge and daily burden. Can we create knowledge systems that move beyond the hegemonic ideas of progress, development, and rationality? Can we refuse the current system of knowledge-making that does not benefit the larger humanity? Epistemological decolonization is necessary for undertaking global structural decolonization. We cannot delink unless we know how "psychological imperialism" in the past has contributed to colonialism, Whiteness, and coloniality and how it continues to act as a dominant global model for understanding humanity (Smith, 2012).

Third, we need situated and complex accounts of decolonial projects and struggles. Epistemological decolonization does not mean we unleash a master plan of decoloniality worldwide without regard to region. We need site-specific and local projects of decoloniality that take into account incommensurabilities and compatibilities between approaches. Homing in on the specific challenges of coloniality within the subdisciplines of psychology is required. For example, cross-cultural psychology has attempted to tackle the psychological differences and similarities across a range of regions around the globe. Although cultural psychologists have thoroughly critiqued cross-cultural psychology for taking a static, homogenizing view of culture, my research (Bhatia, 2018) shows how coloniality in psychology is reflected in new forms of knowledge that can be characterized as global corporate cross-cultural psychology. This type of cross-cultural psychology is primarily based on Eurocentric culture and ideas, but is often used by transnational corporations to understand people's actions, stories, and performances in outsourcing industries and businesses across Asia (Bhatia, 2018). When corporate cross-cultural psychological science merges with the neoliberal language of enterprise, then structural inequality, cross-cultural racism, mental health issues, and ethnocentrism become camouflaged as simple problems of cross-cultural difference and cultural misunderstandings that can be solved through individual effort, self-help, therapy, importation of Western mental health taxonomies, and diversity training (Bhatia, 2018; Bhatia & Priya, 2018). Historians of psychology must systematically account for its epistemic violence and map the "pluriversal knowledge" (Escobar, 2020) suppressed and erased in the name of modernity and science. This is not an attempt to revive some form of pure, refined precolonial knowledge but to begin to revitalize, reclaim, and rebuild knowledge systems that may be better than the one we have now. One question for historians of psychology to study is the forms of psychological knowledge lost, conquered, buried, and made irrational and dangerous in the process.

DECOLONIZING THE HISTORY OF PSYCHOLOGY: A VIEW FROM THE SOUTH: WAHBIE LONG

In the late 1990s and early 2000s, I trained as a psychologist at two of the African continent's leading universities. However, on completing a year's mandatory community service, I applied to have my name removed from the Health Professions Council of South Africa register. I was 24 years old, and seven years of training had left me cold. Perhaps I was too young, but I still did not see how the profession of clinical psychology could be of any use in a racially and materially divided society such as South Africa. I went traveling in the Sahara desert instead.

When I returned to university life in 2010, I was determined to make sense of this problem of relevance—that is, the relationship between psychology and the wider public—which I soon discovered was not a uniquely South African one: it had afflicted the discipline since its earliest days, including in its North American and western European heartlands (Long, 2016). Indeed, the stubbornness of the relevance issue reveals itself today in a different yet related idiom known as the decolonial turn. Across the social sciences and humanities in post-apartheid South Africa, it is rare to find scholars who are not thinking about the decolonization of their respective disciplines. From research strategies to funding applications to course descriptions, everyone—managers, researchers, and students alike—appears engaged in one or other form of discourse about the need to dismantle the colonial character of a decidedly European American canon.

In the so-called Global South, these efforts have assumed different—yet related—forms (Jansen, 2019). In Latin America, for example, the focus has tended to fall on epistemological strategies for reimagining what are understood to be the universalizing, objectifying, and hierarchical modes of knowing that still preponderate in formerly colonial societies. Critical theorists have described this "interestedness" of knowledge—its value-ladenness—for a very long time. Accordingly, in the sciences of social action "those whom the laws are about" develop a reflective consciousness that is capable of transforming "ideologically frozen relations of dependence" (Habermas, 1972, p. 310).

By contrast, at the southernmost tip of the African continent, decolonial praxis has concerned itself primarily with ontological markers of identity. The organizing principle here centers on voice and, specifically, the question of the right to speak. "Nothing about us, without us" is an increasingly common refrain, prescribing not only who may speak but also who may not. For example, at the height of the Fallist protests that rocked South African universities between 2015 and 2017, students demanded that statues, fees, and science fall (UCT Scientist, 2016). One student claimed that the enterprise of "science as a whole is a product of Western modernity and the whole thing should be scratched off. . . . We have to restart science from . . . an African perspective." In particular, the discovery of gravity attracted special scorn—not because it was argued not to exist, but because it was a European scientist who formulated that universal law, "whether people knew Newton or not, or whether whatever happens in western Africa, northern Africa [sic]."

The trouble with the term decolonization is that it does not—and cannot—mean one specific thing. It is understood differently not only across geographical regions but even within institutions of higher learning. Although most South African students, I would imagine, do not subscribe to the view that science in toto must fall, the foregoing episode raises the vexing question of how—for this chapter—one can settle on the parameters of a project for decolonizing a field such as the history of psychology. Scholars who argue for the importance of identity may deem it as simple as changing the racial demographics of historians of psychology in the country. Precious few Black scholars are in the field, not only in South Africa but also internationally. If one is to improve this situation through reverse engineering, one essential strategy will involve heightening the field's visibility within the undergraduate and postgraduate curricula, where it continues to occupy a position that fluctuates between marginality and nonexistence. Equally important is incentivizing postgraduate studies in the field by creating dedicated scholarships, mentorship programs, and tenure track positions, the combination of which will have to happen against the backdrop of a higher education landscape—in South Africa—that is operating under increasingly stressed economic conditions.

By contrast, a different sort of historian may opt for the epistemological route. Among other things, they will insist on interrogating the very question of the archive: its constitution, its possible forms, its modes of analysis, its prior readings, its presentation and dissemination, and its relationship to current imperatives within both academic and broader social life. Crucially, when it comes to modes of analysis, what is nowadays referred to as lived experience must be interrogated alongside the more established—if heavily discursive— ways of knowing. At stake is the prospect of a "pluriversity" that will demand a "horizontal strategy of openness to dialogue among different epistemic traditions" (Mbembe, 2019, p. 241). But it is also at this point that identity enters the fray, mainly because of its diffraction of lived experience in unique ways. The main implication is that the distinction between the epistemological and ontological approaches to decolonization is slightly artificial though indeed of heuristic value. To be sure, the former implies the latter: as Rutherford points out, the archival record can appear to be constituted scientifically even as it obliterates the existence of whole communities. Decolonial forms of praxis—for example, archival stretching—are then required to illuminate such hidden presences.

The problem with setting up rival ways of knowing—even if they are potentially complementary—is that the knowledge-making project is inherently conservative and operates according to a logic of accretion. Kuhnian paradigm shifts are uncommon events. As any decolonizer knows, powerful institutional forces are ranged against such attempts—not necessarily out of bad faith but simply because institutional trajectories and therefore inertias are consequential. Like the formation of disciplines, reimagining a field such as the history of psychology will necessitate sustained engagement with established knowledge producers (Danziger, 1990). In the absence of a willingness to burn institutions to the ground—which is not a hypothetical in South Africa (Dentlinger, 2018)—one must communicate in the *lingua franca* of administrators and the broader university community. However, for many decolonizers, standard academic discourse is like dice loaded in favor of an immovable and hostile European American rationality (Long, 2021).

The apparent power asymmetries that assail the global academy bear this out. The cold truth is that efforts at intellectual decolonization in the Global South are constrained unavoidably by entire fields of knowledge that have been imagined, constructed, and naturalized elsewhere and then exported everywhere (Auerbach et al., 2019). The rhetoric of decentering the academic project is praiseworthy. Still, for intellectuals on the periphery, the stubborn reality is that their local knowledge is only ever transformed into Knowledge with a capital K when endorsed by the European American center (Naudé, 2019). For the time being, talk of a "glocal" academy will prove largely aspirational as long as the globalized (and globalizing) neoliberal approach to higher education remains the only show in town.

Indeed, any disciplinary regime reflects how a specific society perceives, dissects, and solves its problems (Long, 2018). Therefore, a suitably decolonial question is whether psychology—and, by extension, the history of psychology—makes sense as an independent field of inquiry in previously colonized parts of the world. This is fundamentally an interrogation of psychology's cultural, social, and political credentials—a debate well known to historians of the discipline, reinvented under different monikers over the decades, including relevance (Long, 2016), indigenization (Brock, 2006), and now decolonization. Answering this question, however, requires venturing beyond both the discipline and the broader academy—because the call for intellectual decolonization cannot be separated from the larger project of political decolonization, the goals and methods of which, though beyond the scope of this chapter, must vary from one setting to the next.

There is an old joke about the exceptional bitterness of academic politics—that it derives from the stakes being so desperately low. Decolonizing knowledge, that is, does not count for much in contexts where, for example, people are dying of hunger. Intellectuals have earned special notoriety for mistaking the gown for the town (Mamdani, 2019), habitually underestimating the distance from their ivory towers to the streets below. Academic decadence can be a blind spot, and intellectual decolonization—especially of the identitarian kind—can breed a narcissism entirely at odds with its radical posturing. Suppose the decolonial turn is to prove more than just a passing moment. In that case, building concrete alliances with ordinary people and their everyday struggles becomes essential as per the aphorism "nothing about us, without us" (Charlton, 1998).

DECOLONIZING HISTORICAL PRAXIS: ALEXANDRA RUTHERFORD

The stories about psychology's origins, history, and contributions that I have studied and most often contributed to are deeply imbued with and powerfully enforce coloniality, simultaneously making it invisible. To write a decolonized history of psychology requires demonstrating that disciplinary psychology is itself a colonial project, as we have already highlighted. This is the first task of decolonizing history of psychology, a task that is under way but far from finished (e.g., Bhatia, 2002; Schmidt, 2019). History-writing and teaching, though, are also powerful tools in creating altogether new psychologies, what Pickren (2021), drawing on the work of scholars in the decoloniality tradition, termed "psychologies otherwise." To imagine such psychologies otherwise, we must forge histories otherwise, histories that center the cultural forms, ways of being, subjectivities, ontologies, and epistemologies of those not only excluded from the European-origin academic discipline but forcibly oppressed by it.

My ongoing and incomplete shift toward a decolonial consciousness began when I took up gender as a category of analysis to make sense of histories of psychology that excluded women or made them miraculous exceptions to a White, androcentric norm. Gradually I became aware of the ways that psychologists have participated quite overtly in constructing a gender system that enforces patriarchy and colonization, and have come to appreciate more thoroughly that gender was just one vector through which power—and coloniality—were enacted to privilege some forms of knowledge and knowers and suppress others. As a White, settler-colonial feminist scholar working across Canadian and U.S. contexts, my thinking about history and historical practice have been influenced by historians who have written about the enslavement of Afro-descent people in the United States, as well as scholars writing about the histories—and presence—of ongoing genocide against Indigenous people (First Nations, Métis, and Inuit) in the Canadian context. For me, the challenge of doing history differently—in ways that foreground colonizing power and its effects—has become central to my teaching, training, and writing.

In this section, I take up the call Long outlined earlier to interrogate the methodological foundations on which histories of psychology are based—to imagine what it might mean to decolonize historical practice itself. This is more than an abstract, intellectual exercise. Many scholars have written about the power and violence of the imperial and colonial archive and have long highlighted the necessity of attending to power in the production of history (e.g., Fuentes, 2016; Hartman, 2008; E. Said, 1993; Trouillot, 1995). In exploring what this means for constructing narratives of slavery, specifically in her work on slavery in the Caribbean, Marisa Fuentes (2016) asked,

> What would a narrative of slavery look like when taking into account "power in the production of history?" That is, how do slaveholders' interests affect how they document their world, and in turn, how do these very documents result in persistent historical silences? What would it mean to be critical of how our historical methodologies dependent on such sources often reproduce these silences? There is not a paucity of sources about slavery in the Caribbean from the words and perspectives of white authorities and slave owners. (p. 5)

To paraphrase Fuentes in the context of the history of psychology, what would a narrative of psychology's history look like when taking into account "power in the production of history?" How do psychologists' interests affect how they document their work, and in turn, how do these very documents result in persistent historical silences? What would it mean to be critical of how our historical methodologies dependent on such sources often reproduce these silences? Sources about psychology in Anglo European countries told through the words and perspectives of White, European or European-origin (and often male) scholars are legion.

Here I propose that to create histories of psychologies otherwise we need to start by transforming historical praxis. As Ghaddar and Casswell (2019) wrote in their reflection on decolonizing the archive, "Effective decolonization requires a radical transformation that can only be realized through a radical praxis" (p. 71). I present some ideas for how to enact such a radical praxis. To do so, I draw from the work of historians who have grappled with how to tell radically (as in "proceeding from the root") different stories about the past, stories that center the experiences of the colonized, the dispossessed, the enslaved, and the marginalized. What is essential to keep in mind is that the repositories of sources that historians typically draw on to reconstruct the past (e.g., archives of various kinds), the methods they use to interpret them, and the credibility of their resulting interpretations are all products of relations of power: colonizer over colonized, enslaver over enslaved, scientist over subject, doctor over patient. They thus have inherent—and insidious—limitations. As Saidiya Hartman, in her luminous reconstruction of the intimate, rebellious lives of young Black women at the turn of the 20th century in the United States, wrote,

> Every historian of the multitude, the dispossessed, the subaltern, and the enslaved, is forced to grapple with the power and authority of the archive and the limits it sets on what can be known, whose perspective matters, and who is endowed with the gravity and authority of historical actor. (2019, p. xiii)

The challenge of transcending these limitations is at the heart of decolonizing praxis.

Decolonizing Praxis: Archives, Interpretation, and Process

Historians often look to primary sources, such as archival documents, to construct stories about the past. In this process, they are guided by their a priori decisions about what—and who—is important to know about. When a historian of psychology working from a decolonizing framework approaches such sources, they may very well find that the sources themselves absent, silence, or distort the subjects (as in topics, but also as in—literally—people) in which they are most interested, reenacting the violence against these subjects that was— and is—part of the colonial project. In a word, traditional archives are almost always, already, colonial.

In the case of psychology, many formal archives are structured by and about scientific and, perhaps to a lesser degree, professional psychology, as enacted by those who have historically held the power in these disciplines and defined the parameters of what is acceptable psychology and what is not. Moreover, archives of the experiences of those on the receiving end of psychological science and practice—First Nations children subjected to psychological tests to commit them to residential schools and other eugenic schemes in Canada; Black incarcerated inmates involuntarily enrolled in prison token-economies in the United States; the "native" subjects of British colonial rule in India, and so on—are either absent or, when present, are discredited by the rigorous gatekeeping of the colonial academy. Concerning this gatekeeping, Tanana Athabascan feminist scholar Dian Million noted that the personal stories of Indigenous women that express, through their emotional knowledges, the gendered, racialized, and sexualized nature of their colonization, do exist, but are dismissed through this process: "Our felt scholarship continues to be segregated as a "feminine" experience, as polemic, or at worst as not knowledge at all. . . . Academia repetitively produces gatekeepers to our entry into important social discourses because we *feel* our histories as well as think them" (Million, 2009, p. 54). What might an archive of feeling offer historians of psychology?

Where textual accounts from the marginalized, dispossessed, enslaved, and colonized do exist in formal archives, they are often so heavily redacted and anonymized—usually in the name of ethics or because their identities (humanity) were not considered necessary or thinkable from the start—that the ability to pursue systematic lines of inquiry, to humanize, and to flesh out their experiences is, at best, highly impoverished, or at worst nearly impossible. To redress this, some scholars have practiced what historian Tiya Miles (2021) called "restrained imagination" and what Saidiya Hartman (2008), relatedly, called "critical fabulation." This is a twofold method in which the historian uses imaginative reconstruction to fill archival fissures partially, and in doing so, forcefully reveals the fissures that render such rebuilding impossible. Critical fabulation might involve rearranging basic elements of a story, combining elements or events from different stories, and engaging in transtemporal weaving together of past, present, and future to produce a "recombinant narrative" (Hartman, 2008, p. 12). The intent is not to "give voice" or reconstitute the displaced historical subject but rather to imagine the alternative realities and subjectivities that can never be fully reconstituted. As Hartman wrote, "It is a history of an unrecoverable past; it is a narrative of what might have been or could have been; it is a history written with and against the archive" (2008, p. 12; for examples, see Hartman, 2019; Miles, 2021).

Fuentes (2016) practices what she calls reading the archive "along the bias grain." Here she invokes the metaphor of a textile or piece of fabric that affords its greatest tensile flexibility along the bias—the diagonal formed where axes of horizontal and vertical weaves come together. Fuentes wrote that this is a methodology "in which the archival record is stretched to accentuate the figures of enslaved women whose presence influences ontological conditions of others but who are not mentioned in particular archives" (p. 153). The intent is not to challenge the factual veracity of the existing archival documents themselves but rather to doggedly collect and analyze them to reveal the imbalance of records and modes of recording that deaccentuate certain figures, requiring us to stretch to reveal their form.

For an example, a number of years ago, four of my graduate students and I engaged in a reading course exploring the links among gender, sexuality, and madness in the late 19th century. As we collected readings and primary source documents, the lives and experiences of the women committed to asylums for purported insanity emerged largely through the accounts of the neurologists who treated their nervous conditions, the gynecological surgeons who took out their ovaries and wombs, and the barristers who kept them committed to asylums. The archive was replete with information on these women through these sources, but the women themselves remained in the background. They were shadowy figures whose experiences could only be reconstructed through the perspectives of those whose official positions and power privileged their presence in the archive. As a final assignment for the course, the students staged an archivally reconstructed dramatic reenactment of a case conference to discuss a troubling case of a woman with nymphomania. The woman herself was represented as a shadow on the wall of the performance hall, and the students took on the dramatic personae of those whose voices we did have access to, including Dr. Lawson Tait, a gynecological surgeon who pioneered the ovariotomy as a treatment for women's emotional distress, and Dr. James Jackson Putnam, one of the most distinguished nervous disease specialists in the late 19th-century United States. By representing the woman herself as a shadow, whose form was revealed and accentuated through the ensuing dialogue, we were what Fuentes would call reading the archive "along the bias grain."

A final method to reimagine archival practice is to engage with things rather than texts. Even though art historians and archaeologists are versed in interpreting objects, historians of psychology are likely not. How to interpret things owned, made, used, or carried by the colonized, the dispossessed? How to interpret the carefully embroidered jacket of German asylum inmate and seamstress Agnes Richter, who literally stitched her experiences into her institutional uniform (Hornstein, 2009)? Or the humble—and heartbreaking—cloth sack bequeathed from the enslaved Rose to her daughter Ashley on the eve of their violent separation at slave auction (Miles, 2021)? In reconstructing histories of psychologies otherwise, what can objects such as these tell the historian about the subjectivities of the mad, the enslaved, the colonized? As Miles (2021) noted in her sustained analysis of Ashley's sack and its contents, "using the object responsibly as a source for historical enquiry means asking questions of it and, as uncomfortable as it may feel, maintaining a willingness to poke holes into it". (p. 16). She recommended (and practices) placing the object in conversation with other sources and considering its various and diverse historical contexts. For example, Miles used the "tattered dress" noted as one of the contents of Ashley's sack to inspire a deeply researched examination of the role of clothing in the lives of enslaved peoples, including its relationship to artistry, creativity, protection, honor, status, and bodily integrity, at the intersections of race, gender, and status.

"Nothing About Us Without Us" and the Practice of Participatory History

The scholars whose work I highlight have developed ingenious strategies to navigate the limits of existing archives that have been constructed under—and replicate—systems of subjugation and domination that persist in the present. In employing these strategies, they have constructed what Indigenous scholar Eve Tuck (2009) called "desire-centered" rather than "damage-centered" narratives about the subjectivities and experiences of enslaved and colonized people. In reimagining historical practice in the present, we would suggest possibilities available to historians of psychology to disrupt the ongoing violence of the archive and ensure that it does not continue ad infinitum. In the spirit of "nothing about us without us," historians can work in alliance with dispossessed and historically marginalized communities to create archives—and write histories—that do not reproduce these circuits of dispossession and colonization.

Public historians are at the forefront of using community-based participatory methods to collect, document, and preserve experiences through oral history, art, facilitated dialogue, events, films, exhibits, and so on that then become not only the archives of the future, but also and perhaps more important, sources for self-determination in the present. For example, in the Canadian context, critical efforts to reconstruct the history of eugenics and its effects on both Indigenous people and people with disabilities have centrally involved, as full collaborators and architects of the archival record, those who have survived eugenics or been targeted by eugenic practices (see Dyck, 2021; Kelly et al., 2021).

As we think about creating histories otherwise, whose stories, told in what ways, would inform our efforts? How and why do the particulars of the process matter? How can attending to these particulars help decolonize the archive, decolonize history? Assuming the university and the products of its disciplinary regimes, including psychology and history, persist in some form, questions such as these need the full force of our attention.

DECOLONIAL TURN TO PSYCHOLOGIES OTHERWISE: WADE PICKREN

> What is particularly needed is a psychology guided by emancipatory interests.
> (Paranjpe, 2002, p. 29)

History as a modernist project has been an instrument of coloniality of being and knowledge intended to retain the right of intellectual authority over what counts as truth regarding events, people, and ideas of the past (Maldonado-Torres, 2007). Such claims extend to judgment about what practices and which countries or societies are modern, Europe serving as the measure of modernity (Goody, 2006; W. D. Mignolo, 2011). History of psychology, though a minor field, has sought its place in this project.

I have my own history in the history of psychology. I was educated and trained in psychology, its history, and in history of science. Throughout my career, I have focused on questions of oppression and liberation with special emphases on race, ethnicity, indigeneity, and, most recently, ecological impact. Once I became aware of the decolonial turn, new understanding and insights followed. I now think of my work as seeking to understand and meliorate the enduring impacts of coloniality of being and knowledge on human thought and practice. This is what guides my contribution to this chapter.

Much of the historiography of psychology has followed the what is referred to as the WEIRD (Western, educated, industrialized, rich, and democratic) template in terms of subject matter and emphasis. Recent years have brought some change toward engagement with justice, with equity, with White privilege, with history as a colonizer's right. Still, the underlying assumption is often that the White Euro-U.S., especially Anglo-U.S., approaches grounded in European enlightenment rationality form the acceptable foundation for "real" historical scholarship. As Māori educator and scholar Linda Tuhiwai Smith (1999) noted regarding histories of Indigenous peoples, such histories hold that Indigenous peoples are not the "final arbiters of what counts as the truth" about their histories (p. 34). History, she argued, was made into a modernist project in the Western Enlightenment. The result has been that it is those who are modern, traditionally White, male, and of a certain social class, who reserve the right to name lands, make official maps, set compass directions, determine what is history and what is tradition or myth (see also Chakrabarty, 2008; W. D. Mignolo, 2011). But, she argued, history is "part of the critical pedagogy of decolonization. To hold alternative histories is to hold alternative knowledges. The pedagogical implication of this access to alternative knowledges is that they can form the basis of alternative ways of doing things" (Smith, 1999, p. 34). The implication is that such alternative histories are powerful weapons to combat inequities, injustices, and the grip of the colonizer or oppressor on the psyche and selfways of the oppressed (Fellner, 2018). They form counterstories or counternarratives that not only empower themselves but also function as tools to undermine colonialist settler histories and decolonize dominant canons of knowledge (Solórzano & Yosso, 2002). Beyond the primacy of their work to counter the coloniality of being and knowledge of the oppressed, they may also serve, as Tuhiwai Smith argued, as pedagogical tools for those historians and psychologists who aspire to develop decolonial strategies regarding psychology and its history.

Decolonial strategies make it possible to delink from the frame of hegemonic psychology dominated by Eurocentric notions of rationality, ontology, and epistemology that enforce the coloniality of knowledge in ways both subtle and violent—epistemological, geophysical, interpersonal, intercultural violence (Pickren & Tasci, 2022). The decolonial turn holds out a possibility that histories of psychology can be developed not constrained by Global North sensibilities of modernity regarding historical praxes. Developing and using such strategies would bring new ontological, epistemological, and methodological options to the historiography of psychology. Doing so would create new *reals*, psychologies otherwise as part of the pluriverse, a world where many worlds are possible (Escobar, 2020; Pickren, 2021). Practically, the delinking brought by decolonial strategies would make it possible to create psychologies and their histories that are true to their place, to the people whose psychology it is, and most important, a way to live that does not depend on neoliberal strategies of domination, self-promotion, or destructive exploitation of the earth and its beings, human and more than human.

Rutherford suggests new historical methodologies developed by Fuentes (2016), Hartman (2019), and Miles (2021) that are striking examples of decolonial historiographical tools. Bhatia calls for a thorough examination of the colonialist and modernist origins of hegemonic psychological science; the beginnings of such a history can be found in James and Lorenz (2021), Adams et al. (2018), Pickren (2021), and Bhatia (2018, 2019), among others. These studies, and now others, are revealing that what hegemonic psychology portrays as the optimal human psychological characteristics have their origins in the same matrix as neoliberal capitalism, racism, sexism, and the full span of inequities. This matrix created the "conditions of possibility for modern individualism" (Adams et al., 2018, pp. 13–14) and all the ills that have accompanied it. Such conditions of possibility include the sense of separation from Earth, as though humans are somehow exceptional and superior to other forms of life and being on the planet. This sense of separability has fostered practices of destruction on the material life of the planet and underlies many of the crises we now face, such as climate chaos, biodiversity loss, and poisoning of the soil with pesticides and herbicides that portend a future of being unable to feed ourselves (Oliveira-Andreotti, 2021).

Bhatia, in his 2019 article on Indigenous psychologies, articulated the crux of the matter. His argument should have resonance for the historiography of psychology as well:

> One reason why we do not have detailed intellectual and social histories of indigenous psychology is because it has often been considered as *deeply rooted in local practices and relegated to the realm of the mythological, collective, religious, traditional, philosophical, irrational, primitive, imaginative, and cultural.* Against this narrative of marginalization, the Euro American narrative of psychology is seen as having a teleological arc that goes from the cultural, to the scientific, to the universal, and the unit of analysis simultaneously moves from the community to the individual and eventually to psychological processes as localized in the brain. The latter narrative of psychology has become our stock story, from which we have extracted our canonical stories of identity, personhood, emotions, cognition, and *methods about how psychological knowledge ought to be created.* (Bhatia, 2019, pp. 111–112, emphasis added)

I bring attention to his word: primitive. This is what modernity says is not acceptable, that primitive is the very thing that is counter to the project of modernity. A decolonial strategy for history of psychology is to embrace what modernity—John Law (2011) called it the One World World—calls the sign of the primitive, that which is "deeply rooted in local practices and relegated to the realm of the mythological, collective, religious, traditional, philosophical, irrational, primitive, imaginative, and cultural" (Bhatia, 2019, p. 111). Such an embrace can draw the sting of hegemonic psychological science because it grounds the psychological in the local, makes it place based, and thus resonant with how people live.

We must ask why hegemonic psychology is so dismissive of local knowledge. From a decolonial perspective, we can see local practices and the so-called irrationality of the mythological, the collective, the primitive as the foundation of what creates the psychological. Such knowledges threaten the hegemon. Ashis Nandy, an Indian psychologist and prominent intellectual, posited that many in Eurocentric modernity are afraid that giving any credence or place to local, traditional, Indigenous knowledges would destabilize the bases of Eurocentric rationality and epistemology (cited in Rose, 2008, p. 166).

For those psychologists whose fundamental commitment is to hegemonic psychology, the mythological, the local, the collective, and so on are unacceptable because they are Other than the sources of true psychological science and practice. To paraphrase Hegarty and Pratto (2001), such sources are "that which needs to be explained" because they do not fit within the standard narrative of contemporary psychology. Then, we should ask, why is the contemporary hegemonic variety of psychology so skittish, so leery, as Nandy argued?

As Kurt Danziger (1990) pointed out some years ago, psychological science was constructed on a "narrow social basis. That entailed a very considerable *narrowing of epistemic access to the variety of psychological realities*" (p. 197, emphasis added). It is that variety of psychological realities that then becomes interesting. The practitioners of hegemonic psychological science in much of Europe and North America have stoutly resisted acknowledging psychological science's roots in spiritual ideas, myths, religion, mind science, custom, commerce, and, in the case of the United States, intense individualism, as numerous authors have shown (Albanese, 2007; Cooter, 1984; Schmit, 2010; Taylor, 1999; Thomson, 2006). Those who practice scientific psychology prefer to chart the history of psychological science as moving from the local cultural base of knowledge to the claim of the universal, the endpoint being positivist research data that show their point of origin in neural processes (Vidal & Ortega, 2017). Hegemonic psychological science claims that its findings are factual of all people (and even animals), everywhere, at all times (Bhatia, 2019), despite its WEIRD evidentiary database (Henrich et al., 2010; Pickren & Tasci, 2022).

Perhaps the occlusion of hegemonic psychology's mythic, religious, and commercial past is an example of what Santos calls a sociology of absences (2014). One consequence is that many of psychology's knowledge claims are divorced from the daily experiences of most human beings (Escobar, 2020; Santos, 2014). A decolonial strategy of drawing on the local, making psychology and its history place based and directly related to lived experience, would create a psychology that belonged to the people it developed among and thus useful in daily life. An excellent example of this kind of historical scholarship is the recent history of the Mi'gmaq community of the Gaspe Peninsula in Canada: *Nta'tugwaqanminene: Our Story, Evolution of the Gespe'ge-wa'gi Mi'gmaq* (Gespe'gewa'gi Mi'gmawei Mawiomi, 2016). It is members of the community writing their history based on oral histories, archives, and genealogies. The community was assisted by non-Mi'gmaq scholars, lawyers, archivists, historians, and others. It is history told without the colonizer's gaze, without the blinders of the coloniality of knowledge.

The work presented here can help historians of psychology make the decolonial turn and delink from the dominant psychology of our time. Making such a turn will require that scholars and activists develop a habit of ontological and epistemological disobedience to create a psychology linked to the reality of place, which is to say, to life. It will require us to rethink our histories as beginning with the lives of the nonelites in a framework that is not individualistic and that considers relationality and life in common as central to healthy living. That is, to rethink our histories "from the bottom and to the left" (*desde abajo y a la izquierda*), as the Zapatistas say (cited in Escobar, 2017, p. 174).

BRINGING OUR VOICES TOGETHER

To decolonize the discipline of psychology we must center the experiences and knowledges of those who have been erased or marginalized in our histories. This is not a mere recovery project. As we have shown, this recentering necessarily reveals the grossly uneven flows of power that characterized colonization and that continue to be enforced through the coloniality of being and knowledge. The project of decolonizing history will help psychologists interrupt this coloniality of being and knowledge by both exposing these power dynamics and giving psychology entirely new historical footings. In this chapter we have brought forward our diverse perspectives on how to do this, perspectives influenced by each of our unique histories, social positions, experiences, and geopolitical locations. We have stressed that the new histories that emerge from the decolonial turn must be plural, local, situated, coexisting, nonelite, relational, and nonhierarchical. Out of our multivocality comes, we hope, a harmonious expression of our shared commitment to decolonizing psychology and its history.

RESOURCES

Adichie, C. N. (2009, July). *The danger of a single story* [Video]. TEDTalk. https://www.ted.com/talks/chimamanda_ngozi_adichie_the_danger_of_a_single_story?language=en

Eugenics Archive. (2017). *Surviving Eugenics* [Film]. https://www.eugenicsarchive.ca/our-stories

Said, W., & the Media Education Foundation. (1998). *On Orientalism: Western attitudes towards the Middle East* [Video]. YouTube. https://www.youtube.com/watch?v=3MYYDEj4fIU

REFERENCES

Adams, G., Estrada-Villalta, S., & Gómez Ordóñez, L. H. (2018). The modernity/coloniality of being: Hegemonic psychology as intercultural relations. *International Journal of Intercultural Relations, 62*, 13–22. https://doi.org/10.1016/j.ijintrel.2017.06.006

Albanese, C. L. (2007). *A republic of mind and spirit: A cultural history of American metaphysical religion.* Yale University Press.

Arnett, J. J. (2008). The neglected 95%: Why American psychology needs to become less American. *American Psychologist, 63*(7), 602–614. https://doi.org/10.1037/0003-066X.63.7.602

Ashcroft, B., Griffiths, G., & Tiffin, H. (1995). General introduction. In B. Ashcroft, G. Griffiths, & H. Tiffin (Eds.), *The post-colonial studies reader* (pp. 1–4). Routledge.

Auerbach, J., Dlamini, M., & Anonymous. (2019). Scaling decolonial consciousness? The re-invention of "Africa" in a neoliberal university. In J. Jansen (Ed.), *Decolonisation in universities: The politics of knowledge* (pp. 116–135). Wits University Press.

Bhatia, S. (2002). Orientalism in Euro-American and Indian psychology: Historical representations of "natives" in Colonial and postcolonial contexts. *History of Psychology, 5*(4), 376–398. https://doi.org/10.1037/1093-4510.5.4.376

Bhatia, S. (2018). *Decolonizing psychology: Globalization, social justice, and Indian youth identities.* Oxford University Press.

Bhatia, S. (2019). Searching for justice in an unequal world: Reframing indigenous psychology as a cultural and political project. *Journal of Theoretical and Philosophical Psychology, 39*(2), 107–114. https://psycnet.apa.org/doi/10.1037/teo0000109. https://doi.org/10.1037/teo0000109

Bhatia, S. (2020). Decolonization and coloniality in human development: Neoliberalism, globalization and narratives of Indian youth. *Human Development, 64*(4–6), 207–221. https://doi.org/10.1159/000513084

Bhatia, S., & Priya, K. R. (2018). Decolonizing culture: Euro-American psychology and the shaping of neoliberal selves in India. *Theory & Psychology, 28*(5), 645–668. https://doi.org/10.1177/0959354318791315

Brock, A. C. (Ed.). (2006). *Internationalizing the history of psychology.* New York University Press.

Bulhan, H. A. (1985). *Frantz Fanon and the psychology of oppression.* Plenum Press. https://doi.org/10.1007/978-1-4899-2269-4

Chakrabarty, D. (2008). *Provincializing Europe: Post-colonial thought and historical difference.* Princeton University Press. https://doi.org/10.1515/9781400828654

Charlton, J. (1998). *Nothing about us without us: Disability, oppression, and empowerment.* University of California Press.

Cooter, R. (1984). *The cultural meaning of popular science: Phrenology and the organization of consent in nineteenth-century Britain.* Cambridge University Press.

Dados, N., & Connell, R. (2012). The Global South. *Contexts, 11*(1), 12–13. https://doi.org/10.1177/1536504212436479

Danziger, K. (1990). *Constructing the subject: Historical origins of psychological research.* Cambridge University Press. https://doi.org/10.1017/CBO9780511524059

Dentlinger, L. (2018, August 8). #FeesMustFall damage costs soar to nearly R800m. *Eyewitness News.* https://ewn.co.za/2018/08/08/feesmustfall-damage-costs-soar-to-nearly-r800m

Dyck, E. (2021). Doing history that matters: Going public and activating voices as a form of historical activism. *Journal of the History of the Behavioral Sciences, 57*(1), 75–86. https://doi.org/10.1002/jhbs.22069

Escobar, A. (2017). *Designs for the pluriverse: Radical interdependence, autonomy, and the making of worlds.* Duke University Press.

Escobar, A. (2020). *Pluriversal politics: The real and the possible.* Duke University Press.

Fellner, K. D. (2018). Embodying decoloniality: Indigenizing curriculum and pedagogy. *American Journal of Community Psychology, 62*(3–4), 283–293. https://psycnet.apa.org/doi/10.1002/ajcp.12286

Fuentes, M. J. (2016). *Dispossessed lives: Enslaved women, violence, and the archive.* University of Pennsylvania Press. https://doi.org/10.9783/9780812293005

Gespe'gewa'gi Mi'gmawei Mawiomi. (2016). *Nta'tugwaqanminene: Our story, evolution of the Gespe'gewa'gi Mi'gmaq.* Fernwood.

Ghaddar, J. J., & Caswell, M. (2019). "To go beyond": Towards a decolonial archival praxis. *Archival Science, 19*(2), 71–85. https://doi.org/10.1007/s10502-019-09311-1

Gone, J. P. (2021). Decolonization as methodological innovation in counseling psychology: Method, power, and process in reclaiming American Indian therapeutic traditions. *Journal of Counseling Psychology, 68*(3), 259–270. https://psycnet.apa.org/doi/10.1037/cou0000500. https://doi.org/10.1037/cou0000500

Goody, J. (2006). *The theft of history.* Cambridge University Press.

Grande, S. (2015). *Red pedagogy: Native American political and social thought* (2nd ed.). Rowman and Littlefield.

Habermas, J. (1972). *Knowledge and human interests.* Beacon Press.

Hartman, S. (2008). Venus in two acts. *Small Axe, 12*(2), 1–14. https://muse.jhu.edu/article/241115

Hartman, S. (2019). *Wayward lives, beautiful experiments: Intimate histories of riotous Black girls, troublesome women, and queer radicals.* Norton.

Hegarty, P., & Pratto, F. (2001). The effects of social category norms and stereotypes on explanations for intergroup differences. *Journal of Personality and Social Psychology, 80*(5), 723–735. https://psycnet.apa.org/doi/10.1037/0022-3514.80.5.723

Henrich, J., Heine, S. J., & Norenzayan, A. (2010). The weirdest people in the world? *Behavioral and Brain Sciences, 33*(2–3), 61–83. https://doi.org/10.1017/S0140525X0999152X

Hornstein, G. (2009). *Agnes's jacket: A psychologist's search for the meanings of madness.* Routledge.

James, S., & Lorenz, H. (2021). Do your first works over. *Journal of the History of the Behavioral Sciences, 57*(4), 319–335. https://doi.org/10.1002/jhbs.22118

Jansen, J. (2019). On the politics of decolonisation: Knowledge, authority and the settled curriculum. In J. Jansen (Ed.), *Decolonisation in universities: The politics of knowledge* (pp. 50–78). Wits University Press. https://doi.org/10.18772/22019083351.8

Kelly, E., Manning, D. T., Boye, S., Rice, C., Owen, D., Stonefish, S., & Stonefish, M. (2021). Elements of a counter-exhibition: Excavating and countering a Canadian history and legacy of eugenics. *Journal of the History of the Behavioral Sciences, 57*(1), 12–33. https://doi.org/10.1002/jhbs.22081

Kessi, S. (2017). Community social psychologies for decoloniality: An African perspective on epistemic justice in higher education. *South African Journal of Psychology, 47*(4), 506–516. https://doi.org/10.1177/0081246317737917

Kiguwa, P., & Segalo, P. (2018). Decolonizing psychology in residential and open distance e-learning institutions: Critical reflections. *South African Journal of Psychology, 48*(3), 310–318. https://doi.org/10.1177/0081246318786605

Law, J. (2011, September 19). *What's wrong with a one-world world?* [Paper Presentation] Center for the Humanities, Wesleyan University. http://www.heterogeneities.net/publications/Law2011WhatsWrongWithAOneWorldWorld.pdf

Long, W. (2016). *A history of 'relevance' in psychology.* Palgrave Macmillan. https://doi.org/10.1057/978-1-137-47489-6

Long, W. (2018). Decolonising higher education: Post-colonial theory and the invisible hand of student politics. *New Agenda, 69*(May), 20–25. https://hdl.handle.net/10520/EJC-e68710363

Long, W. (2021). *Nation on the couch: Inside South Africa's mind*. Melinda Ferguson Books.

Macleod, C., Bhatia, S., & Liu, W. (2020). Feminisms and decolonizing psychology: Possibilities and challenges. *Feminism & Psychology, 30*(3), 287–305. https://doi.org/10.1177/0959353520932810

Maldonado-Torres, N. (2007). On the coloniality of being. *Cultural Studies, 21*(2–3), 240–270. https://doi.org/10.1080/09502380601162548

Maldonado-Torres, N. (2011). Thinking through the decolonial turn: Post-continental interventions in theory, philosophy, and critique—An introduction. *Transmodernity: Journal of Peripheral Cultural Production of the Luso-Hispanic World, 1*(2), 1–15. https://doi.org/10.5070/T412011805

Mamdani, M. (2019). Decolonising universities. In J. Jansen (Ed.), *Decolonisation in universities: The politics of knowledge* (pp. 15–28). Wits University Press. https://doi.org/10.18772/22019083351.6

Mbembe, A. (2019). Future knowledges and their implications for the decolonisation project. In J. Jansen (Ed.), *Decolonisation in universities: The politics of knowledge* (pp. 239–254). Wits University Press. https://doi.org/10.18772/22019083351.17

Mignolo, W. D. (2010). Introduction: Coloniality of power and decolonial thinking. In W. Mignolo & A. Escobar (Eds.), *Globalization and the decolonial option* (pp. 1–21). Routledge.

Mignolo, W. D. (2007). Introduction: Coloniality of power and decolonial thinking. *Cultural Studies, 21*(2–3), 155–167. https://doi.org/10.1080/09502380601162498

Mignolo, W. D. (2011). *The darker side of Western modernity: Global futures, decolonial options*. Duke University Press.

Mignolo, W. D., & Walsh, C. E. (2018). *On decoloniality: Concepts, analytics, praxis*. Duke University Press.

Miles, T. (2021). *All that she carried: The journey of Ashley's sack, a Black family keepsake*. Random House.

Million, D. (2009). Felt theory: An Indigenous feminist approach to affect and history. *Wicazo Sa Review, 24*(2), 53–76. https://doi.org/10.1353/wic.0.0043

Naknanuk, E. K. (2021). Decolonizing history and Mother Earth's story. *Cultural Survival Quarterly, 45*(3), 12–13.

Naudé, P. (2019). Decolonising knowledge: Can Ubuntu ethics save us from coloniality? In J. Jansen (Ed.), *Decolonisation in universities: The politics of knowledge* (pp. 217–238). Wits University Press. https://doi.org/10.18772/22019083351.16

Ndlovu-Gatsheni, S. J. (2013). *Empire, global coloniality and African subjectivity*. Berghahn Books.

Oliveira-Andreotti, V. (2021). *Hospicing modernity: Facing humanity's wrongs and the implications for social activism*. North Atlantic Books.

Paranjpe, A. C. (2002). Indigenous psychology in the post-colonial context: A historical perspective. *Psychology and Developing Societies, 14*(1), 27–43. https://doi.org/10.1177/097133360201400103

Pickren, W. E. (2021). Psychologies otherwise/Earthwise: Pluriversal approaches to crises of climate, equity, and health. In I. Strasser & M. Dege (Eds.), *The psychology of global crises and crisis politics: Intervention, resistance, decolonization* (pp. 143–168). Palgrave. https://doi.org/10.1007/978-3-030-76939-0_7

Pickren, W. E., & Rutherford, A. (2010). *A history of modern psychology in context*. Wiley.

Pickren, W. E., & Tasci, G. (2022). Indigenous psychologies: Resources for future histories. In D. McCallum (Ed.), *The Palgrave handbook of the history of the human sciences* (pp. 1065–1085). Palgrave. https://doi.org/10.1007/978-981-16-7255-2_80

Quijano, A. (2000). Coloniality of power, Eurocentrism, and Latin American. *Nepantla, 1*(3), 533–580. https://muse.jhu.edu/article/23906

Richards, P. (2014). The Global South and/in the Global North: Interdisciplinary investigations. *Global Society, 8*(2), 139–154.

Rose, D. B. (2008). On history, trees, and ethical proximity. *Postcolonial Studies, 11*(2), 157–167. https://doi.org/10.1080/13688790802004687

Said, E. (1993). *Culture and imperialism.* Chatto and Windus.

Said, E. W. (1979). *Orientalism.* Vintage.

Santos, B. S. (2014). *Epistemologies of the South: Justice against epistemicide.* Routledge.

Schmidt, H. (2019). Indigenizing and decolonizing the teaching of psychology: Reflections on the role of the non-Indigenous ally. *American Journal of Community Psychology, 64*(1–2), 59–71. https://doi.org/10.1002/ajcp.12365

Schmit, D. T. (2010). The mesmerists inquire about "Oriental mind powers": West meets East in the search for the universal trance. *Journal of the History of the Behavioral Sciences, 46*(1), 1–26. https://doi.org/10.1002/jhbs.20393

Seedat, M., & Suffla, S. (2017). Community psychology and its (dis) contents, archival legacies and decolonisation. *South African Journal of Psychology. Suid-Afrikaanse Tydskrif vir Sielkunde, 47*(4), 421–431. https://doi.org/10.1177/0081246317741423

Smith, L. T. (1999). *Decolonizing methodologies: research and Indigenous peoples.* Zed Books.

Smith, L. T. (2012). *Decolonizing methodologies: research and Indigenous peoples* (2nd ed.). Zed Books.

Solórzano, D. G., & Yosso, T. J. (2002). Critical Race methodology: Counter-storytelling as an analytical framework for education research. *Qualitative Inquiry, 8*(1), 23–44. https://doi.org/10.1177/107780040200800103

Spivak, G. C. (1988). "Can the subaltern speak?" In N. Cary & L. Grossberg (Eds.), *Marxism and the interpretation of culture* (pp. 271–313). University of Illinois Press.

Taylor, E. (1999). *Shadow culture: Psychology and spirituality in America.* Counterpoint.

Teo, T. (2011). Reconstructing the critique of ideology: A critical-hermeneutic and psychological outline. *Annual Review of Critical Psychology, 9*(1), 20–27.

Tharoor, S. (2017). *Inglorious empire: What the British did to India.* C. Hurst and Co.

Thomson, M. (2006). *Psychological subjects: Identity, culture, and health in twentieth-century Britain.* Oxford. https://doi.org/10.1093/acprof:oso/9780199287802.001.0001

Trouillot, M.-R. (1995). *Silencing the past: Power and the production of history.* Beacon Press.

Tuck, E. (2009). Suspending damage: A letter to communities. *Harvard Educational Review, 79*(3), 409–428. https://doi.org/10.17763/haer.79.3.n0016675661t3n15

Tuck, E., & Yang, W. (2018). Born under the rising sign of social justice. In E. Tuck & K. W. Yang (Eds.), *Toward what justice: Describing diverse dreams of justice in education* (pp. 1–17). Routledge. https://doi.org/10.4324/9781351240932-1

UCT Scientist. (2016, October 13). *Science must fall?* [Video]. YouTube. https://www.youtube.com/watch?v=C9SiRNibD14

Vidal, F., & Ortega, F. (2017). *Being brains: Making the cerebral subject.* Fordham University Press.

Watkins, M. (2019). *Mutual accompaniment and the creation of the commons.* Yale University Press.

PART **II** SCIENCE, METHODS, AND EPISTEMIC JUSTICE

4

DECOLONIZING AND BUILDING LIBERATORY PSYCHOLOGICAL SCIENCES

HELEN A. NEVILLE, B. ANDI LEE, AND AMIR H. MAGHSOODI

Decolonial psychology is a commitment to the political transformation of the discipline and its institutional place, challenging not only what counts as "psychology" (its epistemic foundations) but also, how it is practised, where it is located, and who has access to it.

—Kessi & Boonzaier, 2018, p. 304

Eurocentric psychology has a history of maintaining racial and other forms of oppression. For example, the discipline of psychology explicitly supported White supremacist projects through theories, research, and practices, including eugenics in the United States and Europe (Guthrie, 2004), apartheid in South Africa (Duncan et al., 2001), and deficit models undermining Indigenous people's sovereignty in Australia (Duckett, 2021). Mainstream academic psychology shows no signs of reversing course, through its entrenchment in investigating purported racial differences, lack of critical exploration

---

Correspondence concerning this chapter should be addressed to: Helen A. Neville, Department of Educational Psychology, 1310 S. Sixth Street, Champaign, IL 61820, or hneville@illinois.edu.

https://doi.org/10.1037/0000376-005
Decolonial Psychology: Toward Anticolonial Theories, Research, Training, and Practice,
L. Comas-Díaz, H. Y. Adames, and N. Y. Chavez-Dueñas (Editors)

of scientific racism, and "a persistent naïve empiricism that demands openness to any empirical question, no matter how conceptually unfounded or discredited" (Winston, 2020, p. 438). Standing on the shoulders of Global Majority scholars over the past century who have challenged the racist underpinnings of psychology, we agree with the assertion of South African researchers Kessi and Boonzaier (2018) in the epigraph that a decolonizing project is warranted; such a project would entail a complete transformation of the discipline. By Global Majority we mean people from the Global South and Black, Indigenous, and People of Color in the Global North.

In this chapter, we propose a framework for decolonizing psychological sciences (DPS) as one step toward transforming the disciplines. The purpose of the DPS framework is to guide psychologists and the profession in decolonizing knowledge production; the framework outlines key processes needed to center Global Majority ways of knowing. We use the plural form of sciences to acknowledge the multiple psychologies practiced around the world; this helps decenter the normativity of Eurocentric psychology (Ratele et al., 2018). The framework focuses on research and incorporates training and practices with respect to creating and disseminating new knowledge. Much like Kessi and Boonzaier (2018), we are most interested in interrogating what counts as data, knowledge formation, and the practice of sciences. To contextualize DPS, we first define complementary literatures in decolonizing psychological sciences and psychologies for liberation. After introducing the key tenets of the DPS framework, we outline current exemplar practices.

DECOLONIZING PSYCHOLOGICAL SCIENCES

> Decolonization means fighting, undoing, and overcoming received colonial ways that have shaped economic, political, and social structures; knowledge practices (which includes psychology and other natural, health and human sciences); interpersonal relationships; and the self. (Ratele et al., 2018, p. 340)

Decolonial psychology consists of intentional efforts to challenge a hegemonic psychology that maintains racist and oppressive myths about the superiority of people of European descent and the inferiority of the Global Majority through the "coloniality of power, being, knowing, and feeling" (Ciofalo et al., 2022, p. 2). As observed by South African scholar Ratele et al. (2018), decolonizing psychology is thus the undoing of coloniality in psychology. Among the legacies of colonialism (e.g., dispossession of land, sovereignty, labor, and resources by another nation) are the persistent erasure of knowledge produced by people who have experienced imperialism and the implementation of deficit or pathologizing research paradigms (i.e., the Global Majority). Eurocentric psychology has legitimized a dominant narrative of humanity reflected in their own image. This includes pushing for universal theories and research in myriad areas such as personality traits, performance evaluations, intelligence testing, psychopathology, and self-actualization (Bhatia & Priya, 2021). Scholars have named the intentional or inadvertent harm caused by coloniality, or more specifically, the theories, research, and corresponding applications on the Global Majority, as epistemic violence (Adams et al., 2015).

We conceptualize decolonizing psychological sciences as practices that (a) uncover and dismantle the epistemic violence against the Global Majority and (b) center the lived experiences and epistemological positions of those most affected by oppression. By center, we mean highlighting the subjectivities and humanity of the Global Majority from their perspective. Numerous scholars have written about and engaged in DPS (Fine, 2018). We highlight three of them to outline the interplay between ontology (what is real), epistemology (what knowledge is) and methodologies (what the procedures to collect and analyze information are). Somaliland scholar Bulhan (2015) provided an analysis of coloniality in his critical article that appeared in the special issue on decolonizing psychological science in the *Journal of Social and Political Psychology*. Bulhan raised ontological concerns within Eurocentric psychology, with its focus on individuals as central to "legitimate" areas of study. Bulhan called for psychology to answer new questions, instead of "promoting individual happiness" the field should "cultivat[e] collective well-being" (p. 239). Decolonizing psychology thus includes shifts from "a concern with instinct to promotion of human needs, from prescriptions for adjustment to affordances for empowerment, from treatment of passive victims to creation of self-determining actors, and from globalizing, top-down approaches to context-sensitive, bottom-up approaches" (p. 239).

Māori scholar Smith (2012/2018) analyzed the role of power in designing and conducting research in her groundbreaking text *Decolonizing Methodologies*. She detailed the ways in which social science delegitimizes Indigenous ways of knowing (epistemology) and erases the voices of people who are being researched. She also described Kaupapa Māori research projects that include Māori researchers, embrace an Indigenous research agenda, and implement associated methodologies: "When Indigenous peoples become the researchers and not merely the researched, the activity of research is transformed. Questions are framed differently, priorities are ranked differently, problems are defined differently, and people participate on different terms" (Smith, 2012/2018, p. 196).

Aaniiih-Gros Ventre scholar Gone (2021) provided a life narrative of Bull Lodge's healing career as a decolonizing method to reclaim American Indian therapeutic traditions in counseling psychology. From his perspective, Indigenous approaches to knowledge that incorporate resistance help to "recover communal meaning systems, and motivate collective action in communities that continue to grapple with coloniality" (p. 267). By centering the epistemological positions of Indigenous peoples, Bulhan (2015), Smith (2012/2018), and Gone demonstrated the importance of context-based, local knowledges in decolonizing (psychological) sciences.

PSYCHOLOGIES FOR LIBERATION

> We must work and fight with the same rhythm as the people [the masses] to construct the future and to prepare the ground where vigorous shoots are already springing up. . . . The problem is to get to know the place that these men [sic] mean to give their people, the kind of social relations that they decide to set up, and the conception that they have of the future of humanity [after colonialization]. (Fanon, 1967, p. 44)

DPS is aligned with psychologies whose aims are consistent with promoting political, economic, and psychological self-determination, including liberation of people in the afterlives of colonialization or slavery. These psychologies grew out of struggle—struggle for independence, sovereignty, and freedom—and include Black psychology in the United States (Williams, 1974), postrevolution Cuban Psychology (Lacerda, 2015), contemporary African psychologies (Ratele et al., 2018), Indigenous psychologies (Ciofalo, 2019), and Filipino psychology (Yacat, 2013), to name a few. These psychologies not only are defined by struggle, but also incorporate undoing coloniality while embracing Indigenous ways of knowing. Many of these psychologies benefit from the writings of revolutionary psychiatrist Frantz Fanon. As one of the first to describe the role of colonization on the psyche of both the colonized and the colonizer, Fanon (1952/2008, 1967) documented the psychological trauma of racism and colonialism, theorized about internalized oppression, and described internal and political struggles for liberation. We began this section with a quote from Fanon's *Wretched of the Earth* to show the potential of psychologies for liberation to extend individual level processes to incorporate the understanding and cultivation of a shared, more humanistic vision of society.

Ignacio Martín-Baró is credited with defining and popularizing liberation psychology. Writing during the Salvadoran civil war in the 1980s, Martín-Baró (1994) urged psychologists to recognize the "main problems burdening" peoples; he called for psychology to delineate how the field could contribute to the resolutions of these problems (p. 45). Martín-Baró was clear about the scope of psychology in addressing injustices; it is unrealistic to expect psychology, he reasoned, to resolve societal issues such as economic or armed conflict. Instead, psychology can help "intervene in the subjective processes that sustain those structures of injustices and make them viable" (p. 45). Martín-Baró proposed several enduring tenets of liberation psychology to assist in individual and collective liberation, such as recovering historical memory, or reclaiming past identity, beliefs, and practices to aid survival in the present and conceptualization of possible futures; de-ideologizing everyday experiences, or becoming conscious of and dismantling the collective lie blaming people for their own oppression; and utilizing people's virtues, or accessing people's commitment to the collective good and a sense of hope in a better, more humane future (see Comas-Díaz & Torres Rivera, 2020, for a longer discussion).

In sum, we argue that there is no one liberation psychology but instead multiple psychologies whose goals are consistent with mental liberation from dominant tropes that reinforce a false sense of inferiority among people who are most oppressed in society. These psychologies investigate and identify practices that can promote individual and collective awareness of the root causes of oppression. Psychologies of liberation are concerned both with the manifestations and consequences of structural inequalities and strategies individuals and collectives use to promote well-being by reclaiming their power and taking action to challenge inequalities. Thus DPS requires a shift in not only how researchers engage in knowledge production, but also the questions they ask, who participates in collecting and analyzing the data, and the outcomes of the sciences.

FOUNDATIONS OF THE DECOLONIZING PSYCHOLOGICAL SCIENCES FRAMEWORK

We first defined the core tenets of DPS and liberation psychologies to provide the foundation for the proposed DPS framework. By understanding the ontological, epistemological, and methodological approaches to knowledge production among those most affected by colonialization and slavery, we have a better sense for the scope of psychological sciences that counter training in traditional psychology departments around the globe. With the overview of liberation psychologies, we introduced the scope of potential topics and aims of DPS. Grounded in these traditions, we present the DPS framework, which builds on our previous scholarship on a Public Psychology for Liberation Training Model (PPLTM; Neville et al., 2021) and healing research methodologies (Lee et al., 2021). In this section we outline each of these approaches. We operate from the core assumptions that it is impossible to decolonize psychological sciences methods without transforming the entire ways in which Western-centered psychologies are practiced. The purpose of the DPS framework focuses on methods to honor, disrupt, and build new ways of knowing for the purposes of mental, physical, spiritual, and economic liberation. We first describe the general PPLTM and later apply principles of the model to DPS knowledge generation, more specifically.

Public Psychology for Liberation Training Model

In our earlier work, we conceptualized public psychology as a field of, for, and with the people, aligning with psychologies for liberation traditions (Neville et al., 2021). We argued that a public psychology for liberation centers the knowledge and wisdom of peoples from the Global Majority to inform and apply psychological knowledge that is explicitly antiracist and dismantles oppressive systems that stem from structural racism, seeking justice and equity for all. The PPLTM is visually represented as a spider web comprising five interrelated foundational domains related to psychological disciplines, and ten lifelong practices that connect these foundational domains. Briefly, these foundational domains are as follows: (a) facilitate human and community relationships (i.e., engage in relationships that prioritize cohesion and collective values), (b) promote ethical consciousness (i.e., adopt an ethics of social responsibility), (c) create empowering learning sites (i.e., infuse culturally-sustaining pedagogies in training), (d) generate reciprocal knowledge and translation (i.e., ensure knowledge sharing is bidirectional), and (e) increase structural equity (i.e., develop structural competencies and policies). The 10 lifelong practices (e.g., cultural humility and care and compassion) incorporate elements of at least two of the aforementioned foundational domains and are adapted from Carjuzaa and Fenimore-Smith's (2010) recommendations of decolonizing research with Indigenous communities, as well as a set of behaviors and conditions that support healing and equity within psychologies (see Neville et al., 2021, for further details). Later we elaborate on the aspects of the PPLTM that have been adapted in DPS4L.

Given its intended use across many subfields, the PPLTM is a developmental model in its training content and its training levels. The training content is meant to be applied in a developmentally appropriate manner for psychologists at any stage of their career (e.g., students, trainees, faculty, professionals), and can be adapted to at least three levels of competency: novice, intermediate, and expert. This developmental aspect of the model affords flexibility in which practitioners of the model may develop in each domain and/or practice at their own pace, and accounts for a continued, iterative process in the application of and learning within the training model.

Finally, in addition to the foundational domains, the underlying principles woven throughout the training model are a commitment to social justice, account for intersectionality, a sense of connection, and the responsibility for fostering radical healing. At the core of liberation is a commitment to social justice, or an equitable and fair distribution of resources to meet the needs of society (Bell, 1997). Within society, social factors and identities may differentially affect people in unique conditions of being multiply marginalized due to race, ethnicity, gender, class, sexual orientation, religious beliefs, and ability. Intersectionality (Crenshaw, 1989) is therefore exceedingly important to consider for a public psychology for liberation to best counter the interlocking oppressions that individuals and communities, particularly those in the Global Majority, may face. Third, a sense of connection, or sense of belonging, emphasizes the connection between those in the field of psychology and our surrounding communities—it reminds psychologists that we have a duty to promote mutual and reciprocal relationships with each other as a collective working for the social good. Finally, radical healing is a key goal of the PPLTM in its emphasis on wholeness and thriving (French et al., 2020). Radical healing moves beyond the role of victimhood for Global Majority members and instead centers individual and collective methods and traditions of healing in the face of oppression and harm, challenges the existing structurally racist systems, and amplifies stories of triumph and joy in the healing journey (Adames et al., 2023).

Healing Research Methodologies

Aligned with the goal of promoting radical healing, the healing research methodologies framework (Lee et al., 2021) is a model developed for Global Majority members that offers guidance on increasing research on healing as well as research that heals. This framework incorporates numerous methodologies that center liberation and social justice, such as critical race theory, decolonizing, feminist, and emancipatory methodologies (Huber, 2008;

Seedat et al., 2017; Smith, 2012/2018). Visually represented in the shape of a flower, the healing research methodologies framework honors the iterative process of healing, generosity, and regrowth that flowers undergo, modeling our understanding of Global Majority members' resistance and restoration in face of historical and present processes of harm in the face of racial and structural oppression. The flower has six petals that represent core dimensions, with three main mechanisms that nourish the healing research flower from the center: reflexivity, intersectionality, and emotion. Briefly, reflexivity is defined as a critical self-reflection on the impact of our values and beliefs on our perceptions and actions in relation to the research process. Intersectionality, to echo the PPLTM, accounts for the overlapping contexts and ways social identities may uniquely oppress and interact with racial identity for Global Majority members (Crenshaw, 1989). Third, our healing research flower allows emotion to be present throughout—we emphasize the need for delight, love, and triumph as well as rage, grief, and anguish as authentic engagements and responses to the healing process.

The healing research methodologies flower petals represent commitments that researchers who use the framework agree to. First, healing research maintains social justice ethics, upholding radical ethical consciousness that sustains equity and fairness in deciding who is centered in the research, who can participate, and who has access to the research. Second, healing research adopts liberation methodologies—explicitly critiquing and dismantling oppressive systems at the individual and structural levels (Comas-Díaz & Torres Rivera, 2020). Liberation methodologies aim to empower Global Majority researchers, emphasizing the cultural strengths and creativity that are embedded in our collective histories and hearts. Third, healing research implements methods that rely on cultural knowledge, wisdom, and spirituality (Dillard, 2008). Fourth, healing research embraces interdisciplinary approaches to promote novel and holistic methods for conducting research on healing and research that is healing. Fifth, healing research catalyzes critical action; it ensures that you want to do something in response to the conditions that necessitate healing and liberation. Stemming from Freire's (1970) *concientización*, critical action extends traditional notions of activism to collective participation in healing research. Finally, petal six charges healing research with promoting community accessibility. Inspired by disability justice activists (Berne et al., 2018) and echoing our understanding of public psychology, the goal of healing research methodologies is to not only promote sustainable practices for justice, solidarity, and collective struggle, but also make certain that it is led by those most marginalized to ensure maximum participation in and benefit from the research. Healing research methodologies thus not only aim to decolonize psychological practice but also light the way for liberation.

DPS FRAMEWORK

The DPS framework incorporates elements of PPLTM and the healing research methodologies models within a contextual framework (see Figure 4.1). Drawing on the healing research methodologies model, the center of the model is represented by a flower, each petal reflecting one of the five PPLTM foundational domains. In this sense, psychologies that contribute to the psychological sciences for liberation: facilitate human and community relationships, promote critical ethical consciousness, generate reciprocal knowledge and translation, create empowering teaching-learning sites, and increase structural equity. DPS consists of multiple systems like many contextual models. Specifically, the concentric circles surrounding the flower are an adaptation of the four levels of what Panamanian-born researcher Causadias et al. (2021)

FIGURE 4.1. DPS Framework

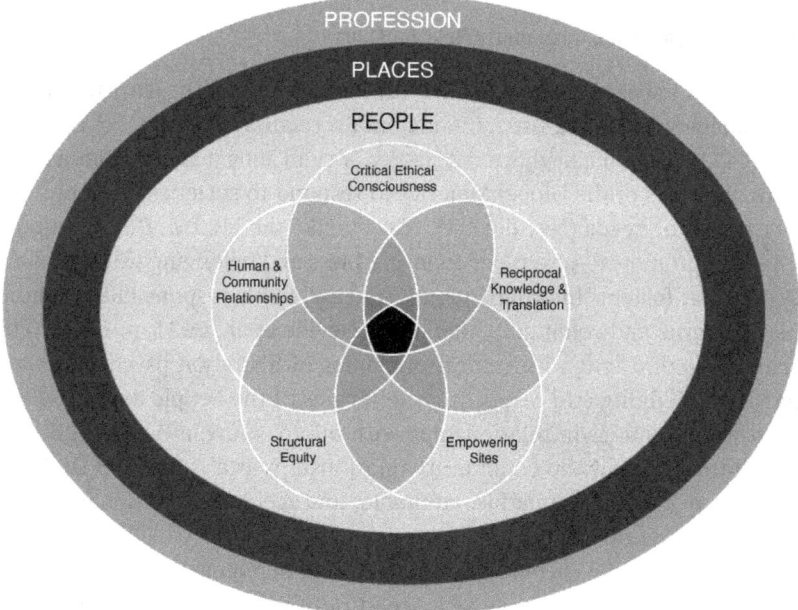

Note. Each of the five domains of the DPS framework can be enacted in each of the three proximal systems represented in the figure (i.e., people, places, profession). DPS = decolonizing psychological sciences.

identified as the cultural research system (people, places, practices, and power). We have adjusted the levels to consider both the ways in which science is produced and the aspirational goals of sciences for liberation. From our perspective, DPS must increase freedom, wellness, and equity across people (individuals within the field of psychology, members and communities affected by the science that is produced), places (settings in which we teach, engage with, and practice psychology), and the profession and practices (including policies, professional practices, systems of knowledge dissemination). DPS thus consists of implementing any combination of the five domains (i.e., flower petals) across each level of the system (i.e., people, places, profession and practices). See Table 4.1 for definitions of the five domains and example practices and recommendations across each level. We do not represent power as a separate system because issues of power are infused throughout the entire model from the foundational domains to the spheres of influence. Although the domains appear static, they are in fact interrelated and thus recommendations may apply to multiple foundational domains. To reduce redundancy, the examples and recommendations in the text compliment as opposed to restate those that are listed in Table 4.1.

Facilitate Human and Community Relationships

Rejecting a science conducted within the insular walls of the ivory tower, DPS instead invokes a humanized, fundamentally relational science. For example, the PPLTM model highlights the necessity of cultivating authentic partnerships with members of the Global Majority to respond to societies' most pressing psychological needs (Neville et al., 2021). Like the PPLTM, DPS is founded on—and promotes—a sense of connectedness and belonging (Stone Brown, 2014) that fosters "interdependence and collective responsibility" among psychologists and community members (Neville et al., 2021, p. 1254). This science is consistent with central principles of liberation psychology, such as acknowledging and respecting the virtues of the People and attending to power dynamics in relationships with others (Burton & Guzzo, 2020). Facilitating human and community relationships as a strategy of DPS thus involves prioritizing empathic, equitable, and reciprocal relationality in all aspects of scientific work.

At the individual (people) level, facilitating human and community relationships involves centering social relationships in everyday professional interactions. Conducting ethical, decolonizing research demands care and meaningful engagement with the communities in which researchers cocreate knowledge. People must be socialized into the importance of relationship

TABLE 4.1. Foundational Domains and Examples of DPS Practices and Recommendations

Foundational domains (definitions)	People	Place	Profession and practices
Facilitate human and community relationships *The obligation to develop reciprocal, affirmative relationships with people and communities that humanizes all members and reorients psychological science to the needs of those most oppressed in society*	• Engage in social justice mentoring that centers relationality (Heppner, 2017; Inman, 2018; Neville, 2015) • Employ healing and culturally responsive research practices (Lee et al., 2021) • Learn about, train in, employ, and promote antiracist, emancipatory communitarian approaches to conducting scientific work (Miller et al., 2019; Prilleltensky, 1997)	• Adopt standards of critical and learner-centered pedagogies that reject the nonreciprocal banking method typically found in classrooms (Freire, 1970) • Establish ethical, reciprocal partnerships with antiracist and social justice–oriented community organizations • Provide opportunities for students to receive regular instruction and training in developing sustaining community partnerships as scientists (e.g., Flores et al., 2014)	• Require scientific research teams to employ community-based individuals as research team members or paid consultants on research projects • Require (and provide access to) antiracist, transformational leadership training for research mentors and educators • Adopt liberatory definitions and models of psychological science (e.g., Public Psychology for Liberation; Neville et al., 2021)

(continues)

TABLE 4.1. Foundational Domains and Examples of DPS Practices and Recommendations (*Continued*)

Foundational domains (*definitions*)	People	Place	Profession and practices
Promote critical ethical consciousness *The responsibility to engage in research practices that center and amplify the voices of the people, honor the knowledge and expertise of community members, and promote wellness and equity*	• Adopt a stance of cultural humility—self-reflection and critique, cultural sensitivities and openness, and commitment to individual and collective well-being—when conducting research (Abe, 2020) • Conduct interdisciplinary research using diverse epistemological approaches (Lee et al., 2021) • Initiate discussions with and honor decisions made by community partners about research design, data collection, and dissemination (e.g., the focus of the study, methods used, "ownership" of the data, shared authorship)	• Incorporate training on how to center the context of Global Majority (GM) knowledges and avoid universal assumptions associated with Western research (e.g., honor Indigenous knowledges and ways of knowing) • Change university tenure and promotion requirements to include dissemination of findings to GM communities • Create university-funded communiversities that focus on healing and liberation research and practice free of charge for community members	• Fund and coordinate regular conferences on "Southern" research to showcase the diverse research methods and practices of scholars from the Global South (e.g., International Congress of Liberation Psychology; Burton & Guzzo, 2020) • Create national funding opportunities for community-based, participatory, or transformative research on topics related to GM healing and liberation (Lee et al., 2021) • Transform professional ethics codes and IRB protocols to create flexibility and adherence to cultural practices in all phases of the research process (Higgins & Kim, 2019; Pope et al., 2021)

Generate reciprocal knowledge and translation

The duty to adopt a bottom-up, collaborative approach to knowledge creation and to disseminate findings in culturally grounded and accessible ways

- Listen to GM communities about their experiences and research priorities (what do they want to study?; Ratele et al., 2018)
- Encourage full participation of all research team members and reinforce mutual learning (Neville et al., 2021)
- Model respect for community expertise and critical reflection of personal and field knowledge gaps (Neville et al., 2021)

- Offer methods courses in decolonial and liberation psychologies to center GM understandings of data and research (e.g., story science; Indigenous methodologies; decolonial big data science; Duran & Firehammer, 2015; Montiel & Uyheng, 2021; Smith, 2012/2018)
- Create training opportunities in media psychology, with an emphasis on accessibility and cultural relevance in disseminating findings (Lee et al., 2021)
- Pay GM community consultants to critique and offer suggestions on curriculum (e.g., topics covered, teaching methods, readings)

- Implement journal policies to acknowledge community members' contributions to scholarship or encourage community members as coauthors
- Collaborate with GM communities or institutions to write data-driven policies based on local knowledges
- Provide free access to journal articles and ebooks to peoples in the Global Souths; eliminate paywalls restricting access to knowledge

Create empowering teaching-learning sites

The need to adopt engaged pedagogies in which teachers and learners operate from a stance of love, practice healing work, and decolonize curriculum and how research theory and methods are taught

- Foster liberation learning spaces in which healing work is prioritized as a topic of investigation and an outcome of learning (e.g., Lee et al., 2021)
- Encourage storytelling as a method of community building and learning (Masinga et al., 2016)
- Affirm and encourage exploration of GM learners' ideas about liberation, antiracism, and healing

- Center writings by GM people in courses, especially research methods courses
- Offer GM community-based learning internships (Trager, 2020)
- Conduct transformative evaluation of training site (e.g., department, clinic; Dhaliwal et al., 2020)

- Implement collaborative, community-centered organizational decision-making practices and abandon hierarchical models (e.g., Robert's Rules of Order)
- Establish decolonizing and liberation teaching, research, and praxis journal
- Create national collaborative initiatives between professional psychology associations and community-based organizations

(continues)

TABLE 4.1. Foundational Domains and Examples of DPS Practices and Recommendations (Continued)

Foundational domains (definitions)	People	Place	Profession and practices
Increase structural equity *The necessity to transform research methods to include a focus on the collective, and center the collective's needs, well-being, and access to self-determination to make society more equitable*	• Work with community insiders as coinvestigators to produce culturally grounded knowledge • Normalize transformative research methods in which findings lead to positive social change (e.g., Crockett et al., 2013) • Engage in everyday resistance (e.g., cross-racial solidarity, antiracist efforts; Malherbe et al., 2021)	• Transform the classroom: diversify the syllabus, engage in critical reflection on extant power dynamics, magnify GM voices • Transform academic units: Increase GM faculty and student representation, uphold fair labor practices • Transform the therapy room: practice solidarity (accompaniment) in healing, allowing client to be the expert (e.g., Fernández, 2020)	• Explicitly name White normativity and the epistemic exclusion of GM knowledge (e.g., textbook creation, grant funding, journal submission requirements, job postings; Settles et al., 2020) • Critique and transform exploitive publication practices (e.g., M. Dutta et al., 2021) • Eliminate psychiatric diagnoses and their ties and to access to insurance, health care, and jobs

Note. DPS = Decolonizing Psychological Sciences framework; IRB = institutional review board; GM = Global Majority.

building and development. One socialization tool is social justice mentoring (Heppner, 2017; Inman, 2018; Neville, 2015), an aspirational approach to mentorship that involves "finding ways to provide [mentees] opportunities to develop efficacy in working individually and collectively toward social justice goals" (Neville, 2015, p. 163). This approach is highly generative in facilitating relationships. It not only involves promoting the creation of mentorship networks for mentees, but also requires mentors to engage in social justice action as community members (Neville, 2015). An additional way to engage this strategy at the individual level is to employ healing and culturally responsive research practices (Lee et al., 2021). These practices center the perspectives and strengths of those who are most oppressed, and they seek to transform systems to dismantle oppression. They depend on effective partnerships with key stakeholders in the community. Finally, psychological scientists must learn about, receive training in, employ, and promote antiracist, emancipatory communitarian approaches to conducting scientific work (Miller et al., 2019; Prilleltensky, 1997). Through these actions, individual psychological scientists participate in the relational strategy of a decolonizing science.

At the place level, administrators can establish systems and procedures that promote human and community relationships in psychological science. For example, departments can adopt standards of critical pedagogy (Freire, 1970), which is relational and reciprocal in nature, and they can provide training, teaching evaluations, and incentives to educators for employing such practices. Additionally, institutions can establish ethical, reciprocal partnerships with antiracist and social justice–oriented community organizations. These partnerships must be structured to ensure accountability of the university; they also provide opportunities for community-engaged research and other involvement. Relatedly, institutions should also provide opportunities for students to receive regular instruction and training in developing sustaining community partnerships as scientists. In the context of sustained university–community partnerships, this can take the form of service-learning experiences (Flores et al., 2014).

Examples of this strategy at the profession and practices level involve issues of policy, licensing and accreditation guidelines, and profession-wide definitions. Regarding policy, institutional review boards (IRBs) and psychological ethical principles can require scientific research teams to employ community-based individuals as research team members and/or paid consultants on research projects. Second, accreditation and licensing boards can require (and provide access to) antiracist, transformational leadership training for research mentors and educators. Such trainings would also promote individual engagement in the decolonizing relational strategies at other levels (e.g., social justice mentoring). Finally, national organizations in the United States, such as the American Psychological Association and the Association for Psychological Science, among others, can adopt liberatory definitions and models of psychological science (e.g., the PPLTM model).

Promote Critical Ethical Consciousness

At the core of DPS is critical ethical consciousness. Moving beyond the value of nonmaleficence, scholars must conduct research that humanizes the people and communities at the center of the work (Pope et al., 2021). Researchers develop ethical consciousness by interrogating the theoretical underpinnings of the work, the questions asked, methods used, data analysis employed, interpretation of the findings, and dissemination of the results. At every stage, researchers within and outside the academy work collaboratively to generate knowledge that enhances the well-being of individuals and communities from a strength-based framework that builds on community-based knowledge and expertise. Critical ethical research thus consciously promotes epistemic justice, which counters epistemic violence by shifting the focus on the knowers and producers of knowledge from those in power to those who have been most marginalized in society (U. Dutta et al., 2021).

We use the example of story science to illustrate the implementation of critical ethical consciousness across multiple levels. According to Native American scholars Duran and Firehammer (2015), *story science* is an "approach to understanding issues in communities and within individuals and a way of achieving insight through narrative" (p. 91). Story science embodies an ethical consciousness because oral tradition is integral to imparting knowledge among Indigenous peoples in North America; people are humanized through the stories they share; and this methodology demands that the story scientist walk with participants in narrating and analyzing the story. Conducted properly, story science inquiries represent epistemic justice by placing the power of data generation in the hands of the storyteller; narrators take the lead on the content and form of the narrative. The telling of counter stories that uplift Indigenous resistance and survivance can recenter those who have been dehumanized through colonial research (U. Dutta et al., 2021). Additionally, these data have the possibility of transforming "beliefs of participants, researchers, and audiences of practitioners" including awareness of the root causes of the identified need or concern (Duran & Firehammer, p. 93).

Individual researchers (people) such as Gone (2021) in his life narrative with Bull Lodge described earlier in the chapter and Native American scholar Jillian Fish's OrigiNatives digital storytelling project reflect the core dimensions of story science. For example, OrigiNatives emerged from a researcher–community partnership to challenge coloniality through cultivating stories by everyday Indigenous people (Fish & Counts, 2021). These visual narratives provide healing opportunities for narrators as they develop and produce personal stories about their histories or culture. Further, narrators are consulted in the meaning-making and knowledge emerging from the stories.

Just as with any research methodology, story science cannot be picked up by reading an article. The multiple methods to this approach must be learned and practiced within the context of its application. A course could be offered on campus and in the community (places). An interdisciplinary lens including knowledge from inside and outside the academy would enable students to learn about the history of oral narratives within a specific cultural context, possible structures of storytelling, the nuance of storytelling as an interaction between participant and researcher, the meaning of silences and other nonverbal communication, and story interpretations and meaning-making. Changes within university IRB and professional ethics boards (profession and practices) are required to incorporate practices that are flexible and adhere to the cultural values of the communities participating in new knowledge, especially through a story science methodology. These practices should ensure that everyone involved in the research process is humanized and that the data collected will be used to promote wellness. It seems important to invite paid community experts to provide input on the policies. This honors the knowledge within communities and may help uncover the perpetuation of epistemic violence before research has been conducted and identify ways to ensure that knowledge creators are recognized for their contributions.

Generate Reciprocal Knowledge and Translation

Consistent with story science methodology, generating reciprocal knowledge mandates that researchers understand their knowledge gaps and acknowledge the expertise of community members. Building a bottom-up science centers the people and the communities to which they belong. This includes identifying critical questions to investigate, possible interpretations of the issue at hand, the types of data that may be helpful to gather, and designing ethical, nonexploitive research. Researchers learn with and from communities and not just about communities. Throughout the research process, the people and communities gain access to available resources and information that unearths and amplifies community strengths, exposes structural factors shaping lived experiences, and stimulates action. Action is multilayered and can imply action within individuals (e.g., behaving differently based on one's increased awareness of internalized oppression), groups (e.g., deciding to implement interventions to address a need), or communities and society (e.g., creating new policy to promote increased freedom and equity based on the findings).

In the words of the National Association of Black Studies, research of, by, and with the people should embrace academic excellence and social responsibility. This includes translating knowledge to accessible formats. DPS includes sharing findings with not only academic audiences but also the people and communities that can use insights from the studies to improve their individual and collective well-being.

We marvel at the ingenious ways collaboratives (people) share findings through art, postcards, infographics, community forums, novellas, etc. For example, South African immigrant Sonn and his colleagues (2017) developed a strong collaboration with a community-based organization in the Narrogin area of Australia. In their investigation of collective hope after community loss, the scholars along with representatives from the Noongar community (i.e., staff and community researchers), created a soundscape of the stories they collected about the identified concern, a film to accompany the audio, and a set of playing cards with common themes or quotations from the stories as a culturally identified way to share results. These arts-based research components were part of a larger community storytelling effort. The findings were launched at a fireside community gathering in which a traditional meal was prepared by community members.

Funds are needed to support bottom-up approaches to generating and translating reciprocal knowledge from a decolonizing and liberatory frame. Thus, local and national funding agencies (places) should offer grants to cover the costs of data collection and dissemination, including paying community researchers to help with data collection and community members to produce arts-based representations of the findings, sponsoring community gatherings to discuss results, assisting in the development of policy briefs to share with community leaders. Additionally, knowledge is public and should not be hidden behind paywalls, especially for members of the Global South. At the very least, journals should make available community-based research with implications for wellness and liberation of members of the Global Majority should be available to readers at no cost (profession and practices; M. Dutta et al., 2021); journals and not authors should absorb the costs associated with ensuring the articles are open access.

Create Empowering Teaching–Learning Sites

DPS requires liberatory teaching practices; it is impossible to teach, and learn, and create culturally embedded knowledge within a traditional Eurocentric classroom and research lab. Empowering teaching-learning sites center subjugated knowledges, or knowledges created by Global Majority members about the conditions of their lived experiences, that have been omitted or distorted in texts and learning sites. Thus an aspect of creating empowering sites involves decolonizing the curriculum. This includes assigning texts by members of the Global Majority and also critical works uncovering the legacy of colonialism and exploitation in the topic of study (Diab et al., 2020; Zembylas, 2018).

The goals of decolonizing, liberatory teaching include more than increasing cognitive comprehension; they also incorporate self-actualization and critical action. The African American feminist theorist and educator bell hooks described empowering teaching as embracing an engaged pedagogy in which educators adopt a holistic approach to teaching and learning. In part, this means that "teachers must be actively committed to a process of self-actualization that promotes their own well-being if they are to teach in a manner that empowers students" (hooks, 2014, p. 15). For teachers to be effective, they must be committed to exploring the influences of their life experiences and socialization on them as people and consequently as professionals. This is in line with the popular phrase, "hurt people, hurt people." A commitment to one's healing and honoring their own humanity, in turn, provides space for teachers to view themselves as learners along the journey and to see students as complete beings (mind, body, spirit). Additionally, engaged pedagogy can help foster liberatory scholarship by both critiquing existing "legitimized" paradigms and developing theories that can be tested and applied in freedom movements. According to hooks (2014), "while we work to resolve those issues that are most pressing in daily life . . ., we engage in a critical process of theorizing that enables and empowers" (p. 70).

Empowering sites are ones in which everyone within the space is viewed as teachers and learners, albeit with differing roles. At the individual (people) level, teachers and learners can engage in deep healing work. This includes honest and ongoing reflection of their (a) positionality within existing hierarchies—how were they socialized, what areas of oppression and privilege might they occupy, and how have these influenced their lived experiences and interactions with others—and (b) personal histories of trauma and resilience. Individuals thus operate from a position of love and deep respect for the humanity of others. This means that empowering sites allow for the expression and processing of a range of emotions that include gratitude, hope, fear, and anger (Lee et al., 2021). It also entails the incorporation of empathy from a decolonizing stance, in which people understand the structures that create suffering and one's role in contributing to the suffering of others (Zembylas, 2018).

Palestinian psychologist Diab and colleagues' (2020) applied research in Gaza offers insights to creating empowering sites in decolonizing clinical research (places, profession, and practices; 2020). Their work highlights the concerns with providing empirically supported psychological interventions to a community with few trained mental health professionals; the main contradiction is how to both acknowledge and speak against therapies grounded in knowledge from the Global North (e.g., traditional research on cognitive behavioral therapy that does not consider the role of community experiences or cultural values). One task is to create spaces that honor the voices of those who have been most affected by oppression while encouraging a dialogue with trained professionals. Empowering pedagogy thus requires "constant coordination between trainers and trainees engaged in a dialogical process of exchange and coordination of meanings between the unique clinical experience of the local practitioners and the systematized knowledge of trainers coming from abroad" (p. 7).

Diab et al. (2020) critiqued the concepts of efficacy and effectiveness of psychological interventions and the challenges to ensure that the culture and needs of the people are met:

> We argue that empirically-informed interventions must withstand tests of efficacy and effectiveness in the context of Gaza's culture. Evidence-based interventions that are imported without questioning their relevance could pose a pedagogical challenge as it might be difficult to test their applicability due to limited time, money and resources. Another challenge of this application could be the lack of coordination between local parties and governmental institutions, where priority might be given to certain psychosocial interventions due to shortage of resources, without prioritizing or even testing the real need of the population. (pp. 11–12)

Diab and his colleagues' (2020) work expands the learning context to include training and professional settings. Their case examples illustrate the interconnections among decolonizing teaching, curriculum, clinical practices, and sciences. Building on these insights, we have additional thoughts about the role of psychologists from the Global North in helping cocreate empowering learning sites when partnering with colleagues from the Global South. This requires deep reflection on one's intentions and self-actualization, awareness of one's positionality and the privileges that they may bring to the collaboration, understanding the limitations of their training, and an openness to learn new ways of being and doing and external validity.

Increase Structural Equity

Toni Morrison charged us with a responsibility to redistribute our power: "I tell my students, 'When you get these jobs that you have been so brilliantly trained for, just remember that your real job is that if you are free, you need to free somebody else. If you have some power, then your job is to empower somebody else" (Houston, 2003, para 12). What Morrison highlighted is that, at its heart, structural equity is a concern of power, and subverting the "the logic of assimilation, the default to whiteness" (Omi & Winant, 2014, p. 46) by intentionally moving to "under-stand," or comprehend from below (Bulhan, 2015, p. 240).

Structural equity ultimately aims to address the disparities in health, wealth, housing, employment, and education (Laster Pirtle, 2020). Within DPS, the methodology used in research should work toward increasing structural equity, with the goal of transforming psychology's focus from the individual to the collective, centering the collective's needs, well-being, and access to self-determination. To increase structural equity, we must first examine the barriers prohibiting it. Bulhan (2015) identified three central barriers in the forms of colonial violence that became normalized and global—the world of things (land, gold, commodities), the world of people (labor, exploitation), and the world of meaning (religions, knowledge, culture). Psychology is best suited to address this last barrier, the world of meaning.

Increasing structural equity for the people means centering and recovering the histories and knowledge of the Global Majority. Foucault and Ewald (2003) referred to subjugated knowledges as knowledges that have been disqualified as conceptually valid or scientifically grounded; Colombian sociologist Fals-Borda (2013) urged us to recover repressed historical memory, as well as understanding reality from the view of those most oppressed. Within a DPS framework, psychologists adopt a strategy of decolonization by Indigenization, in which researchers work with community insiders to produce culturally grounded knowledge that reflects local realities to address local community needs (Adams et al., 2015) and engaging in interdisciplinary collaborations (Lee et al., 2021). On the level of interpersonal interactions and relationships, engaging in everyday resistance is key to increasing structural equity. Everyday resistance includes daily commonplace actions that intentionally undermine oppressive structures, including challenging racial microaggressions when we witness them, refusing to be interrupted in voicing our truths, and recognizing our right to expect cross-racial solidarity in the face of racism (Malherbe et al., 2021).

Increasing structural equity means decolonizing practices in the environments we inhabit, which can span a number of settings, including the classroom, the therapy room, and the academy more broadly (places). For example, in light of the 2020 racial uprisings, calls to decolonize the syllabus—rethinking student learning outcomes, textbooks, readings, and supplementary materials to be explicitly antiracist—have multiplied. However, in practice, from the student coauthors, experiences this has looked like mostly White faculty hastily adding citations from BIPOC (Black, Indigenous, and People of Color) scholars with little to no consideration for the relevance of the content, whether the research has been more recently updated, or, perhaps more egregiously, including BIPOC scholar papers only as "optional readings" in contrast to required "core readings" by White scholars. Structural equity in the classroom deliberately challenges epistemic violence perpetrated within Western-centered psychology curricula.

To truly promote structural equity, faculty and psychology scholars need to go beyond diversifying their syllabi and to critically reflect and step back from citational power dynamics, highlight Indigenous knowledge, and magnify Global Majority voices and lessen the power and presence of White voices in the classroom, in meetings, and in the grounding for research. In the United States, this may be accompanied by hiring and increasing faculty of color; according to the latest data available, BIPOC professionals make up only 16% of the psychology workforce, despite the U.S. population being 40% BIPOC (American Psychological Association, 2020). In addition, the academy must introduce, implement, and uphold fair labor practices for Global Majority students, faculty, and staff.

At the broadest level, increasing structural equity for the profession demands a radical transformation of the field (profession and practices). This includes explicitly naming White and Global North normativity and its erasure of Global Majority knowledges and the methods generating such knowledge. Though uncomfortable, psychology needs to reckon with its historical partic- ipation in scientific racism and tradition of privileging White perspectives over those of the Global Majority (Winston, 2020). Although psychologies in multiple countries have begun to address these long-standing issues (e.g., the American Psychological Association's apology to People of Color; Australian Psychological Society's apology to Aboriginal and Torres Strait Islander people), much remains to be done to assume accountability and accept- able resolution in the eyes of Global Majority psychologists, research partici- pants, and communities that would truly increase structural equity (Auguste et al., 2021; Carey et al., 2017; Newnes, 2021).

One form of action may include the field's need to engage critically in self-reflection and critique existing systems of knowledge dissemination practices. Bulhan (2015) problematized the access to psychological publi- cations, such that "any work that one manages to publish will be in media inaccessible to the people the story is about," which again enacts violence on the world of meaning (p. 245). Increasing structural equity for the profes- sion means ensuring all involved in research have access to the information along the way and the benefits that come from their contributions. Another potential action includes explicitly addressing the role of stress and racism as not only burdens on Global Majority members, but also in how psychology understands psychopathology more broadly. Are we diagnosing Global Majority members as "mentally ill" in the face of normal and valid reactions to racism? The field of psychology should consider revisiting the notions of wellness and "functioning" that predicate psychological diagnoses that can affect structural access to housing, employment, and a healthy life.

DPS FRAMEWORK IN ACTION

To illustrate the DPS framework, we use case examples from two interrelated community-based gun violence initiatives. It is important to first contextualize the topic and identify it as a decolonizing project. The effects of colonialization and slavery persist in the United States and are reflected in racial capitalism, or the dehumanization of BIPOC within racist and capitalist systems that result in health, wealth, and other social inequities (Laster Pirtle, 2020). We argue that the disproportionate impact of community gun violence on African American communities is also a result of racial capitalism. The combination of anti-Black racism and the core sources of gun violence (e.g., income inequality, poverty, underfunded public housing, underperforming schools; Educational Fund to Stop Gun Violence, n.d.) fuel alienation and anger; the availability of guns in poor and working-class African American communities further provide means in which to act out the frustrations and marginalization.

For several years, I (Helen Neville) have worked with campus and community researchers to understand community gun violence—its causes, desired interventions, and solutions. The community-based research collaborative C-HeARTS (Community Healing and Resistance Through Storytelling) was initiated by University of Illinois at Urbana-Champaign faculty Shardé Smith and consists of an interdisciplinary team of five Black women academics, three Black community researchers, and Black students. The 3-year youth participatory action research project, #PowerUp was a partnership between mostly Black graduate and undergraduate students, a faculty member, and youth at an afterschool program.

These efforts prioritized building transparent and trusting relationships within the research teams and with community organizations. In C-HeARTS, community and university researchers spent time getting to know one another and creating a common vision for the work. In #PowerUp, university students volunteered first at the site to build trust with potential youth who would join the collaborative. Relationships were nurtured through regular check-ins, process time to discuss goals and working relationships, and community gatherings with food. Each project worked to center the voices of community members from identifying the scope of study, the data to collect, the stories to highlight, and the analysis and meaning-making of the findings (critical ethical consciousness). For example, both projects included focus groups with adult and youth community members to identify the most pressing concern they would like seen addressed in their community and both centered these voices in charting out next steps.

The projects also provided opportunities for all members to share their gifts with the team and contribute to the generation and translation of new knowledge. This included cofacilitating research team meetings, focus groups, and community forums (C-HeARTS). In C-HeARTS, a community researcher designed and facilitated digital storytelling workshops and he produced five community digital stories. These stories were shared at a community gala with food and opportunities to dialogue about emerging project findings. #PowerUp youth researchers presented their stories and findings at community coalition meetings and two national conferences. Data collection and dissemination were designed to promote community healing and policy changes. For example, #PowerUp researchers advocated for more investments in youth including community teen centers and job training and placements (structural equity).

Cultivating empowering teaching-learning sites was a constant negotiation. It is difficult to reflect on the ways that power and privilege manifest themselves in relationships when people share similar racial identities, but have very different lived experiences based on class, gender, and education level. In C-HeARTS, we had to come to terms with ways the group unintentionally marginalized the voices of community researchers; we periodically made adjustments to amplify the leadership from these valued team members. We engaged in many lively discussions among the #PowerUp university researchers about project direction and strategies to center youth perspectives. I initially served in a primary leadership role as a teacher and colearner; as the team developed greater efficacy, I transitioned into a supportive role.

CONCLUSION

DPS is an ongoing lifelong project to unveil and dismantle the epistemic violence against the Global Majority in the aftermaths of colonialization and slavery. Centering Indigenous and local knowledges in research that is conducted of, by, and with those most affected by oppression is the cornerstone of DPS.

Honoring the expertise in communities about the issues most pressing in their lives, researchers should serve as companions in the research journey (Segalo et al., 2015). This process could entail identifying the root causes of concerns, who benefits, and who loses by its continued presence. To foster social change, it is critical to upend the myth of expertise that researchers hold, and to respect participants' and community researchers' expertise to truly engage in research with, rather than research on communities to affect social change. Furthermore, building a relationship with participants allows us to dispel the myth of dispassionate science and encourage us to engage in value-driven, meaningful work that centers the collective and uplifting the numerous cultural strengths and knowledge that participants bring to the research process (French et al., 2020).

We presented the DPS framework to identify core domains in creating richly contextual, strength-based sciences that focus on healing and support transformative changes. DPS adopts a multisystem approach (people, places, profession and practices) and prioritizes human relationships, ethical practices that humanizes participants and communities, culturally syntonic knowledge creation, engaged healing pedagogies, and structural equity.

RESOURCES

Black in Psych. (2021, March 25). *Decolonizing research* [Video]. YouTube. https://youtu.be/Mfl7RoBTQd8

Dirks, L., & the Lumina Foundation. (2021, October 5). *University of Washington: "Decolonizing" research through collaboration and data sovereignty* [Video]. YouTube. https://youtu.be/km65FK2e5Sg

Gone, J. (2019, October 18). *When healing looks like justice* [Podcast]. YouTube. https://www.youtube.com/watch?v=KoPsOf5xI9E

Hesquiaht Language. (2017, April 3). *Indigenous research methodologies: chuutsqa's story* [Video]. YouTube. https://youtu.be/-9HuUDAYqvY

Onyango, J., & Africa Research and Impact Network. (2021, March 19). *Decolonizing methods* [Webinar]. YouTube. https://youtu.be/IhedO3AQDbE

Smith Tuhiwai, L. (2021, October 18). *Decolonizing methods and methodologies* [Webinar]. YouTube. https://youtu.be/vLqr2dsNmXo

REFERENCES

Abe, J. (2020). Beyond cultural competence, toward social transformation: Liberation psychologies and the practice of cultural humility. *Journal of Social Work Education*, *56*(4), 696–707. https://doi.org/10.1080/10437797.2019.1661911

Adames, H. Y., Chavez-Dueñas, N. Y., Lewis, J. A., Neville, H. A., French, B. H., Chen, G. A., & Mosley, D. V. (2023). Radical healing in psychotherapy: Addressing the wounds of racism-related stress and trauma. *Psychotherapy, 60*(1), 39–50. https://doi.org/10.1037/pst0000435

Adams, G., Dobles, I., Gómez, L. H., Kurtiş, T., & Molina, L. E. (2015). Decolonizing psychological science: Introduction to the special thematic section. *Journal of Social and Political Psychology, 3*(1), 213–238. https://doi.org/10.5964/jspp.v3i1.564

American Psychological Association. (2020, November 1). Psychology's workforce is becoming more diverse. *Monitor on Psychology.* https://www.apa.org/monitor/2020/11/datapoint-diverse

Auguste, E., Nobles, W., & Rowe, D. (2021, November). *Why the APA's apology for white supremacy falls short.* NBC News. https://www.nbcnews.com/think/opinion/why-apa-s-apology-promoting-white-supremacy-falls-short-ncna1284229

Bell, L. A. (1997). Theoretical foundations for social justice education. In M. Adams, L. A. Bell, & P. Griffin (Eds.), *Teaching for diversity and social justice: A sourcebook* (pp. 3–15). Routledge.

Berne, P., Morales, A. L., Langstaff, D., & Invalid, S. (2018). Ten principles of disability justice. *Women's Studies Quarterly, 46*(12), 227–229. https://doi.org/10.1353/wsq.2018.0003

Bhatia, S., & Priya, K. R. (2021). Coloniality and psychology: From silencing to re-centering marginalized voices in postcolonial times. *Review of General Psychology, 25*(4), 422–436. https://doi.org/10.1177/10892680211046507

Bulhan, H. A. (2015). Stages of colonialism in Africa: From occupation of land to occupation of being. *Journal of Social and Political Psychology, 3*(1), 239–256. https://doi.org/10.5964/jspp.v3i1.143

Burton, M., & Guzzo, R. (2020). Liberation psychology: Origins and development. In L. Comas-Díaz & E. Torrres Rivera (Eds.), *Liberation psychology: Theory, method, practice, and social justice* (pp. 17–40). American Psychological Association. https://doi.org/10.1037/0000198-002

Carey, T. A., Dudgeon, P., Hammond, S. W., Hirvonen, T., Kyrios, M., Roufeil, L., & Smith, P. (2017). The Australian psychological society's apology to Aboriginal and Torres Strait Islander people. *Australian Psychologist, 52*(4), 261–267. https://doi.org/10.1111/ap.12300

Carjuzaa, J., & Fenimore-Smith, J. K. (2010). The give away spirit: Reaching a shared vision of ethical Indigenous research relationships. *Journal of Educational Controversy, 5*(2), Article 4. https://cedar.wwu.edu/jec/vol5/iss2/4

Causadias, J. M., Korous, K. M., Cahill, K. M., & Rea-Sandin, G. (2021). The importance of research about research on culture: A call for meta-research on culture. *Cultural Diversity & Ethnic Minority Psychology.* Advance online publication.

Ciofalo, N. (Ed.). (2019). *Indigenous psychologies in an era of decolonization.* Springer. https://doi.org/10.1007/978-3-030-04822-8

Ciofalo, N., Dudgeon, P., & Nikora, L. W. (2022). Indigenous community psychologies, decolonization, and radical imagination within ecologies of knowledges. *American Journal of Community Psychology, 69*(3–4), 283–293. https://doi.org/10.1002/ajcp.12583

Comas-Díaz, L., & Torres Rivera, E. (Eds.). (2020). *Liberation psychology: Theory, method, practice, and social justice.* American Psychological Association. https://doi.org/10.1037/0000198-000

Crenshaw, K. (1989). Demarginalizing the intersection of race and sex: A Black feminist critique of antidiscrimination doctrine, feminist theory and antiracist politics. *University of Chicago Legal Forum, 1989*(1),139–167.

Crockett, D., Downey, H., Fırat, A. F., Ozanne, J. L., & Pettigrew, S. (2013). Conceptualizing a transformative research agenda. *Journal of Business Research, 66*(8), 1171–1178. https://doi.org/10.1016/j.jbusres.2012.08.009

Dhaliwal, K., Casey, J., Aceves-Iñiguez, K., & Dean-Coffey, J. (2020). Radical inquiry—Liberatory praxis for research and evaluation. *New Directions for Evaluation, 2020*(166), 49–64. https://doi.org/10.1002/ev.20415

Diab, M., Veronese, G., Jamei, Y. A., & Kagee, A. (2020). The interplay of paradigms: Decolonizing a psychology curriculum in the context of the siege of Gaza. *Nordic Psychology, 72*(3), 183–198. https://doi.org/10.1080/19012276.2019.1675087

Dillard, C. B. (2008). When the ground is black, the ground is fertile: Exploring endarkened feminist epistemology and healing methodologies in the spirit. In N. K. Densin, Y. S. Lincoln, & L. T. Smith (Eds.), *Handbook of critical and Indigenous methodologies* (pp. 277–292). SAGE Publications. https://doi.org/10.4135/9781483385686.n14

Duckett, P. (2021). Re-embedding racism in psychology: Indigenising the curriculum in Australian psychology. In C. Newnes (Ed.), *Racism in psychology: Challenging theory, practice and institutions* (pp. 43–56). Routledge.

Duncan, N. E., van Niekerk, A. E., de la Rey, C. E., & Seedat, M. E. (2001). *Race, racism, knowledge production and psychology in South Africa*. Nova Science Publishers.

Duran, E., & Firehammer, J. (2015). Story sciencing and analyzing the silent narrative between words: Counseling research from an Indigenous perspective. In R. Goodman & P. Gorski (Eds.), *Decolonizing "multicultural" counseling through social justice* (pp. 85–97). Springer. https://doi.org/10.1007/978-1-4939-1283-4_7

Dutta, M., Ramasubramanian, S., Barrett, M., Elers, C., Sarwatay, D., Raghunath, P., Kaur, S., Dutta, D., Jayan, P., Rahman, M., Tallam, E., Roy, S., Falnikar, A., Johnson, G. M., Mandal, I., Dutta, U., Basnyat, I., Soriano, C., Pavarala, V., . . . Zapata, D. (2021). Decolonizing open science: Southern interventions. *Journal of Communication, 71*(5), 803–826.

Dutta, U., Azad, A. K., & Hussain, S. M. (2021). Counterstorytelling as epistemic justice: Decolonial community-based praxis from the global south. *American Journal of Community Psychology*. Advance online publication.

Educational Fund to Stop Gun Violence. (n.d.). *Racial equity impact assessment.* https://efsgv.org

Fals-Borda, O. (2013). La ciencia y el pueblo: Nuevas reflexiones sobre la investigación-acción (participativa) [Science and the people: New reflections on Participatory Action Research]. In N. Herrera & L. López (Eds.), *Ciencia compromiso y cambio social: Orlando Fals Borda: Antología* (pp. 301–319). Editorial Colectivo.

Fanon, F. (1967). *The wretched of the earth* (C. Farrington, Trans.). Grove.

Fanon, F. (2008). *Black skin, white masks*. Grove. (Original work published 1952)

Fernández, J. S. (2020). Liberation psychology of and for transformative justice: Centering acompañamiento in participatory action research. In L. Comas-Díaz & E. Torres Rivera (Eds.), *Liberation psychology: Theory, method, practice, and social justice* (pp. 91–110). American Psychological Association. https://doi.org/10.1037/0000198-006

Fine, M. (2018). *Just research in contentious times: Widening the methodological imagination*. Teachers College Press.

Fish, J., & Counts, P. K. (2021). Justice for Native people, justice for Native me. In K. C. McClean (Ed.), *Cultural methods in psychology: Describing and transforming cultures* (pp. 237–272). Oxford.

Flores, M. P., De La Rue, L., Neville, H. A., Santiago, S., Ben Rakemayahu, K., Garite, R., Spankey, Brawn, M., Valgoi, M., Brooks, J., Lee, E. S., & Ginsburg, R. (2014). Developing social justice competencies: A consultation training approach. *The Counseling Psychologist, 42*(7), 998–1020. https://doi.org/10.1177/0011000014548900

Foucault, M., & Ewald, F. (2003). *Society must be defended: Lectures at the Collège de France, 1975–1976* (Vol. 1). Macmillan.

Freire, P. (1970). *Pedagogy of the oppressed*. Continuum.

French, B. H., Lewis, J. A., Mosley, D., Adames, H. Y., Chavez-Dueñas, N. Y., Chen, G. A., & Neville, H. A. (2020). Toward a psychological framework of radical healing in communities of color. *The Counseling Psychologist, 48*(1), 14–46. https://doi.org/10.1177/0011000019843506

Gone, J. P. (2021). Decolonization as methodological innovation in counseling psychology: Method, power, and process in reclaiming American Indian therapeutic traditions. *Journal of Counseling Psychology, 68*(3), 259–270. https://doi.org/10.1037/cou0000500

Guthrie, R. V. (2004). *Even the rat was white: A historical view of psychology*. Pearson.

Heppner, P. P. (2017). Creating mentoring opportunities to promote cultural competencies and social justice. *The Counseling Psychologist, 45*(1), 137–157. https://doi.org/10.1177/0011000016688781

Higgins, M., & Kim, E. J. A. (2019). De/colonizing methodologies in science education: Rebraiding research theory–practice–ethics with Indigenous theories and theorists. *Cultural Studies of Science Education, 14*(1), 111–127. https://doi.org/10.1007/s11422-018-9862-4

hooks, b. (2014). *Teaching to transgress*. Routledge.

Houston, P. (2003, November). The truest eye. *O, The Oprah Magazine*. https://www.oprah.com/omagazine/toni-morrison-talks-love/all

Huber, L. P. (2008). Building critical race methodologies in educational research: A research note on critical race testimonio. *FIU Law Review, 4*(1), 159–173. https://ecollections.law.fiu.edu/lawreview/vol4/iss1/15

Inman, A. G. (2018). Social justice mentoring and scholarship: Building a community of leaders and advocates. *The Counseling Psychologist, 46*(8), 1040–1054. https://doi.org/10.1177/0011000018817908

Kessi, S., & Boonzaier, F. (2018). Centre/ing decolonial feminist psychology in Africa. *South African Journal of Psychology, 48*(3), 299–309. https://doi.org/10.1177/0081246318784507

Lacerda, F. (2015). Insurgency, theoretical decolonization and social decolonization: Lessons from Cuban psychology. *Journal of Social and Political Psychology, 3*(1), 298–323. https://doi.org/10.5964/jspp.v3i1.154

Laster Pirtle, W. N. (2020). Racial capitalism: A fundamental cause of novel coronavirus (COVID-19) pandemic inequities in the United States. *Health Education & Behavior, 47*(4), 504–508. Advance online publication. https://doi.org/10.1177/1090198120922942

Lee, B. A., Ogunfemi, N., Neville, H. A., & Tettegah, S. (2021). Resistance and restoration: Healing research methodologies for the global majority. *Cultural Diversity and Ethnic Minority Psychology, 29*(1), 6–14. https://pubmed.ncbi.nlm.nih.gov/34291985/

Malherbe, N., Ratele, K., Adams, G., Reddy, G., & Suffla, S. (2021). A decolonial Africa(n)-centered psychology of antiracism. *Review of General Psychology, 25*(4), 437–450. https://doi.org/10.1177/10892680211022992

Martín-Baró, I. (1994). *Writings for a liberation psychology* (A. Aron & S. Corne, Eds.). Harvard University Press.

Masinga, L., Myende, P., Marais, A., Singh-Pillay, A., Kortjass, M., Chirikure, T., & Mweli, P. (2016). "Hear our voices": A collective arts-based self-study of early-career academics on our learning and growth in a research-intensive university. *Educational Research for Social Change, 5*(2), 117–135. https://www.scielo.org.za/scielo.php?script=sci_arttext&pid=S2221-40702016000200009

Miller, A. L., Stern, C., & Neville, H. (2019). Forging diversity-science-informed guidelines for research on race and racism in psychological science. *Journal of Social Issues, 75*(4), 1240–1261. https://doi.org/10.1111/josi.12356

Montiel, C. J., & Uyheng, J. (2021). Foundations for a decolonial big data psychology. *Journal of Social Issues, 78*(2), 279–297. Advance online publication. https://doi.org/10.1111/josi.12439

Neville, H. A. (2015). Social justice mentoring: Supporting the development of future leaders for struggle, resistance, and transformation. *The Counseling Psychologist, 43*(1), 157–169. https://doi.org/10.1177/0011000014564252

Neville, H. A., Ruedas-Gracia, N., Lee, B. A., Ogunfemi, N., Maghsoodi, A. H., Mosley, D. V., LaFromboise, T. D., & Fine, M. (2021). The public psychology for liberation training model: A call to transform the discipline. *American Psychologist, 76*(8), 1248–1265. https://doi.org/10.1037/amp0000887

Newnes, C. (Ed.). (2021). *Racism in psychology: Challenging theory, practice and institutions.* Routledge. https://doi.org/10.4324/9781003119401

Omi, M., & Winant, H. (2014). *Racial formation in the United States.* Routledge. https://doi.org/10.4324/9780203076804

Pope, K. S., Vasquez, M. J. T., Chavez-Dueñas, N., & Adames, H. Y. (2021). *Ethics in psychotherapy and counseling: A practical guide* (6th ed.). Wiley.

Prilleltensky, I. (1997). Values, assumptions, and practices: Assessing the moral implications of psychological discourse and action. *American Psychologist, 52*(5), 517–535. https://doi.org/10.1037/0003-066X.52.5.517

Ratele, K., Cornell, J., Dlamini, S., Helman, R., Malherbe, N., & Titi, N. (2018). Some basic questions about (a) decolonizing Africa(n)-centred psychology considered. *South African Journal of Psychology, 48*(3), 331–342. https://doi.org/10.1177/0081246318790444

Seedat, M., Suffla, S., & Christie, D. J. (Eds.). (2017). *Emancipatory and participatory methodologies in peace, critical, and community psychology.* Springer. https://doi.org/10.1007/978-3-319-63489-0

Segalo, P., Manoff, E., & Fine, M. (2015). Working with embroideries and counter-maps: Engaging memory and imagination within decolonizing frameworks. *Journal of Social and Political Psychology, 3*(1), 342–364. https://doi.org/10.5967/spp.v3i1.145

Settles, I. H., Warner, L. R., Buchanan, N. T., & Jones, M. K. (2020). Understanding psychology's resistance to intersectionality theory using a framework of epistemic exclusion and invisibility. *Journal of Social Issues, 76*(4), 796–813.

Smith, L. T. (2012/2018). *Decolonizing methodologies: Research and Indigenous peoples.* Zed Books.

Sonn, C. C., Kasat, P., & Quayle, A. (2017). Creative responses to social suffering: Using community arts and cultural development to foster hope. In M. Seedat, S. Suffla, & D. Christie (Eds.), *Emancipatory and participatory methodologies, peace, critical and community psychology* (pp. 91–105). Springer.

Stone Brown, S. A. (2014). *Transformation beyond greed: Native self actualization.* The Book Patch.

Trager, B. (2020). Community-based internships: How a hybridized high-impact practice affects students, community partners, and the university. *Michigan Journal of Community Service Learning, 26*(2), 71–94. https://doi.org/10.3998/mjcsloa. 3239521.0026.204

Williams, R. (1974). A history of the Association of Black Psychologists: Early formation and development. *Journal of Black Psychology, 1*(1), 9–24. https://doi.org/ 10.1177/009579847400100102

Winston, A. S. (2020). Why mainstream research will not end scientific racism in psychology. *Theory & Psychology, 30*(3), 425–430. https://doi.org/10.1177/ 0959354320925176

Yacat, J. (2013). Filipino psychology (sikolohiyang Pilipino). *The Encyclopedia of Cross-Cultural Psychology, 2,* 551–556.

Zembylas, M. (2018). Reinventing critical pedagogy as decolonizing pedagogy: The education of empathy. *Review of Education, Pedagogy & Cultural Studies, 40*(5), 404421. https://doi.org/10.1080/10714413.2019.1570794

5
BEYOND DECOLONIZATION
Anticolonial Methodologies for Indigenous Futurity in Psychological Research

JILLIAN FISH AND JOSEPH P. GONE

Engaging in anticolonial strategies for the protection, recovery, and maintenance of [Indigenous Knowledge] systems means that academics, Indigenous Knowledge holders, and the political leaders of Indigenous nations and settler governments must be prepared to dismantle the colonial project in all of its current manifestations. Academics who are to be true allies to Indigenous Peoples in the protection of our knowledge must be willing to step outside of their privileged position and challenge research that conforms to the guidelines outlined by the colonial power structure and root their work in the politics of decolonization and anticolonialism. This Indigenous approach is critical to the survival of Indigenous Knowledge and ultimately Indigenous Peoples.

—Leanne Simpson, Michi Saagiig Nishnaabeg (2004, p. 381)

Over the past few decades, research psychologists have sought to be allies of Indigenous peoples by engaging Indigenous communities in research about

Correspondence concerning this chapter should be addressed to Jillian Fish, Psychology Department, Olin-Rice Science Center, Macalester College, 1600 Grand Ave., Saint Paul, MN 55106, or jfish1@macalester.edu

https://doi.org/10.1037/0000376-006
Decolonial Psychology: Toward Anticolonial Theories, Research, Training, and Practice,
L. Comas-Díaz, H. Y. Adames, and N. Y. Chavez-Dueñas (Editors)

what promotes thriving Indigenous futures for forthcoming generations. However, the path toward such research is an obscure one, especially within disciplinary psychology. This is due in part to the introduction of decolonization as a response to traditional psychological research methods. Given that decolonization entails, first and foremost, the repatriation of Indigenous land and life (Tuck & Yang, 2012), psychologists are starting to grapple with whether decolonial research is even possible. For instance, returning to a presettler past is not (Bhatia, 2013). Thus, possibilities for psychological research to decolonize Indigenous land and life in meaningful ways are constrained. Although decolonization has instigated discussions among psychologists who are seeking to engage in research that reconfigures settler colonial power structures, it runs the risk of perpetuating further harm against Indigenous communities, who more often than not, obtain no direct benefit from psychological research. For research psychologists to be active proponents of robust Indigenous futures, it is imperative that they confront and resist settler colonialism at all phases of knowledge production and follow the lead of Indigenous peoples in doing so. Anticolonialism, which refers to Indigenous resistance and opposition to colonialism (Hartmann et al., 2019), is a potential alternative to decolonization that can circumvent the noted issues by placing the power to challenge psychological research norms, assumptions, and outcomes squarely in the hands of Indigenous peoples.

The purpose of this chapter is to bring research psychologists into conversation with the politics of anticolonialism vis-à-vis Indigenous studies. Given that research psychologists are primarily concerned with the production of new knowledge, we situate our discussion within the context of settler colonialism to demonstrate how it has given way to a societal structure in which colonial knowledge systems have subjugated Indigenous peoples, including in psychology. We propose that anticolonialism can counter psychology's epistemic violence—violence employed against or through knowledge—toward Indigenous peoples, positioning it as an approach to research that resists colonial knowledge systems and offers tangible outcomes to Indigenous communities by promoting the recovery, reclamation, or revitalization of Indigenous Knowledges (IKs). First, we describe the role of settler colonialism and epistemic violence in oppressing Indigenous peoples in psychology. Second, we review the shortcomings of decolonial research efforts. Third, we discuss anticolonialism's historical and intellectual foundations as it relates to anticolonial methodologies. Fourth, we provide a case example of anticolonialism in a modern Indigenous research context from the White Mountain Apache Tribe (WMAT) and Johns Hopkins University (JHU). We conclude with reflections on putting anticolonial methodologies into action in psychology.

ROLE OF SETTLER COLONIALISM

Settler colonialism is a distinct form of colonization that functions through a "logic of elimination" (Wolfe, 2006, p. 387), in which constructing a settler colonial society necessitates eliminating Indigenous peoples from desired lands. Elimination occurs through various strategies that eradicate the Indigenous as Indigenous (e.g., assimilation, blood quantum laws, boarding schools, genocide), and is the underlying structure of settler colonial societies in the present. For example, Canada, Australia, New Zealand, the United States, South Africa, and Latin America. Modern forms of elimination are subtler than those in the past but are nonetheless violent toward Indigenous peoples. In particular, settlers in Canada, Australia, New Zealand, and the United States tend to enact epistemic violence, which is violence conducted against IK practices and/or violence conducted against Indigenous peoples via knowledge (Galván-Álvarez, 2010). IKs are local meanings, rationales, and philosophies stemming from Indigenous peoples' histories with their environments (UNESCO, n.d.). For Indigenous peoples, IKs structure the ins and outs of daily life and are essential to a broader cultural framework of Indigenous existence (i.e., language, spirituality, relationality). Thus epistemic violence can include the systematic denigration, subjugation, and erasure of IKs throughout settler societies (e.g., difficulties accessing learning materials in Indigenous languages, overreliance on universal principles versus local or place-based knowledge, exclusion of elders in educational institutions). Additionally, it includes knowledge systems that subjugate Indigenous peoples (e.g., textbooks describing Indigenous peoples as of the past, research methods that purportedly reveal psychological deficits among Indigenous peoples). Taken together, epistemic violence maintains and perpetuates the settler colonial project, and poses a formidable threat to psychology's role in Indigenous futures.

Epistemic violence occurs in psychology through *psycolonization*, a term that describes several associated tendencies such as therapists pathologizing Indigenous resistance (Todd & Wade, 1994), therapy culture positioning Indigenous peoples as damaged subjects (Gone, 2023), and the circulation of psychological findings from Western, educated, industrialized, rich, and democratic (WEIRD) nations as globally universal (Teo & Afşin, 2020). Each points to psychology as a colonizing force among Indigenous peoples, especially in the context of psychotherapy (Fanon, 2004). We expand the scope of psycolonization here to include the knowledge that psychology values and generates about Indigenous peoples via scholarly inquiry. Psychologists develop knowledge using highly select research methodologies that undoubtedly shapes Indigenous peoples' experiences in psychotherapy (Gone, 2010) and beyond (Duran & Duran, 1995). Consequently, we define psycoloniza-tion as the domination of Eurocentric epistemes in psychological research that results in the subjugation of Indigenous peoples via knowledge and its politics (Gone, 2008). Epistemes define "the conditions of possibility of all knowledge" (Foucault, 1970, p. 409). Although epistemes can coexist with one another, the one that reigns superior in a particular disciplinary discourse will shape knowledge accordingly, as well as disciplinary power structures, subverting other forms of knowledge. Prevailing research paradigms in psychology include positivism, postpositivism, scientific realism and, to a lesser extent, constructivism and critical theory, which reflect Eurocentric ontological, epistemological, methodological, and axiological approaches to various degrees (Wilson, 2001). Thus, for psychologists to be active proponents of Indigenous futures, we must chart a new path forward—one that follows the lead of Indigenous peoples.

SHORTCOMINGS OF DECOLONIAL RESEARCH

In response to the ongoing presence of settler colonial violence in contempo-rary Indigenous life (Comas-Díaz et al., 2019), psychologists have advocated for decolonizing psychology while grappling with whether decolonization is even possible (see Adams et al., 2015; Barnes & Siswana, 2018; Carolissen & Duckett, 2018; Seedat & Suffla, 2017), a question that has occasioned long-standing conversation in Indigenous studies. Simply put, decoloniza-tion "entails the 'undoing' of colonization" (Gone, 2021a, p. 260). In the context of settler colonialism, decolonization would more precisely require repatriating all land to Indigenous peoples while acknowledging that land and relationships to it "have always already been differently understood and enacted" (Tuck & Yang, 2012, p. 7). Other usages of decolonization are meta-phorical and contribute to epistemic violence against Indigenous peoples and knowledge by detracting from and decentering efforts to repatriate Indigenous land and life (Tuck & Yang, 2012). The relationship that Indigenous peoples have with land is fundamental to IKs. However, decolonial rhetoric has no direct impact on land repatriation (i.e., restitution) or even rematriation—the restoration of spiritual and ancestral relations to Mother Earth. The implications are similar for "decolonizing research methods, " which tend to reflect social justice and critical methods (Tuck & Yang, 2012) and emanci-patory and liberation psychology (Gone, 2021b). Although such approaches are laudable, rarely if ever do they result in land being restored to its original conditions (which, as Indigenous peoples note, is impossible) or returned to

Indigenous peoples. As a result, we are primarily concerned with authentic and substantial efforts to heal and restore Indigenous land and lives, relative to token ones that do little for such outcomes. In fact, it is Indigenous peoples who are leading successful decolonizing projects that result in the repatriation of stolen land. In 2018, the Wiyot people reclaimed a significant portion of Duluwat Island after attempting to do so for decades. If so-called decolonial research does not repatriate or rematriate Indigenous land, but instead makes psychologists complicit in colonial efforts through what Tuck and Yang (2012) described as rhetorical "moves to settler innocence," what alternatives are there for engaging in psychological inquiry that advances Indigenous futures and destroys colonial ones?

FOUNDATIONS OF ANTICOLONIAL METHODOLOGIES

One possible alternative to decolonization is anticolonialism, which is the general opposition to imperial and colonial domination (Hartmann et al., 2019) rather than the undoing or unraveling of colonialism as an enduring societal structure—as in the case of decolonization. This includes various forms of defiance and resistance, ranging from political discourse to violent mass protests (Elam, 2017). Because anticolonialism is an eclectic mix of oppositional approaches, it can be difficult to define, given that more specific descriptions can result in a monolithic presentation of colonialism and Indigenous responses to it. As a multifaceted concept, anticolonialism can be understood as a contemporary phenomenon with historical roots and an intellectual tradition that work together to inform Indigenous opposition to colonial rule (Lee, 2018). Some psychologists are dismissive of anticolonialism's potential to develop an Indigenous psychology that resists the norms characteristic of Eurocentric psychology (Hwang, 2005, 2010), whereas others posit that psychology's anticolonial ambitions have not yet been fully realized (Hartmann et al., 2019). However, we contend that anticolonialism can both oppose and dismantle epistemic violence and forge a path for more equitable Indigenous inclusion in psychology. For this to occur, we review anticolonialism as a movement and philosophy to inform what potential anticolonial approaches may entail.

Anticolonialism as a Contemporary and Historical Movement

Anticolonial movements are a long-standing response of Indigenous peoples to settler colonialism, past and present, and have much to offer psychological science. Historically, several movements are prime examples of anticolonialism, such as Gandhi's response to British domination in India, though we highlight those that have occurred in response to settler colonialism. This includes the Tepehuán Revolt (1616–1620) that resisted warrior marginalization and the reorganization of Tepehuán society by the Spanish and Jesuits in Mexico (Gradie, 2000). Efforts of Indigenous resistance also include the Wiradjuri land warfare (c. 1820s) in Australia, in which the Wiradjuri attacked settlers from the United Kingdom and Ireland who were encroaching on sacred land (Read, 1983). More contemporary forms of anticolonialism include the Māori protest movement in Aotearoa in the 1960s, which was influenced by ancestral resistance strategies, resulting in Māori land repatriation (Mutu, 2020). The Kanesatake Resistance (i.e., the Oka Crisis) was a 78-day armed standoff between the Mohawk Nation and the Canadian government due to settler attempts to construct a golf course on Mohawk territory (A. Simpson, 2014). These, along with countless other iterations, such as the 2016 Standing Rock resistance in response to the Dakota Access oil pipeline, demonstrate that Indigenous resistance transcends space and time. Indigenous peoples reclaim what has been and always will be Indigenous. Realizing similar anticolonial ambitions in psychological research requires following the lead of Indigenous peoples in resisting coloniality and refusing research agendas that do otherwise.

Anticolonialism as a Critical Lens

In addition to acts of Indigenous resistance, anticolonialism can be "understood as a political stance and perspective" (Lee, 2018, p. 6). Oppositional thought occurs through diverse mediums (e.g., manifestos, newspapers) and represents a range of views, some more obliging of settler colonialism and reformation, and others more revolutionary (Lee, 2018). Well-known anticolonial thinkers—including Mohandas Gandhi, Frantz Fanon, Albert Memmi, and Aimé Cesairé—reflect a plurality of critical philosophies and moral reasoning. Each was a political leader of anticolonial movements and theorists of oppositional views anchored in social inequities, local knowledge, and settler colonial constructs. Thus anticolonialism is a function of context. For instance, barriers to accessing Māori te reo (the language) ignited Māori leaders to campaign for its use, resulting in the Māori Language Act of 1987 and subsequent guiding philosophies for language revitalization efforts (Mita, 2007). The diversity of anticolonial thought is discernible in the corresponding psychological literature and the field of psychology more broadly. For the former, Hartmann and colleagues (2019) illustrate that anticolonialism can capture overlapping frameworks (e.g., decolonial theory, Adams et al., 2015; tribal nationalism, Deloria, 1969; postcolonial theory, Moore-Gilbert, 1997), depending on the type of colonialism. Given our emphasis on Indigenous responses to settler colonialism, our views align the closest with tribal nationalism resulting from the Red Power movement, which catapulted sovereignty and self-determination to the forefront of discussions on Indigenous opposition (Deloria, 1969). Such philosophies are further reflected in the creation of the Society of Indian Psychologists, which was founded by Indigenous psychologist Carolyn Attneave in 1975 in response to pressing needs for an organization that foregrounded the Indigenous right to self-governance and that prioritized Indigenous well-being (Gray et al., 2012). Indeed, anticolonial philosophies work in concert with anticolonial efforts on the ground, providing psychologists with a framework for conceptualizing Indigenous resistance to epistemic violence as a precursor for Indigenous justice in the future.

Anticolonial Methodologies

Drawing from Indigenous peoples' opposition to settler colonialism via collective, organized efforts and associated understandings, we imagine how psychologists can engage in action-based anticolonial programs of research that shift the focus of the psychological literature away from how Indigenous peoples measure up in terms of putatively universal norms to how they resist dominance and subjugation in everyday life. Given the heterogeneity of anticolonialism, our definition of anticolonial methodologies is also broad: they capture a spectrum of approaches that at a minimum oppose and at a maximum demolish structures that subjugate Indigenous peoples by knowledge and its politics in psychology. These include approaches that dispute, resist, and challenge hierarchical structures that privilege Eurocentric epistemes and produce knowledge about Indigenous peoples that creates, sustains, and even promotes their ongoing colonization. As we describe later, the spectrum of anticolonial frameworks can include established research approaches, such as community-based participatory research (CBPR), but can also open the door for more innovative Indigenous research methods beyond Eurocentric approaches.

To avoid becoming merely a rhetorical device as in the case of decolonization, anticolonial approaches need to offer more than a stance for researchers to take, and instead result in tangible beneficial outcomes for Indigenous communities. Because research psychologists are principally concerned with generating new knowledge, it seems appropriate and within the scope of psychology for such outcomes to be associated with knowledge necessary for building Indigenous futures (including IKs), within both Indigenous communities and psychology writ large. Not only would this provide a deliverable outcome for Indigenous peoples in the form of preservation and recognition of IKs, it would also directly address the epistemic violence Indigenous peoples endure in psychology without detracting from Indigenous efforts toward decolonization. Consequently, for a given research methodology to exist along the spectrum of anti(settler)colonialism, it needs to include theories of Indigenous resistance and corresponding researcher actions that challenge epistemic violence in psychology and its effects in Indigenous communities, which we describe as follows.

Indigenous Resistance as a Critical Lens

An anticolonial approach necessitates that we understand Indigenous peoples as existing, persisting, and resisting (Kauanui, 2016) as a function or in pursuit of tribal sovereignty and self-determination in response to settler colonialism (Deloria, 1969). From project conceptualization to interpretation of findings, anticolonialism requires that researchers recognize Indigenous peoples' right to confront settler colonial violence and to fight for more just and equitable futures. Adopting this critical lens asks research psychologists to engage in a similar confrontation against the weaponization of psychology against Indigenous peoples by following the lead of Indigenous peoples. Accordingly, it is intentional and normative of Indigenous responses to settler colonialism. Moreover, it is focused on Indigenous peoples overcoming rather than being overcome by structures of adversity, lessons that psychology can learn from Indigenous resistance, and researcher accountability.

Anticolonial approaches foreground Indigenous resistance as a guiding framework for understanding action and subsequent change within a modern Indigenous context. For instance, CBPR builds on the strengths and resources of a given community, which does not exclude Indigenous resistance as a critical lens, but is perhaps only the most basic application of it. In contrast, anticolonial frameworks entail greater specificity of Indigenous communities' strengths and resources in a focus on Indigenous resistance. As a result, Indigenous peoples are not simply equitable partners in the research process who provide psychologists with guidance and oversight but also considered the driving force of nation-building that researchers should take great care to follow. Again, this stance is not mutually exclusive with an approach such as CBPR, which makes room for this possibility (see Figure 5.1). However, anticolonial frameworks demand that we recognize Indigenous resistance, tribal sovereignty, and nationhood as particular strengths of Indigenous peoples throughout the

FIGURE 5.1. Original Figure of CBPR in Contrast to an Anticolonial Framework

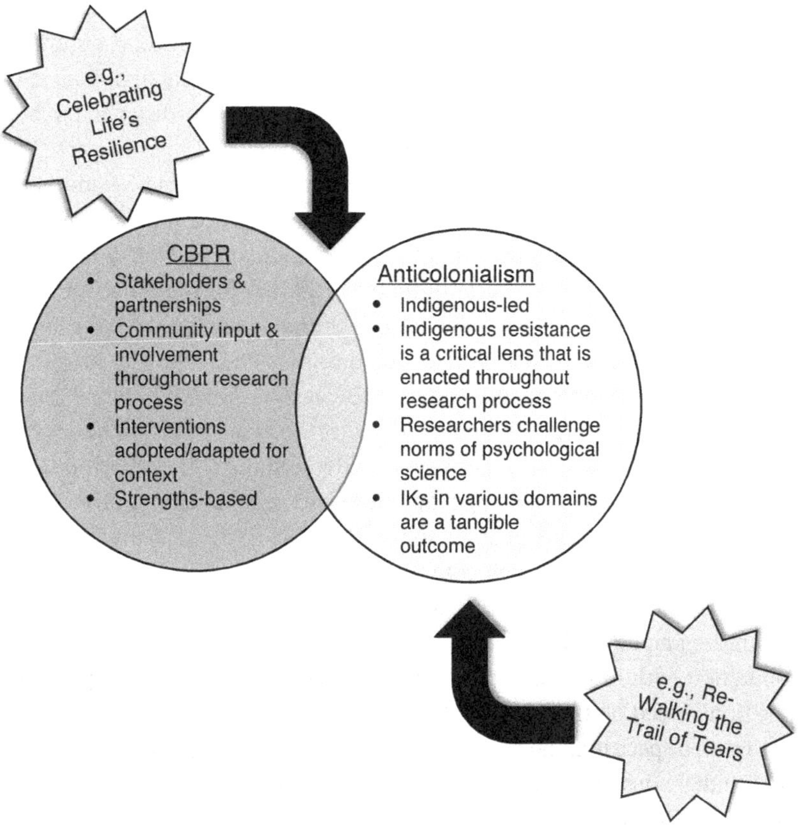

Note. CBPR = community-based participatory research; IKs = Indigenous knowledges.

research process, which we must honor through our actions when it comes to what we as psychologists have to offer Indigenous communities.

Recovery, Reclamation, or Revitalization of IKs

An anticolonial approach also assumes that Indigenous peoples are active agents in recovering, reclaiming, and revitalizing IKs. Anticolonialism recognizes that psychological research cannot accomplish these ends on its own accord or without Indigenous peoples. Anticolonialism entails that research is for and by Indigenous peoples, the result of which is a tangible outcome for local Indigenous communities that promotes the recovery, reclamation, or revitalization of IKs. This principle necessitates that an anticolonial approach has immediate and direct effects that oppose epistemic violence. Refusal plays an integral role in an anticolonial approach, in which researchers refuse Eurocentric assumptions about Indigenous peoples and Eurocentric standards for research as a function of privileging IKs. An anticolonial approach is collaborative, collective, political, action-based, resistant to disciplinary hegemony, and promotes change in real time.

Indeed, an anticolonial approach calls for researchers to do more than include Indigenous peoples throughout the research process, but to have them also lead the way toward the recovery, reclamation, and revitalization of IKs. Frameworks such as CBPR grant greater flexibility for this to occur; to the extent possible, researchers collaborate with Indigenous peoples throughout the various phases of research. The outcome of such is typically sustainable solutions to community needs. Thus, CBPR can be thought of as an existing framework that enables researchers to enact the elements of an anticolonial approach (see Figure 5.1). However, anticolonialism gives permission to psychologists to resist, challenge, and push back against existing frameworks to empower Indigenous peoples to use their IKs to develop an Indigenous scholarship that benefits their communities.

This is the distinction between using an existing framework such as CBPR to legitimize and authorize decisions researchers make on the basis of their collaboration with Indigenous partners and stakeholders or rendering research decisions based on the words of Indigenous peoples alone. If anticolonialism occurs on a spectrum, the latter reflects the more radical approach to research with Indigenous communities, in which psychologists respect the decisions of Indigenous peoples grounded in their knowledges and refuse to validate it through Eurocentric bodies of knowledge. Researcher actions such as these and Indigenous peoples' self-determination are at the crux of anticolonialism, empowering Indigenous peoples to leverage their IKs to promote sustainable Indigenous futures with the support of psychologists at every step of the way.

Summary

The existing literature makes clear that thoughts about and acts of anticolonialism are mutually constitutive. Consequently, the processes underlying Indigenous resistance as a critical lens and recovery, reclamation, or revitalization of IKs are critical to creating larger structural changes that more effectively position research psychologists as allies of Indigenous futures. With this in mind, we describe a resilience curriculum for suicide prevention resulting from a partnership between the WMAT and JHU (Cwik et al., 2019) to more clearly delineate these essential features of anticolonial research.

CASE EXAMPLE OF ANTICOLONIAL METHODOLOGIES

In 2020, the WMAT received the Tribal Nation of the Year Award for their 40-plus year research partnership with JHU to promote the health and well-being of their tribal members (Center for American Indian Health, n.d.). As Cwik and colleagues (2019) noted, the WMAT consists of 17,000 enrolled tribal members located on the Fort Apache Reservation in Arizona. Initially, the WMAT-JHU partnership was established to address behavioral health concerns (Gone et al., 2017), which evolved with the needs of the tribe. The partnership developed within a CBPR framework, which researchers enacted in anticolonial fashion (see Figure 5.1). The partnership entails that the WMAT identifies concerns they would like to address in their community. Following this, JHU partners select what kind of intervention to implement based on risk and protective factors, and gaps in local services (Cwik et al., 2019). Afterward, JHU partners either select an evidence-based intervention to implement with cultural adaptations or "design an intervention from the ground-up" (Cwik et al., 2019, p. 139). Then the WMAT and JHU partners collaborate to refine and enhance the adaptation or intervention design over several months or even years. Although this has resulted in a plethora of notable projects, we focus on a resilience curriculum developed by Apache elders as part of a suicide prevention program as an anticolonial approach to IK revitalization that promotes Indigenous futurity.

Celebrating Life's Resilience Curriculum

Although Cwik and colleagues (2019) do not describe their approach to developing the resilience curriculum with Apache elders as anticolonial, theirs is an excellent illustration. Celebrating Life is a comprehensive suicide prevention program that includes a resilience curriculum developed in response to Apache elders' discussions about the importance of culture and language among tribal members—referred to as *nowhi nalze' dayuweh bee goldoh dolee* ("let our Apache heritage and culture live on forever and teach the young ones"; Cwik et al., 2019, p. 138). According to Apache elders, language enhances tribal members' cultural identities and fosters community connections. Apache elders wanted to teach the language and culture to middle schoolers to prevent increases in suicide risk later in adolescence and adulthood and began doing so in K–8 classrooms at eight schools in 2009. The elders realized there was great variability in the content taught, however, and set out to more intentionally design a language and culture curriculum. Despite some concerns about the inflexibility of the curriculum and the implications of transitioning from the oral tradition, the benefits to what it would provide youth amid the decline of knowledgeable elders in the community were clear. With the support of Celebrating Life staff and JHU, Apache elders developed their resilience curriculum over 4.5 years (see Cwik et al., 2019), which we discuss in terms of Indigenous resistance and revitalization of IKs.

As Indigenous Resistance

The first principle of anticolonial methodologies is using Indigenous resistance as a critical lens. Across all phases of the research process, Indigenous peoples are not relegated to a product of settler colonialism, but instead actively resist it. Thus Indigenous resistance as a critical lens assumes that Indigenous peoples "exist, resist, and persist" (Kauanui, 2016, p. 1) via self-determination and tribal sovereignty, rejecting the settler colonial knowledge structures that attempt to dictate Indigenous relations (Deloria, 1969). This conceptualization maintains that Indigenous peoples know what is best for their communities and make active efforts to combat epistemic violence within them. Thus anticolonialism assumes a particular lens through which action, resistance, change, and sustainability occur. However, Cwik and colleagues demonstrate that this critical lens can be adopted in a CBPR framework. The dialectic of settler colonialism oppressing and Indigenous peoples overcoming is central to this perspective. In research, this means foregrounding the endurance of Indigeneity (Kauanui, 2016), a framing evident in the Apache elders' resilience curriculum. Cwik and colleagues (2019) described risk factors for suicide among Indigenous peoples as a result of settler colonial threats to culture and identity, but indicated several protective factors rooted in culture that have survived settler colonial attempts to eliminate Indigeneity (e.g., values, beliefs). This occurs in opposition to research that creates a deficit-laden and colonial-oriented scholarship of Indigenous peoples by emphasizing the former alone. Instead, Indigenous resistance as a critical lens offers a fuller picture of the Indigenous experience that pinpoints the mechanisms by which Indigenous peoples survive settler colonialism and thrive into the future in culturally continuous ways. For the WMAT, this was the intergenerational transmission of language.

Although Cwik et al. (2019) described their approach as strengths based, we consider their undertaking an anticolonial strengths-based initiative, converging with CBPR's principle of harnessing community strengths and resources and anticolonialism's application of Indigenous resistance as a critical lens. What differentiates a purely strengths-based approach from one that intersects with an anticolonial one is focusing on Indigenous peoples' withstanding settler colonial attempts to erase Indigenous visibility and presence, including IKs.

As Cwik and colleagues (2019) noted, "ensuring cultural beliefs, values, and traditions are passed on represent individual and community solutions against colonialism, historical trauma, and associated mental health and substance use outcomes" (p. 138). Cwik and colleagues (2019) were not simply focusing on Indigenous strengths, but also on Indigenous cultural revitalization as a response to settler colonialism and its effects (Hartmann et al., 2019). Whereas strengths-based approaches accentuate the positive in Indigenous communities, Indigenous resistance as a critical lens understands them as intentional opposition to the violation of Indigenous rights in a move that shifts the conversation about Indigenous peoples in psychological research to be both more accurate and more just. Consonant with Hartmann and colleagues' (2019) description of the anticolonial ambition of practicing "survivance" (Vizenor, 2008), a focus on what contributes to the WMAT's resilience leverages local forms of resistance that counter the erasure of IKs in settler colonial societies (and psychology). Thus Indigenous resistance as a critical lens creates opportunities in research programs and grants permission to ask the following questions: In what ways are Indigenous peoples flourishing in the face of settler colonialism? In what ways can psychological research be an ally in these efforts? Both questions guided the development of the Apache elders' resilience curriculum and the role of researchers within it (Cwik et al., 2019).

Indigenous resistance as a critical lens recognizes that Indigenous peoples are surviving and thriving amid modern settler colonization through self-governance, and decisions made for and by Indigenous peoples. This positions the WMAT, not JHU, as the experts of their own wants and needs. Cwik and colleagues (2019) make clear that the Apache elders are the driving force of language and cultural revitalization efforts to provide tribal members with the necessary resources for resisting the effects of settler colonialism. This can be seen throughout the project, in which JHU prioritized Apache elders' decisions about what the research will address, what content the curriculum will include, who is the designated audience, and how it will be implemented (Cwik et al., 2019). Because tribal sovereignty foregrounds self-determination, it is intuitive that Cwik and colleagues (2019) adopted a CBPR framework, which has been described as a research framework congruent with Indigenous lifeways (Wendt et al., 2019) and one that makes anticolonial ambitions possible. What is remarkable about Cwik and colleagues (2019) approach is that Indigenous peoples are not just collaborators; instead, the Apache elders are leading the entire project with the support of JHU, not vice versa, pushing this project from a CBPR exclusive approach to an anticolonial model of self-determination. Thus Indigenous resistance as a critical lens invites us as research psychologists to similarly resist dominant Eurocentric epistemes (e.g., by merely implementing the latest suicide intervention program tested by psychological scientists) and to instead look to local IKs that can inform how psychological research should unfold (when desired by Indigenous peoples). Rather than adapting a resilience curriculum, the Apache elders constructed one from the ground up from local IKs in a clear example of Indigenous resistance supported by researcher acts of refusal. A. Simpson's (2014) ethnographic refusal is informed by the Kanesatake Resistance and other instances of Mohawk opposition to adhering to settler colonial epistemes of nationhood. Indigenous resistance as a critical lens insists that psychology has much to learn from Indigenous peoples if those in the field are to be champions of Indigenous futures, which must occur via actions conducting research as well.

As Revitalization of IKs

The second principle of anticolonial methodologies is a clear emphasis on the recovery, reclamation, or revitalization of IKs. This does not mean examining IKs for its content (Garroutte, 2006), but harnessing IKs as a legitimate means through which Indigenous peoples know and organize the world. To promote more equitable conditions in psychology and in Indigenous communities, it is necessary that research makes meaningful contributions to the recovery, reclamation, or revitalization of IKs in an anticolonial effort to protect and maintain IKs in the places it matters most (Hartmann et al., 2019). This is also a prerequisite for research psychologists becoming allies of Indigenous futures, which cannot occur if we conduct research with or about Indigenous peoples that centers Eurocentric psychologies and reproduces Eurocentric knowledge that does not contribute to the well-being of local Indigenous communities. What was impressive about Cwik and colleagues (2019) was their focus on Apache elders' language revitalization as a source of resilience as opposed to relying only on Eurocentric understandings of this concept. It is clear that language, along with other aspects of traditional culture, is what Apache elders know to be preventive of suicide for the WMAT. Cwik et al. did not examine the exact content of the resilience curriculum other than noting its themes—which we discuss as an act of refusal—as they prioritized supporting the creation of a practical and relevant curriculum to prevent suicide, which hinges on the revitalization of the Apache language at the direct of Apache elders as a tangible outcome. Although a principle of CBPR is sustainable social change, the exact change that anticolonialism strives for (and can be achieved within the context of psychological research) is the recovery, reclamation, or revitalization of IKs.

The recovery, reclamation, or revitalization of IKs privileges Indigenous peoples as revered knowledge keepers who are already engaging in efforts of recovering, reclaiming, and revitalizing IKs to promote the well-being of their communities. As Cwik et al. (2019) described, elders are the cornerstone of transmitting IKs across generations, which was also true of the Apache elders. Privileging Indigenous peoples as keepers of IKs should be recognized, prioritized, and enacted. Indigenous peoples are not to be considered mere objects of study to include in research, but as valuable leaders guiding the recovery, reclamation, or revitalization of IKs. Like Cwik and colleagues, researchers need to invite Indigenous peoples to be a part of the research process, in which Indigenous peoples are free to determine the extent of their participation and sharing of IKs, if at all. Apache elders were integral to the WMAT-JHU partnership; the resilience curriculum was born out of Apache elders' initiatives to revitalize the language and culture in service to Apache lives (Cwik et al., 2019). For all intents and purposes, Apache elders were the driving force of the resilience curriculum. "It was necessary to develop the intervention from the ground up for several reasons. . . . The intent was for the curriculum to be theirs—created by the elders to be implemented by the elders" (Cwik et al., 2019, p. 140). The recovery, reclamation, or revitalization of IKs is for and by Indigenous peoples, producing real change for local Indigenous communities. What struck us is that the resilience curriculum has been continuously implemented at various Fort Apache middle schools, making anticolonial futures possible for the WMAT.

Cwik and colleagues' (2019) approach to developing the resilience curriculum maps onto the anticolonial tenets of recovery, reclamation, or revitalization of IKs. However, what certifies their undertakings as anticolonial is their acts of refusal (A. Simpson, 2014). One of the formative steps to developing the resilience curriculum involved Apache elders completing qualitative interviews "to decide what traditional values, teaching, and practices, as well as parts of the language, they wanted to pass on to the youth through the curriculum" (Cwik et al., 2019, p. 140). The interviews were transcribed and coded, but were used to develop the curriculum only, not for research. By refusing to use the interview content for research, Cwik et al. protected IKs from circulation outside networks of community accountability. Furthermore, despite the sample lesson plan provided, no additional lesson plans were, in what we construe as an act of Indigenous refusal to share IKs with an audience broader than the one for whom it was targeted. In our appraisal, prioritizing Indigenous peoples and their knowledges, and refusing to disseminate these for academic knowledge, is an investment in Indigenous futures over the settler colonial project in psychology. By refusing the terms of psycolonization (e.g., universal knowledge production, expert role of psychologists, focus on outcomes) on the basis of IKs, Cwik et al. solidified their approach as anticolonial. Ultimately, refusing psycolonization is at the heart of challenging settler colonial power structures that seek to subjugate Indigenous peoples by means of knowledge and its politics in psychology.

Key Takeaways From Celebrating Life's Resilience Curriculum

Our examination of the Apache elders' resilience curriculum revealed several notable qualities about Cwik and colleagues' (2019) approach beyond what could be described. We gave precedence to the elements of curriculum design and implementation that recognized, prioritized, and enacted Apache elders' resistance to colonial threats to Apache adolescents' development through the erasure of IKs. As our analysis suggests, this project materialized at the intersection of CBPR and anticolonialism, with the former providing the conditions for the latter to occur. However, as we mentioned earlier (and will again later), anticolonialism does not have to occur in conjunction with CBPR and can exist on its own. In the context of settler colonialism, the WMAT are the ones who decide the future of their community through their actions in their relationship with Cwik and colleagues. No doubt, the WMAT know the WMAT best, not researchers. This captures the essence of our understanding of anticolonial methodologies; leveraging Indigenous resistance to promote structural changes toward the end of protecting what Indigenous peoples deem sacred.

Cwik et al.'s (2019) position about Indigenous peoples existing, persisting, and resisting settler colonialism, and their enactment of it, was explicit, resulting in a tangible outcome in the form of Apache knowledge that was by and for the community—no one else. Perhaps at the heart of anticolonial projects is refusing one's own disciplinary expertise and instead taking the lead of elders and other community members. Research psychologists acting in an anticolonial ethos should provide Indigenous peoples and communities with resources (e.g., funding, transportation, time, support) to be active proponents of the research process, however that might look to an Indigenous community. Anticolonialism requires psychologists to support Indigenous peoples' efforts to resist epistemic violence as par for the course of a psychology that nurtures Indigenous futurity. Anticolonial research is both generative and destructive; it can help revitalize and maintain IKs at the behest of Indigenous peoples while razing Eurocentric assumptions about the pursuit of psychological knowledge.

ENACTING ANTICOLONIAL METHODOLOGIES IN PSYCHOLOGY

This chapter presents emerging efforts to advance anticolonial research agendas in psychology. We described the Apache elders' resilience curriculum as an anticolonial approach within the context of CBPR that illuminates the role of Indigenous resistance in the revitalization of IKs that promotes Indigenous well-being. Our description of anticolonialism is an excellent fit for researchers engaged in health intervention efforts but can be used in other research contexts as well (i.e., education, policy). For non-Indigenous psychologists who want to adopt or implement an anticolonial framework, it is important to be cognizant of the ins and outs of conducting research in Indian Country (see Gone, 2023), some of which we touched on here. This includes establishing meaningful relationships with Indigenous communities, being aware of Tribal Institutional Review Boards, local terminologies and concepts, tribal histories, cultural norms, resistance efforts, and including Indigenous peoples on the research team itself, among other things.

The case illustration we provided here (Cwik et al., 2019) is one example of an anticolonial approach, and many others remain to be examined as such. Other than Hartmann and colleagues (2019), few resources offer a description of anticolonial methodologies in psychology. Taken together, this is the beginning of anticolonial psychological research—and much remains to be gleaned from Indigenous resistance and its implications for challenging and dismantling epistemic violence in Indigenous communities as well as within our discipline. Although Indigenous studies programs have much to offer anticolonial endeavors in psychology (Hartmann et al., 2019), we would be remiss if we did not highlight that Indigenous communities also have much to offer. As a result, research psychologists should consider local effects of settler colonialism—and attempts to resist it—to ensure that their anticolonial approach is appropriately contextualized.

We have sought to strike a balance between specificity and flexibility to provide psychologists with anticolonial principles that are precise yet broadly applicable, and we encourage researchers to continue to refine what exactly anticolonial approaches are in psychology. Our principles are specific to settler colonialism, but future research could consider anticolonialism in response to other forms of colonization to further explicate psychology's role in creating structural solutions for Indigenous peoples on the ground that simultaneously instigate disciplinary change. The global population of Indigenous peoples is estimated at 370 to 500 million (World Bank Group, n.d.) and it would be a mistake to take a one-size-fits-all approach with anticolonial approaches. Indigenous peoples experience colonization in different ways; a given Indigenous community's history and current affairs should be taken into consideration before applying an anticolonial approach to ensure it is suitable. Researchers who do not do so risk inflicting further harm on Indigenous peoples by way of psychology.

We admit that much is left to elucidate about anticolonialism as an approach to research. To prevent anticolonialism from being used as merely comforting rhetoric, we have been intentional in describing it as a combination of theory and action that results in a tangible outcome for Indigenous peoples in the form of IKs. We invite psychology researchers to continue developing ideas for anticolonial methodologies, but we insist that anticolonialism continue to foreground Indigenous resistance that leads to material action for Indigenous communities. In the case of Cwik and colleagues (2019), this outcome was a resilience curriculum that revitalized and maintained Apache knowledges. This would not only ensure that anticolonial methodologies remain action oriented but also help avoid the pitfalls of decolonizing methodologies that fail to result in the repatriation or rematriation of Indigenous land and life (Tuck & Yang, 2012). Additionally, we look forward to opportunities that refusal offers psychological research by giving researchers permission to resist disciplinary norms and create their own with Indigenous peoples (i.e., Simpson, 2014). Through researcher allowance for Indigenous acts of refusal, we can begin to erode Eurocentric disciplinary dominance in psychology, prevent cultural misappropriation (e.g., by unnecessarily disseminating IKs), and protect IKs.

Finally, although the case illustration was in a CBPR framework (Cwik et al., 2019), we caution researchers against conflating anticolonial methodologies with any approach in particular. Anticolonialism itself is variable and though CBPR is conducive to the anticolonial principles we outlined here, we imagine anticolonialism to offer more exciting possibilities for Indigenous psychological research. Indigenous researchers are engaging in a wide range of anticolonial methodologies that push the boundaries of Eurocentric knowledge by relying on IKs alone. For instance, Walters (2016) rewalked the Trail of Tears in *Yappali: Choctaw Road to Health*, a project in which walking the trail is part of experiential and ancestral knowledge production that promotes Choctaw health in the present and for generations to come. Whereas Cwik and colleagues' (2019) approach occurred at the intersection of CBPR and anticolonialism, Walters' (2016) research framework seems to rely solely on anticolonial principles (see Figure 5.1).

In rewalking the Trail of Tears (i.e., Indigenous resistance as a critical lens), the Choctaw are using their collective and intergenerational experiences as an Indigenous research design to recover, reclaim, and revitalize Choctaw IKs (i.e., solutions for chronic health concerns). As an additional example of what anticolonial possibilities exist for the future, JHU's Center for American Indian Health recently brought together Indigenous social scientists to define what Indigenous strengths-based research is as a way to counter requests of non-Indigenous social scientists to legitimize Indigenous research via Eurocentric bodies of knowledge and approaches, simultaneously building an Indigenous-centered scholarship. These emerging anticolonial trends hold much promise for Indigenous futures. By inviting us to consider Indigenous peoples' past and present resistance to settler colonialism, anticolonialism can better position us as proponents of Indigenous futures, as determined by Indigenous peoples themselves.

CONCLUSION

If the construal of settler colonialism is accurate, then going back to a precolonial nirvana is not possible. However, anticolonialism provides an opportunity to take us forward in lockstep fashion with Indigenous resistance. Through methodologies that attend to and enact Indigenous resistance to settler colonial domination, we can create a more equitable epistemological landscape in psychological research—one that privileges the experiences, knowledge, and judgments of Indigenous peoples. It is crucial that psychologists engage in research at the confluence of resistance and action, taking great care to acknowledge and demonstrate that Indigenous peoples have been leaders in the battle against colonization since the onset of settler encroachment. So long as settler colonialism exists, Indigenous peoples will too, not in terms of merely surviving but thriving. Ultimately, it is up to psychology to decide what role psychologists will play in Indigenous futures. By refusing the terms of Eurocentric disciplinary epistemes, psychologists can engage in knowledge production with Indigenous peoples that produces tangible outcomes and forges structural change. To be clear, Indigenous peoples will remain steadfast in resisting and undoing settler colonialism toward the rise of an anticolonial hereafter, with or without psychology. What remains to be seen is whether psychologists will follow suit. Consequently, we invite psychologists to consider moving forward along with us: Will you be a psycolonizer or a champion of Indigenous futurity?

RESOURCES

Cesairé, A. (2014). *Return to my Native land.* Archipelago.

Erdrich, L. (2020). *The night watchman.* Harper Collins.

Estes, N. (2019). *Our history is the future. Standing Rock versus the Dakota access pipeline, and the long tradition of Indigenous resistance.* Verso.

Flavell, W. (2021). *Ake ake ake* [TV series episode]. TMP & NZ On Air. https://www.rnz.co.nz/programmes/ake-ake-ake

Harjo, J. (2015). *Conflict resolution for holy beings.* Norton.

Makepiece, A. (Director). (2011). *We still live here as Nutayuneân* [Film]. Public Broadcasting Service. https://www.pbs.org/independentlens/documentaries/we-still-live-here/

Memmi, A. (1991). *The colonizer and colonized.* Beacon.

Obomsawin, A. (Director). (1993). *Kanehsatake: 270 years of resistance* [Film]. ACPAV. https://www.nfb.ca/film/kanehsatake_270_years_of_resistance/

Rawal, S. (Director). (2020). *Gather* [Film]. First Nations Development Institute.

Rickard, C. (1984). *Fighting Tuscarora: The autobiography of Chief Clinton Rickard.* Syracuse University Press.

Simpson, L. (2017). *As we have always done: Indigenous freedom through radical resistance.* University of Minnesota Press.

REFERENCES

Adams, G., Dobles, I., Gómez, L. H., Kurtiş, T., & Molina, L. E. (2015). Decolonizing psychological science: Introduction to the special thematic section. *Journal of Social and Political Psychology, 3*(1), 213–238. https://doi.org/10.5964/jspp.v3i1.564

Barnes, B., & Siswana, A. (2018). Psychology and decolonisation: Introduction to the special issue. *South African Journal of Psychology. Suid-Afrikaanse Tydskrif vir Sielkunde, 48*(3), 297–298. https://doi.org/10.1177/0081246318798735

Bhatia, A. (2013). We are all here to stay: Indigeneity, migration, and decolonizing the treaty right to be here. *Windsor Yearbook of Access to Justice, 31*(2), 39–64. https://doi.org/10.22329/wyaj.v31i2.4411

Carolissen, R. L., & Duckett, P. S. (2018). Teaching toward decoloniality in community psychology and allied disciplines: Editorial introduction. *American Journal of Community Psychology, 62*(3–4), 241–249. https://doi.org/10.1002/ajcp.12297

Center for American Indian Health. (n.d.). *White Mountain Apache Tribe receives "Tribal Nation of the Year" award from Blue Cross Blue Shield.* Johns Hopkins University Center for Indigenous Health. https://cih.jhu.edu/white-mountain-apache-tribe-receives-tribal-nation-of-the-year-award-from-blue-cross-blue-shield/

Comas-Díaz, L., Hall, G. N., & Neville, H. A. (2019). Racial trauma: Theory, research, and healing: Introduction to the special issue. *American Psychologist, 74*(1), 1–5. https://doi.org/10.1037/amp0000442

Cwik, M., Goklish, N., Masten, K., Lee, A., Suttle, R., Alchesay, M., O'Keefe, V., & Barlow, A. (2019). "Let our Apache heritage and culture live on forever and teach the young ones": Development of the elders' resilience curriculum, an upstream suicide prevention approach for American Indian Youth. *American Journal of Community Psychology, 64*(1–2), 137–145. https://doi.org/10.1002/ajcp.12351

Deloria, V., Jr. (1969). *Custer died for your sins: An Indian manifesto.* Macmillan.

Duran, E., & Duran, B. (1995). *Native American postcolonial psychology.* Suny Press.

Elam, J. D. (2017, December 27). *Anticolonialism.* Global South studies: A collective publication with the Global South. https://globalsouthstudies.as.virginia.edu/key-concepts/anticolonialism

Fanon, F. (2004). *The wretched of the earth.* Grove Press.

Foucault, M. (1970). *The order of things: An archaeology of the human sciences.* Pantheon Books.

Galván-Álvarez, E. (2010). Epistemic violence and retaliation: The issue of knowledges in mother India. *Atlantis, 32*(2), 11–26.

Garroutte, E. M. (2006). Defining "radical Indigenism" and creating an American Indian scholarship. *Culture, Power, and History, 9*, 169–198.

Gone, J. P. (2008). Dialogue 2008: Introduction: Mental health discourse as Western cultural proselytization. *Ethos, 36*(3), 310–315. https://doi.org/10.1111/j.1548-1352.2008.00016.x

Gone, J. P. (2010). Psychotherapy and traditional healing for American Indians: Exploring the prospects for therapeutic integration. *The Counseling Psychologist, 38*(2), 166–235. https://doi.org/10.1177/0011000008330831

Gone, J. P. (2021a). Decolonization as methodological innovation in counseling psychology: Method, power, and process in reclaiming American Indian therapeutic traditions. *Journal of Counseling Psychology, 68*(3), 259–270. https://doi.org/10.1037/cou0000500

Gone, J. P. (2021b). Recounting coup as the recirculation of Indigenous vitality: A narrative alternative to historical trauma. *Transcultural Psychiatry.* Advance online publication. https://doi.org/10.1177/13634615211054998

Gone, J. P. (2023). Researching with American Indian and Alaska Native communities: Pursuing partnerships for psychological inquiry in service to Indigenous futurity. In H. Cooper (Ed.), *APA handbook of research methods in psychology: Vol. 2. Research designs: Quantitative, qualitative, neuropsychological, and biological* (2nd ed.). American Psychological Association.

Gone, J. P., Hartmann, W. E., & Sprague, M. G. (2017). Wellness interventions for Indigenous communities in the United States: Exemplars for action research. In M. A. Bond, I. Serrano-García, C. B. Keys, & M. Shinn (Eds.), *APA handbook of community psychology: Methods for community research and action for diverse groups and issues* (pp. 507–522). American Psychological Association. https://doi.org/10.1037/14954-030

Gradie, C. (2000). *The Tepehuan revolt of 1616: Militarism, evangelism, and colonialism in seventeenth century nueva vizcaya.* University of Utah Press.

Gray, J. S., Carter, P. M., LaFromboise, T. D., & BigFoot, D. S. (2012). The interrelationship between the Society of Indian Psychologists and counseling psychology. *The Counseling Psychologist, 40*(5), 685–698. https://doi.org/10.1177/0011000012450423

Hartmann, W. E., Wendt, D. C., Burrage, R. L., Pomerville, A., & Gone, J. P. (2019). American Indian historical trauma: Anticolonial prescriptions for healing, resilience, and survivance. *American Psychologist, 74*(1), 6–19. https://doi.org/10.1037/amp0000326

Hwang, K. K. (2005). From anticolonialism to postcolonialism: The emergence of Chinese Indigenous psychology in Taiwan. *International Journal of Psychology, 40*(4), 228–238. https://doi.org/10.1080/00207590444000177

Hwang, K. K. (2010). Way to capture theory of Indigenous psychology. *Psychological Studies, 55*(2), 96–100. https://doi.org/10.1007/s12646-010-0024-3

Kauanui, J. K. (2016). "A structure, not an event": Settler colonialism and enduring Indigeneity. *Lateral, 5*(1). https://doi.org/10.25158/L5.1.7

Lee, C. J. (2018). Anti-colonialism: Origins, practices, and historical legacies. In M. Thomas & A. S. Thompson (Eds.) *The Oxford handbook of the ends of empire* (pp. 1–18). Oxford.

Mita, D. M. (2007). Māori language revitalization: A vision for the future. *Canadian Journal of Native Education, 30*(1), 101–107.

Moore-Gilbert, B. (1997). *Postcolonial theory: Contexts, practices, politics.* Verso.

Mutu, M. (2020). Mana Māori motuhake: Māori concepts and practices of sovereignty. In B. Hokowhitu, A. Moreton-Robinson, L. Tuhiwai-Smith, C. Andersen, & Larkin, S. (Eds.), *Routledge handbook of critical Indigenous studies* (pp. 269–282). Routledge. https://doi.org/10.4324/9780429440229-24

Read, P. (1983). *A history of the Wiradjuri people of New South Wales 1883–1969* [Doctoral thesis, Department of Philosophy, Australian National University]. Open Access Theses. https://hdl.handle.net/1885/109803

Seedat, M., & Suffla, S. (2017). Community psychology and its (dis)contents, archival legacies and decolonisation. *South African Journal of Psychology, 47*(4), 421–431. https://doi.org/10.1177/0081246317741423

Simpson, A. (2014). *Mohawk interruptus.* Duke University Press.

Simpson, L. (2004). Anticolonial strategies for the recovery and maintenance of Indigenous knowledge. *American Indian Quarterly, 28*(3), 373–384. https://doi.org/10.1353/aiq.2004.0107

Teo, T., & Afşin, B. (2020). The impossible conditions of the possibility of an alter-global psychology. In L. Sundararajan, K. Hwang, & K. Yeh (Eds.), *Global psychology from Indigenous perspectives* (pp. 159–174). Palgrave Macmillan. https://doi.org/10.1007/978-3-030-35125-0_10

Todd, N., & Wade, A. (1994). Domination, deficiency and psychotherapy. *The Calgary Participator, 4*, 37–46.

Tuck, E., & Yang, K. W. (2012). Decolonization is not a metaphor. *Decolonization, 1*, 1–40.

United Nations Educational, Scientific, and Cultural Organization (UNESCO). (n.d.). Local and Indigenous knowledge systems. https://en.unesco.org/links

Vizenor, G. (2008). *Survivance: Narratives of Native presence.* University of Nebraska Press.

Walters, K. L. (2016, October 13–14). *Transcending trauma and community health* [Paper presentation]. International Indigenous Health Symposium, Honolulu, HI,

United States. https://native.jabsom.hawaii.edu/docs/hh_2016/presentations/ 13/12.Walters,K.pdf

Wendt, D. C., Hartmann, W. E., Allen, J., Burack, J. A., Charles, B., D'Amico, E. J., Dell, C. A., Dickerson, D. L., Donovan, D. M., Gone, J. P., O'Connor, R. M., Radin, S. M., Rasmus, S. M., Venner, K. L., & Walls, M. L. (2019). Substance use research with Indigenous communities: Exploring and extending foundational principles of community psychology. *American Journal of Community Psychology, 64*(1–2), 146–158. https://doi.org/10.1002/ajcp.12363

Wilson, S. (2001). What is an Indigenous research methodology? *Canadian Journal of Native Education, 25,* 175–179.

Wolfe, P. (2006). Settler colonialism and the elimination of the Native. *Journal of Genocide Research, 8*(4), 387–409. https://doi.org/10.1080/14623520601056240

World Bank Group. (n.d.). *Indigenous peoples.* https://www.worldbank.org/en/topic/ indigenouspeoples#1

6

DISCIPLINARY DISRUPTIONS

Strategies Toward a Decolonial Community Psychology Praxis

JESICA SIHAM FERNÁNDEZ

Psychology emerged in the mid-1800s as a disciplinary area of scientific inquiry focused on the study of the mind, body, and behavior. With foundations in philosophy, specifically the behaviorism and constructivism that were prominent at the time, psychology seeks to better understand the relationship between the mind and body (Jenkins, 2016; Prilleltensky, 1994). Although psychology in general is centuries old, community psychology as a subdiscipline is relatively nascent. Community psychology is concerned with the mind–body relationship as well as the person-environment dynamics that consider power structures, sociocultural practices, and systems level of analysis (Kloos et al., 2012; Levine et al., 2005; Reich et al., 2017; Tebes, 2016; Trickett, 1996). In the United States, community psychology emerged from a place of resistance—struggling to establish itself as a field of study with its set of theories, ethics, paradigms, and approaches to inquiry (Perkins, 2009), community well-being, and liberation.

The author thanks Dr. Christopher Sonn and the anonymous reviewers for their feedback and commentary which helped further develop the ideas featured in this chapter. Thanks to Jadzaí Solis for her editorial guidance.

Correspondence regarding this chapter should be addressed to Jesica Siham Fernández at jsfernandez@scu.edu, or the Ethnic Studies Department, Santa Clara University, 500 El Camino Real, Santa Clara, CA 95053.

https://doi.org/10.1037/0000376-007
Decolonial Psychology: Toward Anticolonial Theories, Research, Training, and Practice,
L. Comas-Díaz, H. Y. Adames, and N. Y. Chavez-Dueñas (Editors)

The sociohistorical and political context that helped form community psychology in the United States accounts for the discipline's core values and theories. Furthermore, this contextualizes why U.S.-based community psychology is distinct from those developed in the Majority World, which emerged and were formed in relation to popular education, feminist and decolonial epistemologies, and movements aligned with community struggles. Instead of emerging from traditional psychological approaches, like clinical psychology, which at the time were oriented toward intervention and individualism, most non–U.S.-based community psychology theory and practice is grassroots oriented, as well as informed by social justice struggles for liberation (Comas-Díaz et al., 1998; Martín-Baró, 1994; Montero et al., 2017).

The genealogy of U.S.-based community psychology is more aligned with traditional psychology, especially positivist and individualistic person-centered approaches to intervention and rehabilitation. This may help explain why the 1965 Swampscott Conference is often credited as the birthplace of U.S. community psychology. Most community psychology programs name the Swampscott Conference as the starting point of the field (Jenkins, 2016). At this gathering, psychologists were urged to expand their engagements beyond mental health toward prevention and the promotion of community empowerment and wellness via an ecological analysis of social issues, and the development of settings that could support processes for empowering individuals and communities to change their lives (Kloos et al., 2012; Levine et al., 2005; Prilleltensky, 1994; Tebes, 2016). The emergence of community psychology is exemplified in the discipline's desire to shift away from traditional, mostly clinical psychology orientations, and as a political response to the 1960s deinstitutionalization movement.

Community psychology sought to affirm and make explicit its commitment to justice, which traditional psychology approaches appeared unconcerned with given the focus on individual-level analyses, intervention, and treatment/rehabilitation. Individualized forms of treatment or care appeared to be the focus of community psychologists and allied professionals in what was and, to a degree, still is an emerging, growing, and evolving discipline. The deinstitutionalization movement along with civil rights struggles were thus pivotal in agitating community psychologists to reimagine psychology: What it is or can be, and who it is for. Community psychologists and allied practitioners were called to be agents of change or dissenters urgently demanding disciplinary transformations. Decades later, we find the discipline engaged in similar calls for change, and a desire to transform itself (Tebes, 2016; Perkins, 2009). The call aligns with a national—perhaps global—racial reckoning of psychology's complicity in reproducing colonial power

(Fernández et al., 2021; Quijano, 2000) at the intersections of oppressions (Moradi & Grzanka, 2017; Rosenthal, 2016).

Reflecting on the histories, and as a response to the present moment, four interconnected strategies are offered and described to decolonize theories and practices in U.S. community psychology. With this intention, the chapter is guided by the question of whether a decolonial community psychology in the United States is possible. By describing the strategies via auto-ethnographic vignettes and featuring writings by critical community psychologists who identify as scholar–activists, we can reimagine a U.S.-based community psychology oriented toward a decolonial standpoint (Reyes Cruz & Sonn, 2011). The strategies are embodied critical reflexivity (Fernández, 2018), *saberes entrelazados* (intertwined knowledge; Bargero, 2004; Ciofalo, 2019; Cusicanqui, 2012), radical relationality (Dutta, 2021), and trans-disciplinarity (Maldonado-Torres, 2019; Serrano-García, 2020). The guiding question, and the vignettes or reflections offered, can help identify values or ethics for decolonial epistemologies and paradigms that can help undo colonial power. The strategies are intended to unsettle the Western Euro-centrism of U.S. community psychology.

Through these strategies, adapting them to serve our particular and unique positionalities, engagements, ethics, and values, a decolonial community psychology is indeed possible. The strategies urge scholars, researchers, educators, and practitioners to reflect, dialogue, and pursue actions toward developing community psychology research with, by, and for peoples. A community psychology that remains oriented toward Western Eurocentric frameworks is complicit in the reproduction of oppression. The complicity is sustained by the unreflexively unexamined application of positivist, deficit-based, and individualistic frameworks. This chapter offers a reflection—indeed an invitation—to enacting disciplinary dissent as a form of necessary radical disruption. The disruption is warranted because it presents the potential to transform and revolutionize the field toward anticolonial and decolonial liberation praxes. The recognition and will to transform community psychology, especially in the United States, is the first step and should be followed by strategies to craft and imagine a decolonial community psychology.

U.S. COMMUNITY PSYCHOLOGY: A BRIEF LOOK TO THE PAST

Despite the initial motivations that animated the discipline's formation and its dissenting approach away from traditional, specifically clinical, psychology approaches, the cannon of community psychology is U.S./Western Eurocentric, and often focused on a critique of clinical psychology (Prilleltensky, 1994; Rappaport, 1977). This critique acknowledges clinical and behavioral psychologies as complicit with structures of oppression, which instead of challenging systems, practices, and discourses of hegemony—such as racism and heteronormativity—often remain uncontested. The psychologies of the 1960s and 1970s were relatively passive in challenging the status quo. In fact, they often unintentionally contributed to deficit perspectives under the assumption of purporting rigorous scientific inquiry for the "betterment" of society. The deinstitutionalization movement, along with civil rights struggles for Black liberation and freedom, were the breaking point and the start of departure for some community psychologists who were driven by the more liberatory and radically emancipatory praxes reflected in the critical psychologies of the Majority World. These critical psychologies were more adequately responding to and supporting community struggles for enfranchisement, justice, and liberation. The emergence of community psychology in the United States was thus accompanied by efforts to craft a field attuned to the needs, strengths, and social conditions of communities on the margins.

Community psychology's purported resistance to the pathologizing of social groups, specifically Communities of Color and people of marginalized genders, constitutes part of the discipline's historical narrative (Fernández et al., 2021). In being critical of traditional psychological research frameworks, especially clinical or medical approaches that are often decontextualized, community psychology has sought to offer a more ecological and systemic analysis of social issues that affect individuals and groups. Yet a more explicit sociohistorical and intersectional analysis that interrogates systems of power is necessary. Considering the sociopolitical context and a critical decolonial standpoint, U.S.-based community psychology is to a significant degree tethered to coloniality, specifically frameworks that reproduce circuits of oppression (Comas-Díaz et al., 1998; Fine, 2015; Reyes Cruz & Sonn, 2011). Despite attempts to craft a more humanizing discipline, U.S. community psychology has yet to explicitly engage in the disruption of structural violence that intersects with systems of oppression that reproduce colonial research, theory, pedagogy, and practice (Dutta et al., 2016).

Over the course of its formation, community psychology has been principally concerned with promoting community empowerment, sense of community and belonging, and with creating settings to support individual and community mental health and well-being. These goals are still central to community psychology despite some limitations and critiques (Boonzaier & van Niekerk, 2019; Ciofalo, 2019; Kessi et al., 2021; Serrano-García, 2008, 2020; Watts & Serrano-García, 2003). Also central to the development of the discipline were the writings of Ignacio Martín-Baró (1994), which helped community psychology orient itself toward a sociopolitical praxis of liberation (Watts & Serrano-García, 2003). These perspectives are still relevant and central to the discipline today, as critical community psychologists underscore and as evidenced in recent publications and special issues (Boonzaier & van Niekerk, 2019; Kagan et al., 2019; Kessi et al., 2021), U.S. community psychology must be expanded. The discipline needs to explicitly attend to the historical, contextual, and structural organization of intergenerational trauma emerging from coloniality and structural violence (Montero et al., 2017). Latin American liberation psychology has helped inform recent perspectives and epistemologies in U.S. community psychology (Comas-Díaz et al., 1998).

The popular education and grassroots movements in South America, such as the literacy programs associated with Paulo Freire's (1970) *conscientização*, or the process of critical consciousness, helped develop new frameworks and theories in community psychology. Equally important is the work of Martinique psychiatrist and political philosopher Frantz Fanon (1967) on the psychology of the oppressed, of people who are dehumanized or treated as subhuman. The perspectives offered by Martín-Baró, Freire, and Fanon continue disrupting U.S. community psychology. The liberation perspectives they offer are cracking the fortress (Pillay, 2017) of colonial power in the psychology of U.S. community psychology and psychologists. The cracks in the discipline are greatly owed to Fanon, as well as critical community psychologists in and outside the United States who incite the discipline toward transformation or to contend with its "identity crisis" (Kagan et al., 2019). Community psychology, especially in Westernized contexts like the United States, is attempting to trace and grow new routes and roots toward decoloniality (Fernández et al., 2021). In fact, in the past decade, writings on decoloniality have increased (Boonzaier & van Niekerk, 2019; Kessi et al., 2021; Seedat & Suffla, 2017), especially in U.S. community psychology journals and professional outlets. In these publications, racial reckonings are a theme that have been engaged by community psychologists who identify as White or hold proximities to structures that uphold Whiteness. U.S. community psychology is in a moment of historical reckoning with coloniality and colonial power. Thus, from this place of critique and dissent, possibilities for reimagining and transforming the discipline are unfolding.

The disruptions that are creating a decolonial shift in U.S.-based community psychology appear to be led by budding community psychologists, some of whom are in the West or Global North—or whose histories, identities, and worldviews, which inform their subjectivities, are implicated in coloniality.

These subjectivities are also informed by their ties or affinities with community struggles for liberation in the Majority World. Furthermore, these changes and shifts are being led by community psychologists who may identify as Black, Indigenous, or People of Color. Among the budding disciplinary dissenters within U.S. community psychology communities who are envisioning an "otherwise" are comrades and coconspirators with whom I share a vision for a more humanizing decolonial critical psychology. Such a psychology entails a disciplinary re/evolution attuned to and conscious of the histories of the coloniality power and structural violence and oriented toward a decolonial feminist praxis—specifically, toward the formation of a critical decolonial community psychology that is responsive and responsible for undoing the structures of Whiteness and White supremacy that remain unshattered yet must be deconstructed. Indeed, we are building toward the formation of a U.S. community psychology that disrupts the racialized regimes that continue to shape how we inquire into the relationship between the body, mind, and environment. Relatedly, how we inquire into our values, ethics and praxis, or the heart of a discipline oriented toward self- and collective determination, liberation, and upholding the power of communities to transform their lives, is necessary for psychology. An extensive history of U.S.-based community psychology is beyond the scope of this chapter (see Perkins, 2009; Prilleltensky, 1994; Tebes, 2016). Yet, it is enough to say that the discipline continues to evolve and develop in response to the urgencies of the current context.

By acknowledging the discipline's history, the tensions along with the possibilities toward a decolonial community psychology, this chapter identifies a set of strategies as disruptions that community psychologists can and must engage to transform the discipline. Strategies, from theories to methodologies, that can help community psychology in the U.S. actualize its liberatory values are urgently needed. To illustrate an emerging yet notable shift in the discipline is its receptivity to feminist methodologies, such as autoethnography. I describe autoethnography as a decolonial feminist methodology that summons us to engage in disciplinary disruptions toward fostering a decolonial liberatory community psychology praxis.

AUTOETHNOGRAPHY: A DECOLONIAL FEMINIST METHODOLOGY

Autoethnography is a methodology and a practice informed by feminist epistemologies and decolonial paradigms (Anzaldúa & Moraga, 1981) that center lived experiences, emotions, and subjectivities in relation to the topic or inquiry guiding the research. The intimate emotions felt in the body that shaped an individual's worldview, and thus are reflected upon and enacted, characterizes an autoethnographic method (Silva et al., 2021). It values experiential and relational knowledge, self-awareness, and introspection (Dutta, 2021). Unlike other methodologies, autoethnography engages self and embodied subjectivities as important sources of knowledge that can guide critical consciousness and research inquiry (Chang, 2008).

Autoethnography is an important practice to develop beyond its methodological implications. The introspective process of autoethnography facilitates the practice of ethical critical reflexivity (Fernández, 2018), which is important to engage in because it can help inform research ethics, standpoints, and praxis. Through an autoethnographic approach, challenges, vulnerabilities, and risks, along with joys, hopes, and imagination, surface to guide the research. Dutta (2021) purported that autoethnography is a critical methodological intervention in research paradigms and approaches aligned with epistemic justice. Important sources of information that emerge through reflexivity can help ground the researcher in a critical understanding of power in relation to positionalities, sociohistorical, and political contexts. Thus, autoethnography calls for a critical examination of power and how we can work for liberation. Fundamentally, it is most concerned with addressing "questions of heart and soul, rather than mind," as Jones wrote (1998, p. 423). Autoethnography is a necessary form of dissent that challenges relations of power, engaging in inquiry from within the body.

ENGAGING DISCIPLINARY DISRUPTION: FOUR DECOLONIAL STRATEGIES

Decolonial feminist values can support humanizing praxes, transformative justice, and individual and collective well-being that can unsettle disciplinary coloniality and colonialism. To demonstrate the possibilities for deconstructing coloniality in community psychology theory, research, and practice, I offer four strategies through autoethnographic vignettes informed by my experiences as a trained community-social psychologist. The vignettes, and where relevant, writings by scholar–activists illustrate the four strategies—embodied critical reflexivity as an ethical reflective practice (Fernández, 2018), intertwined knowledge in action (*saberes entrelazados*; Bargero, 2004; Ciofalo, 2019; Cusicanqui, 2012), radical relationality (Dutta, 2021), and transdisciplinarity (Maldonado-Torres, 2019; Serrano-García, 1984, 2020; Sonn et al., 2017)—toward a critical decolonial community psychology praxis, specifically in the U.S.

Embodied Critical Reflexivity

An ethical practice of embodied critical reflexivity is characterized by an introspective self and relational and sociocultural awareness. Associated with this practice is the process of perceiving or engaging with one's subjectivities, specifically the affectivity or feeling that often surfaces in relation to one's positionalities, identities, and lived experiences including past or present circumstances. An awareness embodied feeling is important to recognize because it can help shape researcher's subjectivities or understandings of issues or tensions to be redressed. The body can often produce a response to a circumstance that may feel unsettling before a cognitive response or label is associated with the emotion embodied. When researchers develop their capacities to link their awareness of their body's response, or embodied awareness, with their reflections in the form of critical social analysis, a consciousness develops. The ability for researchers to engage embodied critical reflexivity is fundamental to addressing tensions in research collaborations, developing ethical interventions, and working toward transformative change and liberation. Because community psychology is concerned with group, societal, and systemic dynamics that are liberatory, researchers and practitioners should strive toward connecting their thoughts or cognitive processes with their body, feelings, and actions. An embodied critical reflexivity practice can help facilitate the development of actions and relationships that can support connectedness within research collaborations.

Informed by Women of Color feminist epistemologies, the concept of a theory in the flesh (Anzaldúa & Moraga, 1981) is fundamental to an embodied critical reflexivity. This is especially the case for Women of Color, who often draw sources of knowledge from their subjectivities and bodies as we engage in inquiry. In other words, rather than being theorized from abstract concepts or ideas, knowledge is situated in and within the body—the flesh. Experiences can shape self-understandings and understandings of others within histories, cultures, and sociopolitical contexts. How we see and understand ourselves, in relation to how others perceive us, and in turn how we interact with others, is constantly shifting in response to our shared experiences of coexisting and cobeing.

To offer an example of what this looks like in practice I share an autoethnographic fieldnote from my collaboration with a Chicanx nonprofit organization, El Centro (The Center). Located in downtown San José, El Centro has been organizing in the city for more than three decades and, as of this writing, seeks to remove colonial representations in the city, such as the statue of Captain Thomas Fallon. The statue depicts Fallon, and several other settlers with a horse, raising the U.S. flag in what is now the city of San José. The statue commemorates Fallon as a pioneer of Western expansion and settler colonialism in a moment in history where the territory was part of México. At present, the statue is in downtown San José, a region commonly known as Silicon Valley. Because of this history of annexation, many Mexican American and Chicanx people, including Ohlone and Muwekman Ohlone communities in the area, have deemed the statue as a representation of coloniality. Because the statue was built in the 1990s, Chicanx and Indigenous communities have organized to remove it and raise awareness about the erasure of Indigenous and Mexican culture and histories. To demonstrate some of the actions communities engaged, I offer a fieldnote from a strategic planning meeting organized by El Centro to produce a statement to share with city and county stakeholders.

> Today's planning meeting was joined by several of the *veteranos*, the Elders (former leaders of the 1960s Chicano movement and grassroots organizing in San José), as they are called by Señora C and "Chale," who since the 1960s, at the height of the Chicano Moratorium, have been mobilizing to remove the Fallon Statue. As they each shared their *testimonio*, reflecting on those past struggles and their relevance and significance to this day, I was noticing how my students were attentively listening, commenting over the Zoom chat, and using emojis to express resonance with the struggles of belonging, representation, and inclusion the Elders were describing. As the Elders continued to share their stories, one of them suggested writing a statement for why they were demanding the statue be removed. They wanted to produce a statement— a manifesto, as one of them commented—and share it with city officials including the Mayor and the Cultural Commission Office. Doña K mentioned that I should write the statement, and several other Elders seemed to agree, adding that I—"*La Profe*" (professor)—could write it. I smiled, feeling humbled and grateful that they would involve me in their actions, yet also feeling out of place to write a statement for a struggle and movement that they had been leading for decades. I questioned my role in the movement and wondered why they were not owning their voice or experience to write the statement themselves. I paused to take in the responses and reactions that I was noticing over Zoom. I responded to Doña K that I could help support the writing of the statement, however, anything that was written must be with and from the perspective and experiences of the communities fighting for the statue's removal. I added that Doña K has the words and *sabiduria* (wisdom) to write, and that I could help edit and frame some of the arguments. Chale added, "we just don't have your fine words Profe!" causing people to laugh. I laughed too but out of nervousness. If we wanted the statement to be a testament, a manifesto, of what the Elders, and allied Chicanx and Latinx communities in San José organizing on this cause wanted, then it needed to reflect the voice of the community. In that moment, I acknowledge my outsider-ness, not as a limitation to my relationship with the collective at El Centro (The Center), but as a strategy that I could utilize to shift the spotlight onto those who were better positioned than I to lead actions toward change.

Although being asked to contribute to the development of the statement was intended to involve me in the process, perhaps because I was perceived as having the "words" or language to speak on these issues, and include me as one of them, I felt that it was not my place to tell the story of struggle, resistance, and movement building that many of the Elders present were a part of.

The community of El Centro—of which I was slowly becoming a part of and felt treated and seen as equal to them yet with a different set of expertise, resources, and privileges—had years of experience in grassroots organizing and movement building in San José that I did not have. Acknowledging the community's funds of knowledge and community cultural wealth (Fernández, Guzmán, et al., 2020) is an essential element of an embodied critical reflexivity oriented toward a decolonial community psychology. Additionally, they had the connections with city and county stakeholders that they could leverage to strategically organize to remove the statue. Producing a statement would complement their actions, along with the histories of struggles they all engaged and experienced still to this day. All of this needed to be a part of the story—the manifesto—they wanted to produce. An embodied critical reflexivity of one's positionalities in relation to and within communities, spaces, and contexts is necessary to ensure the sovereignty and determination of the communities themselves. As researchers, we should have the capacity and, indeed, the will and humility to discern when we are needed and how, and when what we may offer or may be asked to do may limit or minimize the power, determination and agency of communities who can act on their own power and wield resources for themselves.

As feminist scholars write and demonstrate through their work, theory is and must not be disconnected from emotions, and the body. Unlike other forms of knowledge production, which are usually from the top-down, an embodied critical reflexivity guided by one's theory in the flesh is a bottom-up process characterized by situated ways of knowing and orienting oneself in the research process. Knowledge and understanding, along with meaning making and consciousness, is derived from what is felt and lived physically, emotionally, psychologically, and through being in relationships or as part of a community, or both. This may also involve negotiating boundaries or *borderlands*, working through tensions, or sharing risk and vulnerability alongside joy and hope (Dutta, 2021; Reyes Cruz, 2008). Elsewhere I have described the notion of a theory in the flesh along with my own praxis (Fernández, 2018). Other critical community psychologists and feminist scholar–activists have also cited Anzaldúa and Moraga (1981; Bell et al., 2020; Guishard, 2019; Silva et al., 2021) to underscore the importance of engaging reflexivity. The engagement must come from the thoughts of those involved in the research, as well as from the body and feeling experienced by those who are a part of the process. Consistent with decolonial feminist community psychologists (Silva et al., 2021), and as the example I offered illustrates, an embodied critical reflexivity manifests in how ways of knowing, being, and connecting are read and understood by the self and others, and how this in turn shapes knowledge in action. Action is thus guided by what is known or understood. Knowing is fluid, purposeful, intentional, and active, a process of unlearning and relearning toward acting in the world and within communities, with a desire for transformation.

Intertwined Knowledge in Action

Knowledge is most often produced through experiences. What is known and understood is often associated with what is learned, engaged, and shared through purposeful behaviors, actions, and interactions. Varied sources of information are acquired through experiences that shape understanding as knowledge. Thus through these opportunities for interconnected actions, inquiry, and engagement unlearning and relearning take place. The unlearning-relearning cycles that are characteristic of reflection and inquiry resemble those that align with *conscientização* (Freire, 1970) or a critical consciousness. Critically understanding conditions of oppression, including the roots of intergenerational trauma, for example, is necessary to engage in transformative practices toward liberation and healing. Yet awareness of oppression alone is not enough to experience justice, liberation, and healing, nor is it sufficient for transformative systemic change. Critical consciousness should be followed and sustained through actions guided by collective desires to actualize liberation, and as the right to be recognized and cared for in one's fullest humanity (Montero et al., 2017; Watts & Serrano-García, 2003).

Collectively determined community-engaged opportunities for learning often via applied, directed, or purposeful strategies can help develop liberation-oriented interventions and actions. Silvia Rivera Cusicanqui (2012), for instance, described this process as *mestizaje de saberes* (hybridity in knowing or different ways of knowing). The collective and relational ways of creating knowledge is purported to be fundamental to community liberation because people come to know and understand their social condition by interconnecting their stories with place, histories, and movements. In resonance with Anzaldúa's notion of the borderlands and a *mestiza* consciousness, *mestizaje* describes hybridity or blending. It is also often used to describe the process of Spanish and Indigenous colonization that led to a caste system and a multiracial or multiethnic demographic in the Americas. The interwoven interconnected knowledge characteristic of hybrid experiences is a by-product of coloniality. Yet the hybridity of experience that Cusicanqui (2012) described is one in which cultural difference is embraced as fundamental to ways of being and knowing. Rather than viewing *mestizaje* as limiting or exclusionary, *mestizaje de saberes* asserts that the antagonizing or contradicting experiences that are a by-product of coloniality can often complement each other to produce pluriversality, which is diversity in knowing. Thus, when shared and shaped by communities (Ciofalo, 2019), knowledge can be engaged strategically to support collective actions to aid historically and institutionally marginalized communities in their thriving.

Although some knowledge is formally shared and passed down from generation to generation, it is often the informal and experiential knowledge that can lead to action—from resistance to resilience. Knowledge among communities that is co-constructed and dialectical can help shape the present moment, self-awareness, and understandings. Shared knowledge, what Bargero (2004) described as *saberes compartidos* (mutual or shared understandings), help shape institutions, organizations, and structures within existing systems, including those to be reformed. Coexisting with those whose experiences or subjectivities might be different from one's own characterizes the process of *saberes compartidos* as the intertwined knowledge that can inform action. To demonstrate interwoven knowledge in action, I offer a reflection of a research collaboration with a group of Mexican immigrant women, who referred to themselves as *madres* (mothers), and collectively as Madres Emprendedoras (Entrepreneurial Mothers; Fernández, Orozco, et al., 2020).[1]

> In the context of this participatory action research (PAR) project, the *madres* engaged photovoice as a method. Photovoice utilizes photographs, and corresponding narratives about those photos, as tools to help communities develop a critical social analysis about social problems. The *madres* utilized photovoice to help them discern issues in their school, community, and neighborhood, specifically what they wanted to see changed and addressed. Doña Maria proposed developing a project to support students with "special needs" or diversity in learning. She shared her story of struggle with the school district, and tireless advocacy for her child to receive education resources. She spoke powerfully about her experiences, and why this was an important issue for her and other *madres*. She took the mic, and some of the other *madres* joined

---

[1] Readers are encouraged to consult other publications where I have described with greater detail the *Madres Emprendedoras* and our collaborations (Fernández, Guzmán, et al., 2020; Fernández, Orozco, et al., 2020; Fernández & Silva, 2023). To learn more about the mural unveiling event, please see the 2018 Univision media coverage (https://www.univision.com/local/san-francisco-kdtv/revelan-mural-en-honor-de-las-mujeres-en-san-jose).

her in leading this project. Over the course of our months of collaborating, Doña Maria, with support of the *madres,* took the lead in developing an action project centered on addressing the needs of students. Doña Maria became the spokesperson for the project in the county's local radio station Radio La Kaliente, at the mural unveiling event featuring themes from their projects, and at public community and school gatherings. Stepping into her power, Doña Maria acted to demand change and affirmed her knowing. PAR is anchored in an ethic to help uplift individual and collective power forward among community members on the frontlines.

As illustrated in the reflection featuring the agency and leadership of Doña Maria, the knowledge Bargero (2004) described is organized to shape action toward change. Behaviors, like public *testimonio,* are how people come to understand and interact in their worlds and make calls for dignity and justice. It is through the experience of "mattering" that our existence or presence is valued in society (Prilleltensky, 2020), that our humanity is seen in honored and dignified ways when we care for and are being cared for by others in liberatory ways. By weaving and intertwining knowledge—ways of knowing, being, feeling and relating—actions are and can be engaged in what would otherwise be perceived as challenging if considered in isolation.

Intertwined knowledge, or *saberes compartidos,* can help researchers develop the necessary skills or capacities to better understand and therefore meet the needs of communities in ways that align with communities' cultural practices and strengths. Such ways of knowing and being can take multiple forms; however, experimental knowledge is inherited through intergenerational and translocal practices. In other words, interwoven knowledge is the mode of knowing through doing, acting, being, and existing. Reflexivity, in this case, is the collective participation in and the organization of knowledge that is woven, circulated, and shared. Such forms of knowledge may not be self-evident because they are informal parts of everyday experiences or interactions, yet it is here where understanding unfolds, and where the shaping of how people come to acknowledge and perceive such experiences begins. It is the relational knowledge that is formed and shaped through shared experiences, connections, and accompaniment—in essence, learning the value and significance of action for transformative justice through coexisting. New insights or sources of knowledge are acquired through meaningful, intentional, and purposeful engagement with others in context. Knowledge is not constructed or experienced for the sake of knowing, or the accumulation of information; on the contrary, it is experienced as an important fundamental source of information that can guide, facilitate, and animate action. Such understandings shape consciousness, as well as the relationships that are formed with others.

Radical Relationality

Renowned activist Angela Davis, in a speech delivered at the National Women's Conference, remarked that we must "wish to be radical in our quest for change" and "get to the root of our oppression." She added that "radical simply means grasping things at the root" (1988, p. 353). Thus, the term radical in radical relationality describes the capacity, will, and desire to foster relationships that run deep. Radical relationality is about being with and in connection with others through authentic genuine relationships. Instead of surface level or superficial relationships, radical relationality is "a process of simultaneously tracing our dynamic knowing as our experiences transform us" (Dutta, 2021, p. 604). A strategy toward a decolonial community psychology is cultivating or sustaining authentic genuine relationships that are founded on care and solidarity with communities, thus fostering radical relationality.

Radical relationality requires a commitment to be in communion and mutuality with communities in struggle. The relationships formed may involve sharing, cobeing, or coexisting in nontransactional ways. The collective experience of knowing through relating and coexisting in community with others describes a radical relationality informed by shared lived experiences. Although some experiences may be perceived as different or distinct among individuals, threads of connectedness are formed and shared, fostering community. The process of transformation, evolution, and growth toward liberation and thriving necessitates radically being with and among others to allow for transparency and accountability to be enacted.

One goal of radical relationality is to challenge and disrupt the hierarchies, bifurcations, and dichotomies in research, especially within more collaborative or participatory domains. Radical relationality goes beyond the mere expression of having a relationship or interaction with communities. Indeed, it is aimed at challenging and extending research approaches, and paradigms that challenge hegemonic relations informed by and reproduced through colonial arrangements. The colonial relations are often reflected in positivist research perspectives that label researchers as credible experts, and communities as subjects or objects of inquiry. Epistemic violence is reproduced through research paradigms where communities are studied, observed, and examined, or sought out for information, thereby not recognized as holders and producers of knowledge (Dutta, 2021). To illustrate, I offer a fieldnote from a research collaboration with Women of Color student activists at a predominantly White institution where we use participatory action research to support student activists' sociopolitical development.

As the academic year comes to an end and students in the Sociopolitical Citizenship Participatory Action Research (SC-PAR) Project, whom I have collaborated with for the past four years graduate, I am reminded about the power of providing students with meaningful opportunities to engage research, to see themselves as holders and producers of knowledge, and as agents of change who can utilize research as a tool to challenge existing hegemonic discourses at a White neoliberal institution, and to create a care through relational solidarities among ourselves as Women of Color—students, faculty, and staff alike. During the end of year ceremony, two students remarked how through their participation and engagement in SC-PAR they saw themselves as capable of producing knowledge that countered what the administration was consistently purporting yet not fully enacting. The expression "we see you, we hear you," yet nothing being concretely done to redress the racism and anti-Black discrimination that students experience, contributed to students documenting their stories, featuring these in a digital archive under the student voices section of the AntiRacist Teaching Collective website, as well as in their senior capstone projects. Witnessing students come into their power, share experiences of anger alongside the joy, possibility, and radical hope, affirms for me the power of being in community—of being connected and in solidarity with struggles that are differentially experienced. We are bearing witness and acting together to transform the university conditions that challenge our capacities to exist and thrive.

As illustrated, radical relationality involves sharing risks and vulnerabilities, along with the imagination and desire of something different from what is being experienced. The connectivity among us in the SC-PAR collective is characterized by our will to see, hear, and feel as well as to act collectively and with students who, given the culture and history of higher education, are often made to feel excluded, marginalized, unwelcomed, and othered within the university. The relationships of community care, commitment, and mutuality continue and often unfold in other ways even after students graduate or their collaboration in SC-PAR concludes. This sense of mutual commitment and accompaniment with one another underscores a key feature of radical relationality; our relationships are not bound by a project, time, or context, but instead are sustained through shared experiences, relational solidarities, and deep authentic care.

Radical relationality, however, should not be interpreted as a voyeuristic process. In other words, it should not be understood as a naive illusion that by merely coexperiencing life with and in the presence of communities, profound humanizing relationships can be formed or sustained. What sets radical relationality apart from other modes of being in relationship with people is the centrality of sharing the risks, tensions, vulnerabilities, and challenges. As scholar–activists, Dutta (2021) and Atallah (2017) enacted solidarities with communities that aim to build coalitions for healing and transformative justice. To demonstrate radical relationality, Dutta and Atallah each offered reflections from collaborations with Miya and Palestinian communities. Miya communities, for example, engage poetry as a strategy to affirm their humanity and collective power before consistent systemic violence and disenfranchisement (Dutta, 2021).

Similarly, Palestinian communities enact intergenerational resilience through storytelling, narratives, and rituals, which are passed down among families and communities (Atallah, 2017). This practice of "embroidering emotions" through storying fosters relationality and resilience, which are necessary to transgress and challenge conditions of intergenerational trauma, structural violence, and displacement ensued through coloniality and imperial hegemony. Radical relationality, therefore, is characterized as a process of rehumanizing research. The rehumanizing process unfolds through affective bonds and connections grounded in shared storying, refusal, and decolonial praxes. Indeed, Atallah (2017) and Dutta (2021) showed the importance of being human together, sharing hope alongside struggles while taking collective risks. In pursuit of community liberation, they intentionally and purposefully embody radical relationality. Through actions and values oriented toward radical relationality, creative coalitional building is thus possible.

Knowledge as a process and outcome of being with others, in what is characterized as a relational experience, is constructed through an intentional iterative and consistent practice of coexistence. By cocreating knowledge through relationships, people invite a sense of openness to complexity, listening with critical compassion and curiosity, as well as introspection or reflection. When done collectively, this can facilitate experiences for reimagining and embracing change, uncertainty, and complexity, which often comes with a degree of tension. Related to these challenges are experiencing possibilities to enact equity and justice so that liberation can be actualized. Thus enacting liberatory values can lead to a mutual responsibility to bring freedom into reality. Bell et al. (2020) described this as decolonial imaginings, or utopian militant hope for an otherwise, where radical dreaming is possible through shared experiences. When experiences of struggle are examined, they create a desire for something different—for SC-PAR this means a decolonial, humanizing university.

Radical relationality requires being attuned to the complexities of lived experiences. It is the desire to experience life in accompaniment with others through inclusive opportunities for shared reflection, dialogue, risk, and joy. Unique to radical relationality is a commitment to engaging in an embodied critical reflexivity that includes a sociopolitical structural analysis of power, privilege, and oppression, and the subjective affectivities that can lead to deeper ways of knowing and connecting (Dutta, 2021). Radical relationality can be understood as an approach toward accompaniment, which psychologists describe as psychosocial accompaniment (Watkins, 2015). Psychosocial accompaniment as a form of radical relationality is a practice of engaging in critical inquiry through active listening, witnessing, advocacy, and solidarity. As a critical approach toward enacting accompaniment, radical relationality is rooted in liberation and epistemic justice—two interconnected principles that reflect the last strategy: transdisciplinarity.

Transdisciplinarity

Transdisciplinarity aims to expand the ecologies of knowledge, the epistemological paradigms of community psychology toward the goal of epistemic justice and liberation. As a strategy that aligns with decoloniality, transdisciplinarity describes the importance of extending and expanding community psychology to engage other epistemologies, ontological standpoints, and perspectives within and beyond the field. Although U.S.-based community psychology is predominantly grounded in the behavioral sciences, specifically a biomedical paradigm toward the clinical and health sciences, which are concerned with the relationship between the mind and body, other allied disciplines have had an influence as well. As an evolving and growing discipline, sociology, anthropology, and education have contributed theoretical perspectives or methodologies to community psychology in some direct or tangential way.

Reflecting on her professional trajectory as a community psychologist, Serrano-García (2008) stresses the importance of transdisciplinarity, specifically, the importance of approaching community concerns and social problems central to community psychology from multiple perspectives, from public health and policy to education. Community psychologists must engage transdisciplinary, and transnational/regional collaborations, which may extend beyond academe, and the United States. Transdisciplinarity can contribute to expanding existing theory, research, and practice to align with liberation (Serrano-García, 2020; Watts & Serrano-García, 2003).

As critical community psychologists demonstrate, transdisciplinarity strives to purposefully link multiple disciplines to better understand and address community issues. This allows for a structural systems-level analysis complemented by a sociohistorical understanding of social conditions. In relation to the work of Serrano-García (2020), for instance, the structural and sociohistorical analyses facilitate a consciousness of coloniality and colonialism.

Moreover, these understandings inform how colonialism continues to shape Puerto Rican communities' experiences of struggle, resistance, and calls for sovereignty. These threads are made in relation to an embodied critical reflexivity and sociopolitical analysis (Serrano-García, 2008), as well as a disciplinary, epistemic, and theoretical development (Serrano-García, 1984, 2008, 2020). Similarly, Reyes Cruz (2008) described the importance of unsettling the imperial legacies of colonialism to better understand the challenges and social conditions of Puerto Rican communities on the island and the mainland. As community psychologists, Reyes Cruz (2008) and Serrano-García (2008) offer an intersectional perspective of marginalization that renders visible possibilities for transformative justice because social issues are approached from an ecological analysis and a sociohistorical understanding that goes beyond the discipline. Transdisciplinarity is imperative for an in-depth critical, sociocultural, and structural analysis of inequities experienced by communities who live with and resist the coloniality of power.

Community psychology stands to benefit from transdisciplinarity. Considering the histories that formed the discipline's values, the commitment to liberation is not disciplinary but rather epistemic (Sonn et al., 2017). Other disciplines, like ethnic studies for example, have similar trajectories of resistance, applied research, and solidarities tied to social movements. In writing about the foundations and legacies of ethnic studies in the United States, Maldonado-Torres (2019) describes transdisciplinarity as a decolonial strategy that contributes to projects aligned with decolonization that are unbound by disciplinary conventions as determined by the academy. Transdisciplinarity "is an epistemic decolonial turn that suspends methods and disciplines through decolonization as a project and attitude" (Maldonado-Torres, 2019, p. 242). A transdisciplinary strategy is aligned with a decolonial consciousness to deconstruct systems of power that inform praxes that may compromise epistemic justice, freedom, and liberation.

Participatory action research as a transdisciplinary paradigm to support the process of inquiry, knowledge production, and action is often used within U.S.-based community psychology. PAR is multidisciplinary and grassroots oriented and often used by educators, organizers, practitioners, and academics alike. A strength of PAR is that it strives to deconstruct, and even blur the line, between researchers and the researched; the who in the process of knowledge production, the what in the knowledge being produced, and the why or toward what knowledge is the end goal. Although PAR is offered as an example, the unregimented efforts that transdisciplinarity affords can help transform the field of community psychology in ways that can contribute to its goals of liberation, transformative justice, and well-being.

To demonstrate the value of transdisciplinarity I offer some reflections from the Roots and Routes of Decoloniality in Community Psychology (RRD-CP) Project, which is a transnational collaboration with Christopher Sonn, among other colleagues in the Majority World: Garth Stevens and Ronelle Carolissen in South Africa, James Ferreira Moura in Brazil, and Monica Madyaningrum in Indonesia. Through this collaboration, we have engaged in transdisciplinary reflexive dialogues that are informed by critical, decolonial, postcolonial, feminist, and Indigenous epistemologies and by praxes that span a range of disciplines—from traditional fields like education, philosophy, sociology, and anthropology to critical race and ethnic studies, women, gender, and queer studies, as well as Black and Indigenous studies.

> The RRD-CP Project is a transnational collaboration among critical community psychologists engaging in reflections and dialogues on decoloniality within and beyond community psychology, and allied disciplines. Our connections and collaborations are anchored in questions and tensions within community psychology and the direction of the discipline.
>
> We, Jesica and Chris, were brought together by shared questions on the relationship between psychology, specifically community psychology and decoloniality, in relation to and distinct from liberation. In particular, we wanted to learn how community psychology, and community psychologists, engage in the decolonial turn. Furthemore, how a decolonial standpoint informs community psychology theory, research and practice, as well as decolonial critical community psychology praxis.
>
> The purpose of the RRD-CP Project is to document these processes and practices, as well as orientations, standpoints and approaches toward decoloniality and decolonization within community psychology. Hence, the metaphor of the roots and routes, which we reference to underscore the foundations of community psychology that have strived toward de-linking from Western-Eurocentric logics and perspectives, as well as the coloniality of power. In doing so we seek to contribute to the development, cultivation and sustainability of decolonial, decolonizing and anti-colonial praxes within the discipline, and toward a decolonial critical community psychology. (Community Identity Displacement Research Network, 2016, para. 1–3)

Although our collaboration is grounded within the discipline of community psychology, we are located across varied geographies and regions, each with our unique history, and within different institutions, departments, and affiliations. What we share is the process and practice of transgressing disciplinary boundaries, of moving and shapeshifting between disciplines as we are in conversation with each other, guided and informed by our colearning process that is inclusive of varied epistemologies and theories. We are engaged in a pluriversal psychology where many psychologies, or approaches to knowing and understanding the self, others, and our world, can fit.

Community psychology stands to benefit from this process of blurring the line as it purports a commitment to community determination and power to create conditions that can actualize justice, liberation, and sustained well-being. Fundamental to transdisciplinarity is the symbiotic relationship of knowledge, politics, and activism, as well as art and innovation—that is, the blurring of what is described as "spheres of knowledge production" (Maldonado-Torres, 2019) with the goal of creating a fluid way of thinking: a dissident and dissenting attitude. Moreover, a critical inquiry praxis that is unbounded by the perspectives or expectations of any discipline to facilitate creative innovation, radical imagination, and freedom dreaming (Bell et al., 2020). A transdisciplinary approach is best characterized by borderland theory, which Anzaldúa described via disciplinary and nondisciplinary orientations, including, and perhaps most important, her lived experience. The borderlands that describe the liminality of being and knowing is a site of power. Standing at the crossroads of multiple forms of knowing can produce tension. Yet, from a decolonial liberation standpoint, this can foster a radical imagination or creative potential to foster epistemic justice for transformation and emancipatory liberations. Transdisciplinarity involves crossing, bridging, and connecting differential, perhaps contradictory or opposing disciplinary orientations, perspectives, and paradigms (Fernández et al., 2021; Sonn et al., 2017), as well as histories of coloniality and epistemic violence (Comas-Díaz et al., 1998). The crossing or tension is not intended to set disciplines apart or create divisions, but instead to provide practitioners with theories, practices, tools, skills, and approaches for a community psychology that is inclusive of alternative forms of knowledge. Transdisciplinarity as a decolonial psychological praxes can thus work to support liberation.

CONCLUSION: TOWARD A DECOLONIAL COMMUNITY PSYCHOLOGY

To support the development of a decolonial U.S. community psychology practice, four proposed interconnected strategies are described in this chapter. In calling for a decolonial community psychology praxis, I provide a historical overview of the discipline, locating the initial disruptions of the field; specifically, the rupture from conventional, more traditional approaches in psychology, such as clinical psychology, toward social or applied political and critical psychologies. The community-oriented psychology of decades past did not respond sufficiently to the urgencies of the 1960s sociopolitical movements. Against this backdrop, four strategies are described through autoethnographic vignettes.

In briefly tracing the dominant narrative of U.S.-based community psychology, I have sought to describe how this history, and the discipline's genealogy, accounts for the tensions or disruptions in the field. Community psychology strives to be a responsive and responsible discipline, yet it continues to often fall short of actualizing its values and principles because it still demands recognition and validation from the broader general field of psychology. By acknowledging the past, the historical sociopolitical context that led to establishing community psychology in the United States more than five decades ago, and how this differed from how it developed in the Majority World, has at its foundation a practice of dissent, specifically, of striving to be something different, transgressive, and critical of the norm and status quo with the goal of aligning with community struggles for freedom and liberation.

Over the past decade interest in a decolonial standpoint has grown. As Communities of Color continue to affirm the rights to belong within varied institutions, and to demand access to resources, opportunities, and enfranchisement, coloniality has become a topic of concern. Coloniality continues to structure societies, including ways of knowing, being, and relating to the world. Coloniality outlives colonialism, and community psychology with its attentiveness to context is not absolved from colonial relations of power (Fernández et al., 2021). We need to approach the decolonization of the discipline with a stronghold commitment to reckoning with critical histories in the United States. This is especially important for those of us in the United States, where genocide, settler violence, and slavery led to establishing a hegemonic imperial nation-state responsible for the inequities experienced globally—from climate change to economic precarity to militarized violence, displacement, and occupation.

How can we cultivate a critical decolonial community psychology that is attuned to the local in relation to the historic and contemporary, to the national and transnational, to the individual and the collective? We need to engage in and develop strategies that can help deepen the discipline to support decolonial community liberation, specifically, cultivating the sovereignty of communities to determine the conditions of their living and well-being by practices that affirm their humanity. The movements that have continued to resurface on racial freedom, gender justice, and economic equity are relevant today as they were decades ago. These strategies are an offering, a proposal, and an invitation to consider what can be, and to reimagine and retool the field so that it may more adequately, ethically, socioculturally, and relationally attend to social issues and critical inquiries for epistemic justice that can actualize liberation.

RESOURCES

Concordia University. (2016, March 20). *Decolonizing methodologies: Can relational research be a basis for renewed relationships?* [Video]. YouTube. https://www.youtube.com/watch?v=rqYiCrZKmOM&t=190s

Data Center. (2013, July 22). *Decolonizing knowledge* [Video]. YouTube. https://www.youtube.com/watch?v=7Ib7edhWghY&t=4658s

Society for the Psychological Study of Social Issues. (2019, February 22). *Toward a decolonial psychology: Three scholars in North American settings* [Video]. YouTube. https://www.youtube.com/watch?v=IVUgdCmianU&t=102s

REFERENCES

Anzaldúa, G., & Moraga, C. (1981). *This bridge called my back: Writings by radical women of color.* Kitchen Table: Women of Color Press.

Atallah, D. G. (2017). A community-based qualitative study of intergenerational resilience with Palestinian refugee families facing structural violence and historical trauma. *Transcultural Psychiatry, 54*(3), 357–383. https://doi.org/10.1177/1363461517706287

Bargero, M. (2004). Saberes compartidos, entendimiento mutuo, instituciones y ordenamientos Sociales [Shared knowledge, mutual understanding, institutions and social regulations]. *VI Jornadas de Sociología.* Universidad de Buenos Aires.

Bell, D., Canham, H., Dutta, U., & Fernández, J. S. (2020). Retrospective autoethnographies: A call for decolonial imaginings for the new university. *Qualitative Inquiry, 26*(7), 849–859. https://doi.org/10.1177/1077800419857743

Boonzaier, F., & van Niekerk, T. (Eds.). (2019). *Decolonial feminist community psychology.* Springer. https://doi.org/10.1007/978-3-030-20001-5

Chang, H. (2008). *Autoethnography as method.* Left Coast Press.

Ciofalo, N. (2019). Indigenous psychologies: A contestation for epistemic justice. In N. Ciofalo (Ed.), *Indigenous psychologies in an era of decolonization* (pp. 1–38). Springer Nature. https://doi.org/10.1007/978-3-030-04822-8_1

Comas-Díaz, L., Lykes, M. B., & Alarcón, R. D. (1998). Ethnic conflict and the psychology of liberation in Guatemala, Peru, and Puerto Rico. *American Psychologist, 53*(7), 778–792. https://doi.org/10.1037/0003-066X.53.7.778

Community Identity Displacement Research Network. (2016). *Roots & Routes of Decoloniality in Community Psychology (RRD-CP) project: A transnational survey of decolonial discourse in community psychology praxis.* https://www.community-identity.com.au/portfolio/roots-routes-of-decoloniality-in-community-psychology-rrd-cp-project-a-transnational-survey-of-decolonial-discourse-in-community-psychology-praxis/

Cusicanqui, S. R. (2012). Ch'ixinakax utxiwa: A reflection on the practices and discourses of decolonization. *The South Atlantic Quarterly, 111*(1), 95–109. https://doi.org/10.1215/00382876-1472612

Davis, A. Y. (1988). Let us all rise together: Radical perspectives on empowerment for Afro-American women. Address to Spelman College. *Harvard Educational Review, 58*(3), 348–354. https://doi.org/10.17763/haer.58.3.32147541624550x3

Dutta, U. (2021). The politics and poetics of "fieldnotes": Decolonizing ethnographic knowing. *Qualitative Inquiry, 27*(5), 598–607. https://doi.org/10.1177/1077800420935919

Dutta, U., Sonn, C. C., & Lykes, M. B. (2016). Situating and contesting structural violence in community-based research and action. *Community Psychology in Global Perspective, 2*(2), 1–20.

Fanon, F. (1967). *Black skin, white masks*. Grove.

Fernández, J. S. (2018). Toward an ethical reflective practice of a *theory in the flesh*: Embodied subjectivities in a youth participatory action research mural project. *American Journal of Community Psychology, 62*(1–2), 221–232. https://doi.org/10.1002/ajcp.12264

Fernández, J. S., Guzmán, B. L., Bernal, I., & Flores, Y. G. (2020). *Muxeres en acción*: The power of community cultural wealth in Latinas organizing for health equity. *American Journal of Community Psychology, 66*(3–4), 314–324. https://doi.org/10.1002/ajcp.12442

Fernández, J. S., Orozco, A. R., Rodriguez, P., Cermeño, I. E., & Nichols, L. (2020). *Madres emprendedoras*, entrepreneurial mothers: Reflections from a community-based participatory action research course with Mexican immigrant *madres* in the Silicon Valley. *Peace and Conflict, 26*(2), 181–191. https://doi.org/10.1037/pac0000403

Fernández, J. S., & Silva, J. M. (2023). Is there room for more?: Considering the need for a decoloniality community psychology core competency. *Global Journal of Community Psychology Practice, 14*(1), 1–21.

Fernández, J. S., Sonn, C., Carolissen, R., & Stevens, G. (2021). Roots and routes toward decoloniality within and outside psychology praxis. *Review of General Psychology, 25*(4), 354–368. https://doi.org/10.1177/10892680211002437

Fine, M. (2015). Global provocations: Critical reflections on community based research and intervention designed at the intersections of global dynamics and local cultures. *Community Psychology in Global Perspective, 1*(1), 5–15.

Freire, P. (1970). *Pedagogy of the oppressed*. Continuum.

Guishard, M. (2019). Dear Barbara T. y Gloria E.: Autoethnographic letters to Blacktina Nepantla acrobats. In G. Y. Acosta (Ed.), *Latina outsiders remaking Latina identity* (pp. 129–139). Routledge. https://doi.org/10.4324/9780429401558-20

Jenkins, R. A. (2016). Clinical community psychology: Reflections on the decades following Swampscott. *American Journal of Community Psychology, 58*(3–4), 269–275. https://doi.org/10.1002/ajcp.12040

Jones, S. H. (1998). Turning the kaleidoscope, re-visioning an ethnography. *Qualitative Inquiry, 4*(3), 421–441. https://doi.org/10.1177/107780049800400307

Kagan, C., Burton, M., Duckett, P., Lawthom, R., & Siddiquee, A. (2019). *Critical community psychology: Critical action and social change*. Routledge. https://doi.org/10.4324/9780429431500

Kessi, S., Suffla, S., & Seedat, M. (2021). *Decolonial enactments in community psychology*. Springer.

Kloos, B., Hill, J., Thomas, E., Wandersman, A., & Elias, M. J. (2012). *Community psychology: Linking individuals and communities*. Cengage Learning.

Levine, M., Perkins, D. D., & Perkins, D. V. (2005). *Principles of community psychology: Perspectives and applications*. Oxford University Press.

Maldonado-Torres, N. (2019). Ethnic studies as decolonial transdisciplinarity. *Ethnic Studies Review, 42*(2), 232–244. https://doi.org/10.1525/esr.2019.42.2.232

Martín-Baró, I. (1994). *Writings for a liberation psychology.* Harvard University Press.

Montero, M., Sonn, C. C., & Burton, M. (2017). Community psychology and liberation psychology: A creative synergy for an ethical and transformative praxis. In M. A. Bond, I. Serrano-García, C. B. Keys, & M. Shinn (Eds.), *APA handbook of community psychology: Theoretical foundations, core concepts, and emerging challenges* (pp. 149–167). American Psychological Association. https://doi.org/10.1037/14953-007

Moradi, B., & Grzanka, P. R. (2017). Using intersectionality responsibly: Toward critical epistemology, structural analysis, and social justice activism. *Journal of Counseling Psychology, 64*(5), 500–513. https://doi.org/10.1037/cou0000203

Perkins, D. D. (2009). The death of community psychology (and the development of community research and action) in the United States: Issues of theoretical, methodological, and practical diversity. In C. Vazquez Rivera, D. Perez Jimenez, M. Figueroa Rodriquez, & W. Pacheco Bou (Eds.), *International community psychology: Shared agendas in diversity* (pp. 285–314). Activitidades de Formacion Communitaria.

Pillay, S. R. (2017). Cracking the fortress: Can we really decolonize psychology? *South African Journal of Psychology. Suid-Afrikaanse Tydskrif vir Sielkunde, 47*(2), 135–140. https://doi.org/10.1177/0081246317698059

Prilleltensky, I. (1994). *The morals and politics of psychology: Psychological discourse and the status quo.* SUNY Press.

Prilleltensky, I. (2020). Mattering at the intersection of psychology, philosophy, and politics. *American Journal of Community Psychology, 65*(1–2), 16–34. https://doi.org/10.1002/ajcp.12368

Quijano, A. (2000). Coloniality of power and Eurocentrism in Latin America. *International Sociology, 15(2),* 215–232. https://doi.org/10.1177/0268580900015002005

Rappaport, J. (1977). *Community psychology: Values, research, and action.* Holt, Rinehart & Winston.

Reich, S. M., Bishop, B., Carolissen, R., Dzidic, P., Portillo, N., Sasao, T., & Stark, W. (2017). Catalysts and connections: The (brief) history of community psychology throughout the world. In M. A. Bond, I. Serrano-García, C. B. Keys, & M. Shinn (Eds.), *APA handbook of community psychology: Theoretical foundations, core concepts, and emerging challenges* (pp. 21–66). American Psychological Association. https://doi.org/10.1037/14953-002

Reyes Cruz, M. (2008). What if I just cite Graciela? Working toward decolonizing knowledge through a critical ethnography. *Qualitative Inquiry, 14*(4), 651–658. https://doi.org/10.1177/1077800408314346

Reyes Cruz, M., & Sonn, C. C. (2011). (De)colonizing culture in community psychology: Reflections from critical social science. *American Journal of Community Psychology, 47*(1–2), 203–214. https://doi.org/10.1007/s10464-010-9378-x

Rosenthal, L. (2016). Incorporating intersectionality into psychology: An opportunity to promote social justice and equity. *American Psychologist, 71*(6), 474–485. https://doi.org/10.1037/a0040323

Seedat, M., & Suffla, S. (2017). Community psychology and its (dis)contents, archival legacies and decolonization. *South African Journal of Psychology. Suid-Afrikaanse Tydskrif vir Sielkunde, 47*(4), 421–431. https://doi.org/10.1177/0081246317741423

Serrano-García, I. (1984). The illusion of empowerment: Community development within a colonial context. In J. Rappaport, R. Hess, & C. Swift (Eds.), *Studies in empowerment: Steps toward understanding the psychological mechanisms in preventive interventions* (pp. 173–200). Haworth Press.

Serrano-García, I. (2008). To be different: The challenge of social-community psychology. *Journal of Prevention & Intervention in the Community, 35*(1), 45–59. https://doi.org/10.1300/J005v35n01_04

Serrano-García, I. (2020). Resilience, coloniality, and sovereign acts: The role of community activism. *American Journal of Community Psychology, 65*(1–2), 3–12. https://doi.org/10.1002/ajcp.12415

Silva, J. M., Fernández, J. S., & Nguyen, A. (2021). "And now we resist": Three *testimonios* on the importance of decoloniality within psychology. *Journal of Social Issues, 78*(2), 1–25.

Sonn, C., Arcidiacono, C., Dutta, U., Kiguwa, P., Kloos, B., & Maldonado Torres, N. (2017). Beyond disciplinary boundaries: Speaking back to critical knowledges, liberation, and community. *South African Journal of Psychology. Suid-Afrikaanse Tydskrif vir Sielkunde, 47*(4), 448–458. https://doi.org/10.1177/0081246317737930

Tebes, J. K. (2016). Reflections on the future of community psychology from the generations after Swampscott: A commentary and introduction to the special issue. *American Journal of Community Psychology, 58*(3–4), 229–238. https://doi.org/10.1002/ajcp.12110

Trickett, E. J. (1996). A future for community psychology: The contexts of diversity and the diversity of contexts. *American Journal of Community Psychology, 24*(2), 209–234. https://doi.org/10.1007/BF02510399

Watkins, M. (2015). Psychosocial accompaniment. *Journal of Social and Political Psychology, 3*(1), 324–341. https://doi.org/10.5964/jspp.v3i1.103

Watts, R. J., & Serrano-García, I. (2003). The quest for a liberating community psychology: An overview. *American Journal of Community Psychology, 31*(1–2), 73–78. https://doi.org/10.1023/A:1023022603667

7

DECOLONIZING IN A TRANSNATIONAL FEMINIST COMMONS PERCHED PRECARIOUSLY BETWEEN THE ACADEMY AND MOVEMENTS FOR JUSTICE

ADREANNE ORMOND, PULENG SEGALO, MARÍA ELENA TORRE, AND MICHELLE FINE

Dedicated to the little girl in Cornwall, South Africa, with "unpresentable hair."

We write as a quartet of decolonial feminists, scholars, activists, family, and friends dedicated to critical, community-based inquiry rooted in movements and communities close to our hearts: Puleng in Pretoria, South Africa; Adreanne in Mahia, New Zealand; María and Michelle in New York City, United States. We have been deeply connected for decades, with winds blowing our ideas back and forth across oceans and national borders, and most recently over Zoom. We meet, in the stretchy simultaneous space of Zoom, splintering time zones and datelines, time-traveling instantly between the northeastern coast of the United States, Pretoria, and Mahia, to share insights and incites, wisdoms and questions, dilemmas and ethical quandaries, and lately our beleaguered sense of "Is our work enough?" We study and engage with concerns of the global environmental crises, acute in Aotearoa, Mahia, and state and intimate violence against women and femicide, and the brutal impact of the carceral state on Women of Color and those surviving in poverty, in both South Africa and the United States.

https://doi.org/10.1037/0000376-008
Decolonial Psychology: Toward Anticolonial Theories, Research, Training, and Practice,
L. Comas-Díaz, H. Y. Adames, and N. Y. Chavez-Dueñas (Editors)

In this chapter, we sketch our emergent decolonizing feminisms in research and pedagogy (Fanon, 1961; Lugones, 2007, 2010; L. Smith, 2012), making visible, with humility, how we root our teaching and psychological inquiries in historical and contemporary struggles (Anzaldúa, 1987; Bryant-Davis & Comas-Díaz, 2016; Dutta et al., 2016; Fine & Torre, 2021; Martín-Baró, 1994; Segalo & Fine, 2020). We unpack how we engage epistemic justice (de Sousa Santos, 2014) in our research collectives and our classrooms—centering, with fierce commitment, knowledges well beyond the academy and collective wisdoms borne in social movements. In our home spaces, we collaborate with youth climate activists in Aotearoa, women in and out of prison in New York and women in an embroidery collective in South African townships. In this chapter, we try to show how we conjure a homegrown, transnational feminist commons (Butler, 2011; Ticktin, 2020), where we share ideas, tensions, readings, struggles, despair, and radical creativities across our varied sites of work. Over the last two decades, we have visited each other's communities, Zooming across, sharing students, writing together, always trying to decipher what critical geographers have called the *glocal*—that what is locally constituted on and by those most affected by injustice, and what stretches across geographies, in terms of both brutal oppressions and vibrant forms of collective resistance. We consider both an obligation of the university: To align with local movements and to reach across transnational borders to trace the brutal vestiges of oppression and the vibrant forms of resistance and reimagination.

Collectively, we aim to provoke a liberatory praxis (Ayala et al., 2018; Bryant-Davis & Comas-Díaz, 2016; Comas-Díaz, 2020; Fernández et al., 2021; Mosley et al., 2020), rooted in collectives of inquiry, aligned with movements for justice, attentive to power inequities, and ignited by radical liberatory imaginations. Even as, or especially because, we sit in academic spaces, we organize to pierce the walls of the ivory tower, disrupt notions of objectivity as distance, introduce analyses from the radical margins into our scholarship and syllabi, and take seriously the responsibility—and joy—of decolonizing academic work with public science. As we link our home spaces, we grow theory, methods, ethics, epistemologies, and radical pedagogies through and within a created transnational space.

As you might imagine, our worlds and her-stories are very different, but we share deeply held values and ethics that makes our solidarity meaningful and possible. Our research collectives in classrooms, schools, prisons, and communities are built on and nourish an understanding of *nos-otras*, a "we" made of us and others (Anzaldúa, 1987; Torre, 2009) and are rooted in epistemologies that bend toward the wisdom of those most affected by structural, historic, environmental, gendered, or racial violence (Martín-Baró, 1994).

Our ethics stretch well beyond informed consent, into the messy spaces created in solidarity and care (Guishard et al., 2018). Our designs take many forms—quantitative, qualitative, aesthetic, archival, and performance based, and always hold history, intersectionality, and multiplicities (Anzaldúa, 1987; Ayala et al., 2018; Cole, 2009; Crenshaw, 1991; Du Bois, 1903; Fanon, 1961; Weis & Fine, 2012). Our praxis is accountable to those who came before, those who still struggle, and those who have yet to come. The results of our inquiries materialize into journal articles and embroideries, legal briefs, community zines, murals, and white papers, with a humble hope to "be of use" to communities and movements under siege (Piercy, 1982).

With this chapter, we unpack the intimate details of our decolonizing praxis. We ask ourselves, and you, in these days of COVID-19 and racial reckonings, rising White nationalisms and authoritarian regimes, to whom your scholarship or praxis is accountable (Uzwiak & Bowles, 2021). Indeed, when María and Michelle begin a new research project, with community partners who are coresearchers and eventually usually friends, we take the time—all of us—to write letters of accountability, that begin simply. Each person in the research collective—traditional researcher, youth activist, woman in prison or recently out, young person in foster care, elders in a community saturated in police violence—is asked the question, "Let's think about for whom or to whom (y)our work is accountable. Who sits in your heart as you take up this inquiry? It could be a future child, a mountain, an elder, your younger self, someone you see but do not yet know, a river, someone recently passed, a spirit . . . and write for 15 minutes." The letters read like this: "Dear XXX: I think of you often, and I want you to know. . . ."

These letters of accountability begin the decolonizing praxis; reminding each and all of us that research does not have to be an abstract activity designed to gather a degree or get tenure, it can be an intentional act of love with and for, inquiry launched alongside and in support of movements, nourished by the words, actions and courage of elders long gone that echo in our being. People write to once pristine rivers now polluted, a grandmother who has passed, relatives left behind in war-torn countries, neighborhoods gentrified, men and women who remain in prison, children who have died of drug overdoses or police violence. . . . In this way the research allows for entangled relations between humans, the natural world, and the systems that surround and shape us, and in so doing endows the work with a multiplicity of connections that provide a rich sense of purpose.

And so we ask you, the reader, to do the same. We invite you into our intimate space where both our homegrown and well-studied versions of decolonizing feminisms unfold and are always debated, where our research grows, where friendships and sweet solidarities and care hold us amid global winds of rising violence and injustice, and as the miracle of enduring resistance, caresses.

Adreanne, Puleng, María, and Michelle

****

Freedom's Journal, the first African American newspaper in the United States, issued a call in 1827 urging African people who were violently taken to the Americas and forced into slavery to tell their stories. They published the following statement: "We wish to plead our case. Too long have others spoken for us. Too long has the publick been deceived by misrepresentations in things which concern us dearly" (Alexandre, 2023). The urgency of the words inked in *Freedom's Journal* persist around the globe today as calls for decolonization are advanced and reimagined (Kiddle et al., 2020). Within the academy, decolonizing practices and community-based or engaged work has been commodified and misrepresented, becoming a public-facing, neoliberal university brand. We worry about this slippery trend, which is why we situate ourselves delicately at the dangerous and joyous membrane between university and community and balance ourselves by holding hands across national borders.

In the face of the daunting challenges of our time, it is essential that universities and communities form partnerships of trust and walk hand in hand across the bridge that connects us. We must recognize that knowledge creation is not the sole domain of the academia and embrace the diverse perspectives, experiences, and aspirations of communities. Using cocreative dialogue, we can build bridges between academia and communities, grandmothers and professors, ancestral landscapes, spirits and entities and cocreate knowledge that is grounded in community knowing. This partnering can break down the colonial and western traditions that separate academic research from lived experience and empower individuals, communities, more-than-human entities, and ancestral ecologies to help resolve the issues that threaten life as we know it and build a just and equitable society. In this vision of a future world, knowledge flows freely and openly between the diverse knowledge holders and the perspectives they hold are valued and respected. Together, hand in hand, we can, we must, embark on a transformative journey to cocreate a future of hope.

We call for new and old ways of knowing, being and doing, and look to Indigenous ontological, epistemological, axiological praxis, decolonial feminisms, and critical participatory action research for support. We commit, on very distinct lands, to contest "misrepresentations in things which concern us dearly." We engage what María and others call PAR Entre-mundos— a participatory inquiry praxis nourished in the fragile yet powerful spaces "between worlds," speaking alongside and with communities under siege (Torre & Ayala 2009; Ayala et al., 2018). Sketching a public science (Torre et al., 2012), by and for the people (Martín-Baró, 1994), our projects and our teaching seek to assert the dignity and rights of those most affected to shape policy, build theory, claim legitimacy, educate publics, preserve radical histories, build archives, demand reparations, correct the historic record, disrupt, organize, and transform. Yes, we work in the academy but also well beyond. Yes, we publish in volumes like these, and write poetry elsewhere. We help build online archives of stories untold, go to court with community generated evidence, craft legislation to support those long marginalized by state violence, and contribute to curated displays of embroideries that dare to tell the gendered and racialized stories of apartheid. Yes, we know and adore Suntosh Pillay's reflection (2020) that "the revolution will not be peer reviewed." Still, we are honored to be with you. To begin, let us share from where we come as we spin a story across our works/lives.

REFLEXIVITIES: POSITIONALITIES, COMMITMENTS, AND ACCOUNTABILITIES

Opening with ourselves, in our work, we commit to critical interrogation of how we understand ourselves both as individuals and together, often called reflexivities and, we add, commitments and accountabilities. The question is not simply who we are, but also what we believe in, will fight for, where we are positioned, and to whom we hold our work accountable. We invite readers to move well beyond simple, often essentialist confessionals of race, gender, place, and sexuality. As we craft new inquiry projects, or begin a new course, we open with what Bianca Williams (2016) called radical honesty, elaborating where we came from, what we bring, the harms our communities have endured or perpetrated, the gifts we might offer, our points of vulnerability, the critical perspectives we import to the work, where we feel open to new wisdoms, what we love. We do not stop there. We consider, then, how these biographies nourish our epistemic, political, theoretical, and ethical commitments to varied forms of inquiry. We dive into the points of discomfort or disagreement. We learn alongside and never seek consensus but dignity and appreciation for the differences we bring. And so we begin at our first Zoom meeting.

> *(Buzz Buzz Buzz. . . . I turn my phone alarm off. The temperature is cooler but still unusually warm for autumn in New Zealand. Anthropocene daylight filters out the*

dissipating shards of dark. The white rooster instinctively sensing human movement begins his chorus—"cock-a-doodle-doo human, feed me." I fall out of bed and flick open my laptop. Familiar faces from South Africa and New York appear, and conversation flows effortlessly as we talk, laugh, muse, and love our distant yet interconnected worlds into being.)

ADREANNE: Kia ora, are you there?

MARÍA: Good morning! What time is it?

ADREANNE: It's 7 a.m. of your tomorrow.

PULENG: I'm looking out at the 9 p.m. sky of your yesterday!

WHITE ROOSTER: Cock-a-doodle doo!

MICHELLE: Is that a rooster?

The white male rooster pecks and tries to get in. His loud persistence, his colonial intrusive beak sometimes interrupts us, but we don't stop. He is as real as he is a metaphor of coloniality. As Walter Mignolo argued, "Coloniality is far from over, and so must be decoloniality" (2017).

I (Adreanne Ormond) belong to Aotearoa or New Zealand—a land down-under—a literal geographic Global South of the Pacific. My people are the Indigenous Māori who, because of their skilled deep-sea navigation and ocean explorations, have been referred to as the Vikings of the Sunrise (Buck, 1938). Formed by the belly, muscle, dreams, and future of these ancestors I identify as Indigenous Māori and intentionally privilege the Indigenous in a world deeply wounded by coloniality (Mignolo, 2012). Growing up within my Māori ancestral homeland of Rongomaiwāhine I was raised by my various relations, human, natural world, spirit beings and material entities. I learned that together we coconstituted our ancestral homeland (Ormond & Ormond, 2018). This holistic connection of humanity, ancestors, animals, plant, land, sea, sky, and more is understood as a relationality (Moreton-Robinson, 2017) bespoke to Indigenous peoples; an organic collective from which a life force, intelligence, and energy are generated that nurture all forms of being. From this positionality comes an ontology that the world in its totality is a living being. Mountain, ocean, sky, spirit, animal, human, and plant are comprehended as equally dynamic intelligent beings with energy and agency and which interact with our ancestral landscape to shape and influence it across the various times and spaces in which we exist. It is from this dynamic epistemology of love that I consider young Māori and drawing on a Māori ontology together we radically reimagine what a decolonial future might mean for them.

I (Puleng Segalo) grew up during turbulent times in South Africa. I witnessed police brutality through the eye of a child in the 1980s, I saw buildings go up in flames in what was called the State of Emergency. Black people were constantly protesting and fighting against a brutal apartheid system. Many lives were lost, and constant police surveillance was the norm. We were treated as subhumans; were perceived as what Frantz Fanon (1961) calls the wretched of the earth, the unwanted. This is one of the vivid memories I have of growing up in South Africa. I learned about and saw what injustice looks like when I was a young girl. I grew up with this memory, this knowledge that Black people were unwanted, perceived to be less than. I accompanied my mother, who was a domestic helper, to work—I saw how she felt like a body out of place in the house of her White employer. In these moments, I observed how the macro intersects with the micro in very significant ways. But I also remember communities coming together in solidarity, protecting each other when the police raided homes. I remember feeling safe in an unsafe world. Communities created nests that cushioned children, trying to provide normal lives and families in very abnormal circumstances. This is where I learned about ethics of care.

I (Michelle Fine) am the daughter of refugees from Poland, Jews fleeing pogroms, landing at Ellis Island in the United States in 1921. My mother was the youngest of 18, my father an orphan child. I grew up in the solid White working-class labor sector, witnessing what Karen Brodkin (1998) called "How the Jews became White," lifted by the updraft of White assimilation and socialized into the epistemologies of ignorance, not seeing, and not noticing, even as my mother carried the depression of loss and my father embodied the triumph of Becoming American. Early on, sitting at the margins, my soul was pulled toward political movements, solidarities with others on the margins. I knew entanglements, that gendered stories of loss and depression sat beside stories of merit and progress; in fact, in my house they slept together. As I came to the university, I bathed in feminist, critical race, and Marxist theories. After graduate school, the power of Latin American liberation psychology, braided with socialist feminist commitments, and then critical race theory, stirred me. My work sits alongside others lit by an appetite for justice, bearing witness to the ashes of inequity, dedicated to critical research by and for communities under siege. Always stewing in questions of ethics and privilege, solidarity and ambivalence about "my place," I have leaned on María as we have worked together for decades in prisons, schools, and communities, building spaces for solidarity studies. Feeling always unrooted, I learn so much from and with Adreanne and Puleng, who know, deeply and intimately, where they are from and where they belong even as we each stretch toward one another for epistemic oxygen. I met Adreanne when I was a visiting scholar with Linda Tuhiwai Smith at the Institute for Māori Studies in Auckland, and I was lucky enough to work with Puleng who arrived as a Fulbright scholar and doctoral candidate at the Graduate Center of the City University of New York.

I (María Elena Torre) grew up in an immigrant family that left Galicia, the autonomous region in the northwest coast of Spain, during the years of *la miseria* before and after the civil war. I was raised on stories that came from another place: stories of separation, loss, and longing; stories of hope and a deep sense of responsibility and care; stories of finding any and all available cracks from which to build in community. From these stories I learned laws were not always right, that institutions that commanded respect, like the Catholic church or the government, were organized around power not morals—that they could hold you down and steal your food, arrest, or even kill you if they did not like what you thought or said. My family stories of survivance, told to me in Gallego, Spanish, and English, were filled with a kind of outrage that was layered with a sadness, acceptance, humor, pride, and defiance. "When Abuelo finally made it, he was so covered in coal Vincente didn't even recognize him!" A stowaway on a sugar boat to Cuba, his friend who cooked in the ship kitchen hid him in the coal storage. That part of the story was told with a laugh that no one stopped to analyze. Was it funny because he was covered with coal? Was it funny because he looked Black? We just seemed to move on, in the same way we seemed to not pause to think what it meant for our family to seek refuge in a land we were not from. As a child growing up in the United States, I absorbed lessons about colonization as if it were something that happened elsewhere. It was what the Kings and Queens did, it was what the Church, and later governments, did in South America, in Africa, and to the Islands of the Pacific like New Zealand. . . . Unlike Puleng and Adreanne, it was not until I was in college and graduate school that I developed a deeper understanding of the intricacies of coloniality, my place in it, and of how colonization has shaped all our pasts and presents. Questions of what it means to be an immigrant on stolen land, of the complications of not being able to connect to, or for many, not knowing even where to look for, your ancestral land. My family's experience of survival migration, the discrimination that followed, and the unexamined consequences they, we, and I participate and participated in, produced in me an orientation toward in-between spaces: spaces of "made belonging"—chosen families and communities, spaces where people come together with divergent histories and experience around a common commitment or purpose. It is what drew me to reimagine Pratt's (1991) notion of contact zones—spaces where radically differently positioned people come into contact—as fertile spaces to confront power, build analyses, to grow theory, and to try out new ways of being. Participatory contact zones, places where differently positioned people choose to come together in solidarity as an enactment of decolonial praxis, is an offering for a liberatory psychology. It is what calls me toward Vizenor's (1999) recognition of survivance—a blend of survival and resistance, a reminder of the agency, connection, creativity, and imagination of people grappling with the power and colonial domination, the emergence of new ideas, relations, and cultural productions that can be sparked by and even rise up in the face of brutal contact. This recognition, migrated to participatory inquiry spaces, and opened up epistemological and methodological frameworks for me that center the creative and unimagined possibilities of contact chosen in solidarity, when differences produced by hierarchies of power are analyzed and used as catalysts.

Now that you have met each of us, we want to introduce you to the "we" of us. We do not work alone. In our theorizing in relation, we embrace ideas and enact what feminist philosopher Karen Barad (2007) called entanglements. In her critical study of physics, as if speaking to mainstream psychology, she wrote, "The paradox arises out of the mistaken assumption that there are individually determinate entities from the outset . . . entities are not separately determinate individuals but rather inseparable parts of a single phenomenon" (p. 316). Our ontologies, and our knowledge building praxes, are relational.

Barad (2007) challenged the Anthropocene and the centrality of humanity and seeks to reset this default positioning that has been so hazardous to our planet and lifeforms by uplifting the interconnection between the natural world and humanity. The life-generating and life-sustaining philosophy of the inseparability shared between humanity and the natural world has long been known to indigeneity (Mika, 2017). Adreanne echoed this in her connection with the land-sea-skyscape (Ormond et al., 2020) she belongs to and that belongs to her. Puleng spoke from an African epistemology and reiterated that life is more than just humanity through "sister constructs" wholeness and Ubuntu, notions positioned within an African-centered psychology (Ramose, 1999). Reiterating our collectivity across our geopolitics, worlds, space, time zones, both Adreanne and Puleng contested the individualistic, autonomous, and self-regulating view of being. Puleng, through African-centered psychology and ethics, called for a holistic view of the world. According to Mkhize (2018), "wholeness means that the separation of moral and ethical conduct from people's aspects of life, such as their community, art and lived experiences (participation), is meaningless" (p. 33). Likewise, and with a shared spirit of Anzaldúa's *nos-otras*, Ubuntu acknowledges our connectedness to others, as human beings. As African scholar John Mbiti (1970) argued, "I am because we are, and because we are, therefore I am" (p. 141). Because Indigenous African approaches to ethics are grounded in social and communal life, human and ecological solidarity becomes an important moral and ethical imperative (Mkhize, 2018, p. 38).

These shifts in ethics, epistemologies, and ontologies are crucial to decolonizing as an ongoing and collective process of critical public inquiry. Recently, Michelle was lovingly challenged by Rachel Liebert (University of East London), who with Teah Anna Lee Carlson (kaupapa Māori research, Massey University) is launching the Tipuna Project on intergenerational healing, settler accountability and decolonizing PAR in New Zealand. The Tipuna Project is designed and engaged with ancestors long gone and those still alive, as coresearchers, working on intergenerational healing and settler coloniality in New Zealand. We gathered on Zoom for a seminar in May of 2023, and Rachel opened: "Michelle, we love CPAR but." And (now paraphrasing) perhaps, Rachel added, it is maybe considered a bit colonial, relying only on living coresearchers. The Tipuna Project will invite elders and ancestors, from Pakeha (White European and British descendants of colonial settlers) and Māori communities, as coresearchers to work through the colonial wounds that echo across generations. Indeed, as our ideas travel across worlds and their unique views, they mutate, stretch, and transform—annunciating that decolonizing is more than a reclaiming of what was but includes critical transformation, over time and space, of theory, methods, ethics, and epistemologies.

We are four women, growing up and witnessing social dynamics from the rim of racial, ethnic, or immigrant margins. In our little girl bodies, we were intimately entangled with histories and lands (taken or fled); anchored in gendered dynamics at home, racism and ethnic violence around us, knowing things might be otherwise. Now we are intimately entangled with our local contexts and struggles and also, by design and desire, with each other. To read through the rest of our essay, you need to know that we hold dear our love for and obligation to each other. We do not gesture toward "love" lightly, as the currency of the moment, but as a channel for theorizing in relation, through *sentipensando*, a feeling-thinking (Arendt, 2006; Fernández et al., 2021; Lorde, 1978; Mosley et al., 2020; Peterson, 2021; Rodriguez Castro, 2018). We lean on each other to stabilize our shaky footing; we seek Zoomy hugs after we confront backlash; we strengthen muscles of courage to speak radical truths, as we search for hope when despair envelops.

Now that you have a sense of where we come from and what grounds us—let us share how we frame our work theoretically and epistemically, through decolonial feminisms and critical participatory action research as critical and relational praxes. We will then dip into scenes created from our inquiries and our teaching—where we have stretched toward and stumbled in attempts to create a decolonial practice. Throughout, we will try to model how we work together across disciplines, biographies, genealogies, and nation states, and in our conclusion, we invite you to consider the precious commitments of epistemic justice, decolonizing and liberation that you might bring to your work (see Montero et al., 2017).

Our work meets at the sweet intersection of years of trust, friendship, transnational love and hard conversations as well as readings and writings on decolonial feminism and critical participatory praxis. Linda Tuhiwai Smith (2012) has taken up residence in our collective hands, hearts, and heads:

> The intellectual project of decolonizing has to set out ways to proceed through a colonizing world . . . [with] radical compassion that reaches out, seeks collaboration, and is open to possibilities that can only be imagined as other things fall into place. *Decolonizing Methodologies* is not a method for revolution in a political sense but provokes some revolutionary thinking about the roles that knowledge, knowledge production, knowledge hierarchies and knowledge institutions play in decolonization and social transformation. (p. xii)

It was in this spirit and on the wings of Franz Fanon and Maria Lugones that we write together, humbling our local understandings as they rub against our transnational dialogues, trying to make sense in the immediate and across our places. We notice of course that structural violence travels across, but so does radical resistance. For instance, not long ago Puleng and Michelle published an essay on decolonial feminism (Segalo & Fine, 2020; see also Arvin et al., 2013; Davis, 1981; Mendoza, 2016; Moraga & Anzaldúa, 1981; Runyan, 2018).

> To decolonize is to *dig deep into our histories* and see how colonialism has distorted how we see and engage with the world. Decoloniality is the process of *untangling the knots that suffocate us* and make it difficult for us to breathe, it is to release the shackles that bind us to coloniality. To do this, we need to look back and confront our relationship to the forces of colonial legacies because colonization has made us strangers to ourselves. Chabani Manganyi (2018) articulates this process of making strange in his challenge of psychology and how it is complicit in the process of making people turn away from who they are by labeling and categorizing them. Kenyan scholar, Ngugi wa Thiong'o (2009) asserts that colonialism removed our internal software that carries the content of who we were as a people (speaking specifically about Africa) and inserted a new (European-Western) software that aimed at deleting our histories. . . . wa Thiong'o urge[s] us to delve in the quest for *re-membering the forgotten and erased histories and re-learn our humanity*. (Segalo & Fine, 2020, p. 207)

Decolonizing insists that we theorize contemporary phenomena by tracing the breadcrumbs and narratives across time (Bradbury, 2021), through history and power and chronicling what Puleng has called poison in the marrow (2020), toxic residues of oppressions that live in our bodies even in what James Baldwin called the "after times" (Glaude, 2020). We analyze all of this in order to fully understand the brutality of gendered violence in the United States and in South Africa. With communities and movements, and a sense of urgency to imagine otherwise (Chuh, 2003), we trace the residues and enactments of structural violence but animate vibrant capillaries of desire, joy, and subversion, pulsing toward freedom dreams and projects for collective liberation.

A GLIMPSE INTO OUR INQUIRY AND PEDAGOGICAL SPACES

As an Indigenous Māori of New Zealand, I (Adreanne) am inseparable from the land-sea-sky scape of my ancestral homeland because I am a part of it and it is a part of me. I also live within a colonial society, which means straddling two worlds, including economic systems, social-cultural norms, geopolitical landscapes, knowledge systems, languages, spiritualities, and material phenomena. This requires a double consciousness (Du Bois, 1899)—the ability to live and function within an Indigenous worldview while navigating the colonial world.

My Indigenous worldview recognizes the natural environment as a living, intelligent, and agentic being who nurtures and sustains us. As a child, I grew up with an intuitive connection to the land-sea-sky scape, the animals, plants, waterways, and spiritual and material phenomena that form our ancestral ecology. However, the colonial or Western worldview that I learned at school viewed the natural world as abstract resources with no life or intelligence, thereby alienating Māori from our ancestral ecology. These two worldviews—that of Māori and of colonizer—have caused great emotional and spiritual heartache as well as social and economic inequality for my people. The colonial settler state that colonized my country instigated a Western worldview and enacted their belief system upon my people, leading to alienation from the natural world and landscapes we are a part of. As Māori, our well-being is intertwined with that of the natural environment and this disconnect has had profound consequences for us. It is at the intersection of Māori culture, young Māori, the natural world, and addressing issues of environment degradation caused by coloniality that my recent research has taken me. I explore what it means to be young and Māori, to belong to an ancestral environment and to be aware of the knowledge, aspirations, responsibilities, and futures that can be bought into possibility through decolonization, intergenerational healing, love, and transformation. As sea levels rise, the livelihood of atoll communities in the Pacific are threatened and extreme weather events of floods, cyclones, earthquakes, bushfires, and droughts devastate communities across the globe. Leaders urgently search for solutions to what they identify as climate change; the modern world is turning toward other knowledge systems and ancient ways of knowing, such as are found within Indigenous community. Provoking and challenging the dominant narratives that see the resolution to the chaos caused by natural disaster to lie in technology, laboratories, theory, and government and state alliances, I work with young Indigenous people who are raised to understand the natural world as an extension of their being and deeply connected to all aspects of their well-being. These young Māori are challenging the destructive practices of humanity, which have pushed all life forms, including the planet, to the brink of extinction; both on a national basis and in conjunction with other states and community, they are demanding political, economic, and industrial accountability for the destruction occurring to the world and to their own ancestral ecology. Although I acknowledge their contributions toward the national and international spaces, here I focus on engagement local to our community of Rongomaiwāhine. These young people are mostly seen as problems to be solved (Du Bois, 1899) because their worldview is drawn from Rongomaiwāhine ontology and epistemology, and because of their refusal to conform to colonial or Western ways of knowing and social practices. Drawing on our close ancestral and genealogical relationships, shared identity, and sense of collective belonging I invite them to metaphorically walk hand in hand across the bridge between my academic knowledge and their embodied knowledge and talk, listen, and learn. Sometimes we meet at their homes and talk about nothing waiting for the gem of wisdom to glisten and attract our undivided attention. Other times we meet at one of the main rivers, sitting on the bridge and swinging our legs over the side as we consider the changing river tides and how the area where the river and ocean meet has eroded the land and road away and how this pattern may reflect other significant tidal changes that can potentially impact our community and national coastline. We share stories told to us by our parents and grandparents about how the water of the river was clear aqua, unpolluted, and about the types of fish and creatures that lived there and were caught for food. We discuss how that is changing and, drawing from Rongomaiwāhine knowledge, ways to take action to protect the river. In our walks and talks, we pass the burial grounds of families and usually know those buried there, so we visit and tell our memories of the death and burial ceremony, knowing that in doing so we evoke them as well as other ancestors. We talk about them and to them, what they taught us and how we might use with honor any gifts of knowledge. We talk about our responsibility and duties to our community, ancestral ecology, each other, family, and ourselves. Our discussions are layered with genealogy, the privilege and burden of belonging, references to ancestral landmarks, family, the future, and much more. Topics that come up are not always easy, humor is used to mask awkwardness and sensitive topics can often be left partially explored to be picked up another time or never. All this takes place as we sit on our ancestral land that we protect and that protects us and together, hand in hand, we—young people, ancestors, and myself—try to make sense of us, them, me, our community, and our world together. Through the invaluable Rongomaiwāhine knowledge and wisdom, we understand and how we live alongside and within our ancestral ecology. The knowledge we have collectively encompasses a deep understanding of the natural world and its interconnectedness with human life, as well as the intricate social and cultural systems developed over thousands of years. This knowledge is not static; it is energized and constantly evolving and adapting to the changing world. In my research with young people, we explore how this ancient knowledge can be reexamined and recontextualized today to address the challenges we now face. By recognizing the agency and intelligence of the natural environment and its connection to our well-being, we can begin to understand how we can coexist in a more sustainable and just way. The knowledge these young Indigenous Māori embody and have within our Rongomaiwāhine community provides a blueprint of critical insight into practices of reciprocity, partnership, love, trust, and caring for each other that forms a livelihood that sustains all creation. This may be useful for other Indigenous and non-Indigenous communities to explore, use and challenge their status quo of living with each other and upon this planet.

Puleng

It is with my memories of growing up in apartheid South Africa and the grounding in my community that I come to psychology. Entering the university was almost as if I were getting into a space where I did not belong. I went to the university shortly after South Africa gained its independence from the apartheid regime and was admitted at a previously Whites-only institution, which meant having to navigate a space that was not ready for someone who looks like me. It was within the corridors of the university and encounters with the study materials that I felt alienated. These feelings of alienation persisted from my student days until I became an academic. In 2015, students from various South African institutions of higher learning took to the streets in protest against increases in student fees and things started to shift openly. The students demanded that the government should offer more student funding and that no student should be excluded for an inability to pay fees. These protests led to the formation of what was to be later called #FeesMustFall movement. The students further demanded that the university curriculum should be decolonized and that be centered instead on African ways of knowing and being in the world. This call for decolonization culminated into calls for the statue of Cecil John Rhodes, whom the students believed indicated and represented the perpetual colonial gaze, which was at the center of one of the universities to be demolished or removed. This call for the statue to be removed was known as the #RhodesMustFall movement. These movements brought an awakening in many of us: we felt for the first time that we could challenge the structures of power such as universities more openly. This also meant a rethinking of the material we prescribe and privilege in the lecture rooms. This is where the process of decolonization and Africanization were named as necessary for the true transformation of universities and, by extension, our society more broadly. Acknowledging colonialism's continuous presence through the process of coloniality, I deem it important to be conscious of the need to create platforms and spaces for the reimagining of ways in which knowledge is produced and how it circulates. For me, this is where the possibility for creative research methodologies becomes useful. My work draws from a visual artistic form called embroidery. I focus on historical traumas that Black women in South Africa have gone through and ways in which the making of embroideries offer an avenue for the salving of their past (and sometimes present) suffering (Segalo, 2014, 2018; Segalo et al., 2015; Segalo & Fine, 2017).

I also draw from an African-centered psychology. One may ask why I prefer to speak of Africanizing psychology. African psychology is an epistemological frame of work that rejects exclusion of other ways of knowing. It encourages multimodal understanding of being human and how one navigates the world, taking context into consideration. It came (was birthed) as a result of the need for African people to tell their own stories and not solely rely on imported theories to understand local realities (Nwoye, 2015, 2017). African psychology is interested in understanding the psychological capital of the African people.

I was recently invited to give a lecture on African psychology and decolonization to clinical and community psychology students at a university based in the United Kingdom. The lecture offered a critique of the discipline of psychology, its relationship with colonization, and how the discipline was imported to various parts of the world. The focus was also on what a decolonized and African-centered psychology could offer. The class consisted of a diverse group of students from various parts of the world. Their reflections and experiences of the class included the following:

> Thank you so much for availing this workshop to me. Listening to it made me feel like I have found the key to unlocking a lot of the questions I have grappled with being in the diaspora from Africa, to London, and for the last 20 years in the USA.

> Attending this session was like when time stops and you enter another world for two hours, and come out afterwards like, 'Wow!'

> You have offered so much for us to think with: the construction of knowledge, the possibilities for Psychology and working with the person.

> The session was very interesting and thoughtful, it was purifying and made me feel teary.

My work, which centers the importance of visual methodologies, continues to travel both within and outside academic walls. With the commitment to create spaces for visibilizing gendered injustices and unmuting silenced voices of women who continue to be rendered second-class citizens, the women's narratives stitched onto cloth continue to travel across geographical locations, from Africa, to Europe, and now to North America. The embroidered stories were featured in a 2021–2022 exhibit at the Canadian Museum for Human Rights alongside the Witness Blanket. As the world continues to grapple with various forms of human rights violation, this exhibition serves as a reflection and reminder of where we come from as a people, what we have survived, and the work still to be done if we are to create a just and peaceful world. With the advent of COVID-19 and its immense impact on the world, we were reminded of the intersecting violations that women suffer both within and outside their homes. Gender-based violence became hyper visible and was highlighted on numerous media platforms as if it has not been a cancer that has long eaten away at women across the world. The Intuthuko embroidery collective and myself came together to engage on how we can visually depict the ways in which gender-based violence manifests in our everyday encounters. In early 2021, we came together to brainstorm, collectively come up with themes, and begin work on an embroidery project that focuses on the everydayness of gender-based violence. We aimed at visibilizing how gender-based violence has created what Pumla Gqola (2015) called the fear factory, where women cannot walk freely and safely in the streets. We came together every week through June 2021 and worked together to carve these visual narratives of gendered violence. Our work is a participatory action research project; coming together every week allowed us the opportunity to check in and offer support and solidarity to one another during the difficult time of COVID-19. The pandemic has brought loss, isolation, loneliness, and despair to many; our coming together allowed space for sharing pain, comforting each other, and sharing meals with each other while we reflected and worked on our embroideries. The work is ongoing. We plan to produce an easily accessible booklet based on the project—a booklet that can be shared with community members so that they can reflect on the myriad ways in which gendered violence manifests in communities. We plan to host community dialogues where people on the ground can have conversations alongside the visual reflections we have produced.

María and Michelle

Our work at the Public Science Project weaves together participatory research and praxis, sweet and delicate entanglements of public science with movements for justice and communities under siege. Research with communities, and not on or about, we take seriously a commitment to "no research about us without us." It is no surprise that critical research entwines struggles for justice. The urgency of the present moment requires that we address, at the same time, radical inquiry alongside communities and movements that dissent; legal interventions; popular education; critical theory; and healing, pedagogy, and activism. On most projects, we are invited by community members seeking critical science they can trust or they can produce. This may include women in prison, low-wage working women affected by COVID-19, or communities living with ongoing state sponsored police violence or family separations at the Mexican–U.S. border. At this moment of political–ethical implosion, we build critical participatory action research collectives entwined with struggles, science, inquiry, creativity, rage, law, public education, healing, and joy filled survival.

Consider the Survivors Justice Project (SJP), a research collective we helped build in the aftermath of the 2019 passage of the New York State Domestic Violence Survivors Justice Act (DVSJA). In terms too simple, DVSJA allows judges to resentence survivors to shorter prison terms or program alternatives, if the court finds that at the time of the offense, they were a victim of domestic violence; the abuse was a "significant contributing factor" to their participation in the offense; and a sentence under current law would be "unduly harsh." Once the law was passed, our collective was born: lawyers, advocates, organizers, researchers, university faculty, and social workers; most of us are women who have survived prison or domestic violence. We came together just after passage of the DVSJA, to document, litigate, and build community with women in prison and to advance women's (trans, cis, gender expansive) access to the DVSJA, particularly Black women, immigrant women, and those experiencing poverty. We knew well that this radical law, the outcome of decades of struggle by survivors, would only be as strong as the community-based praxis that would follow. We feared that DVSJA could lie fallow unless activists, lawyers, and researchers could document where, how, and under what conditions women were submitting petitions to be resentenced; being approved and denied for resentencing or release; how race mattered, as well as gender and state county or geography.

We knew that to build a pluralistic and ethical research design, our research collective had to be anchored in the wisdom cultivated inside prison by women who did time as well as the experiences of women who had survived domestic violence or family abuse. We needed legal expertise to litigate and social researchers to document; it soon became apparent that we would need activist feminist social workers to help women inside craft "new narratives" that might enable petitions for resentencing. For two years, every other Thursday, we have been meeting, litigating, inviting newly released women to join the advisory board, dissecting judge's decisions, women's petitions, prosecutors' rebuttals, and painful newspaper accounts. We've had hard conversations about how race and racism influence the forms of evidence women can provide and their perceived credibility. We confronted our mixed feelings when a man was the first person to be released under DVSJA. Among us, the SJP collective carries more than 150 years of carceral wisdom. We have experienced our share of *choques or clashes*, and though our work kindles our internal fires of resistance, we are awash in the residue of despair produced by long-standing injustice.

One particularly heavy Thursday, after an interview with a newly released woman, we had to confront the betrayal of freedom for the woman, who was now living in a homeless shelter, terrified of COVID-19, with her 15-year-old daughter. "If I knew this was what I was returning to I should have stayed inside," she told us. We discussed another woman eligible to be released, who is facing a return to the home of her abuse, with new layers of psychological trauma. We confront the limits of reforms that appear liberatory and are always insufficient. Critical PAR evokes joy and breaks hearts. And new openings, as you will read below, emerge on the winds of critical decolonial yearnings.

In August 2021, our collective met on Zoom with a group of scholars and activists at University of South Africa, including Puleng, a group engaged in inside and outside prison education. For two hours, we shared stories, marveled at our deep differences, and yet cried over shared struggles of women entrapped in the carceral state, losing access to their children, never—even after release—being free. Transnational feminist courage and rage electrified our online space and gave us courage as we returned to our local projects.

EPISTEMIC JUSTICE: CHALLENGING ACADEMIC AUTHORITY AND ACKNOWLEDGING WISDOM BORNE IN STRUGGLE

Across our very distinct biographies and projects, we knew early that the academy has no monopoly on knowledge. We recall the words of Orlando Fals-Borda (1995; Gott, 2008) as he spoke to North American sociologists at the Southern Association of Sociologists:

> Do not monopolize your knowledge nor impose arrogantly your technique, but respect and combine your skills with the knowledge of the researched or grassroots communities, taking them as full partners and coresearchers . . . be receptive to counternarratives. . . . Science should not be necessarily a mystery nor a monopoly of experts and intellectuals.

In ways distinct yet linked, we each came of age with a foot in schools and home communities, bathing in lots of forms of wisdom, stories, and knowledge shared around kitchen tables, community gatherings, funerals, and in quiet conversations with elders. It is no surprise that we commit to epistemic justice as a research practice. We knew our grandmothers' knowledge would carry us forward even as we each excelled in school. We each—in very different spaces—have relied on the knowledges of those most marginalized and discredited (de Sousa Santos, 2014). We have questioned in our academic socialization the pressure to erase, appropriate, or literally white-out cultural knowledges; we resisted the scientific reductionism embedded in the positivistic encoding of human experience, natural world phenomena, and the intelligence that exists outside the rational logic. We take guidance from Adreanne and the Māori culture of habitat (Peña, 2011) that collaborates with multispecies, embodied others, and selves as well as the natural and materialistic environment to generate relations of life, kinship, community, reciprocity and solidarity with humans and more-than-humans alike. Together we speak of the Indigenous lands that are part of the colonial settler conquest our modern societies are constructed on and the life that has been extracted from Indigenous communities by inhuman humanity. We debate and ponder what it means for our transnational decolonial sisterhood in our diverse geopolitics, New Zealand, New York, and South Africa, to more fully comprehend this history in the places/spaces we come from and create. Our quest for epistemic justice is constantly embedded in the decolonial. Even as Puleng reminds us that coloniality thrives as "poison in the marrow."

More concretely, in our research projects and classrooms, we contest the "danger of a single story" (Adichie, 2009; Ayala et al., 2018). We create spaces for the multiple knowledge systems that exist—*nos-otras* (Anzaldúa & Keating, 2000; Torre, 2009); knowledge from the Māori world, *kaupapa* Māori (Pihama, 2010; G. Smith, 2012); *matauranga* Māori (L. Smith et al., 2016); as well as Rongomaiwāhine ontology (Ormond et al., 2020) that arises from Adreanne's ancestral ecology and land—to create radically different knowledges that can pool together, building an alchemy of inquiry other than colonial knowledges. We aim to create spaces where the knowledge of marginalized communities and individuals, who are often silenced and overlooked, seen as below in the Global South can be centered and valued alongside other knowledge systems, creating and celebrating plural perspectives and understandings that enhance the ways we relate to each other and can live together.

This commitment to invite and dialogue among wildly divergent perspectives is more crucial today than even when we first wrote this essay; as the world folds in on itself, polarizes, polices educational curricula, animates authoritarian schooling, and bans controversial discussions. We conjure a critical public science to be "of use" for, with and by communities in struggle. We realize and relish First Nations scholar Shawn Wilson's (2008) insight that research is ceremony, one that arises from and should be navigated in ways that align with the lives of people and the landscape they have loved, become embittered by, survived, and thrived alongside.

For Puleng, this praxis has long involved collaboration with an embroidery collective of Black African women who tell their stories of living through apartheid, stitched onto a Black canvas; for Adreanne, this has involved accompanying Māori youth and their community to engage with decolonization and inviting them to speak their testimonies as a collective ensemble; for María, this has involved critical participatory research with women in prison, women once they have come home, with queer young people, engaged together—across rich differences—excavating and building on knowledges long buried; for Michelle, too, this has involved critical inquiry with Muslim American young people, immigrant youth, women in and out of prison, to build critical knowledge for struggle, from the margins, to transform policy and to tell "another story." Our designs stand on firm ground—no research about us without us—to honor ways of being and ways of knowing, knowledge systems long silenced, censored, or punished, knowledges borne in struggle, at kitchen tables, on long walks, in difficult dialogues and conflicts, behind prison bars, in college classrooms, on grandma's lap, on farms, on the front lines of protests and in shelters far from public view.

In townships, on beaches and in concrete high rises on Fifth Avenue in New York City, we build participatory contact zones (Fine & Torre, 2021; Torre, 2009; Torre & Fine, 2008), nests of inquiry where counternarratives can be assembled and unleashed—with statistics, narratives, arts, and history. Yes, all of these. In our contact zones, we [be]come together. As members of participatory contact zones, we bring in evidence of how we know what we know. Academic articles sit beside hip-hop lyrics, images of coastlines eroding, enraging headlines that blame victims and embroideries of life during apartheid; we are nourished by mother's stories, photographs, textiles, birth records, or grandfather's Bible. We read books, newspaper stories, and peer-reviewed essays and analyze social media together to reveal how we see, what we see, where we fail to see, how we might grow a new collective way of seeing and thinking otherwise.

This process is neither conflict free nor a hegemony-free zone. The white rooster is always lurking around and within us. The dominant narratives and structural violence we seek to undermine, perpetually hover, invade, arrogantly and annoyingly try to peck at the window, and sometimes we peck at each other. The affects in these contact zones can be intense, suffocating, enraging. These are not abstract issues being studied by people from afar. These are crises, interrogated by those most affected. Fears, anxieties, memories, rage, ignorance, shame seep into every project we take up, waiting for us around corners, crawling onto our tongues, into our interpretations (Segalo, 2020), under our skin. Our research collectives—with women in prison, women creatively embroidering life under apartheid, queer youth making homes, young people living on and off their ancestral lands—seek to clear the way for deep inquiry. Without question these predictably unpredictable affects erupt. Thus, in our contact zones, we build in processes to metabolize our differences, address our needs for healing, encourage dissent, and anticipate *choques*—as Gloria Anzaldúa (2000) would call them—difficult clashes, inevitable when working across power lines. When a *choque* occurs, we stop, acknowledge, and build in processes to unearth, engage, learn, and repair without seeking false consensus or silencing. Although painful when they happen, we have found *choques* to be generative and growthful, often leaving us more interconnected than when we started.

Consider the research-teaching space in which Adreanne collaborates with young Indigenous Māori and peers in other nations of the world, as they call out the failure of politicians, teachers, parents, and corporations to create a future in which they, the young, can flourish (Bandura & Cherry, 2020; Moon, 2013; Thunberg, 2019). Young people take to social media platforms (Panaligan, 2019; Wielk & Standlee, 2021) within both liberatory and troubling exchanges, challenge the absence of commitment from the political and economic hubs of the globe, and sound the alarm against climate change (Batabyal, 2014; United Nations Development Programme, 2019) and global warming (Barrett, 2006). They amplify their voices to ricochet around the globe and generate solidarity. In the hands of the young, YouTube (Duran-Becerra et al., 2020), Facebook, TikTok, Twitter, and Instagram become tools of global dissemination that transcend race, culture, community, geographic location, gender, and social class. Following and generating updates about rising sea levels (Simmons, 2021), disappearing islands (Klein, 2017), changing precipitation patterns, longer summers with higher temperatures and shorter warmer winters, disappearing glaciers and shrinking ice sheets, dust storms (Fenton et al., 2007), and so forth, young people keep abreast of trending environmental news. At the cusp of planetary crisis (Duffy, 2011; Gray, 2015), young Indigenous Māori, Pacific Nations, and other concerned communities challenge all to consider the Anthropocene world that for too long has privileged human-centric greed, big business, and profit above other forms of life, intelligence, and ways of doing. They demand less harmful and more inclusive knowledge, environmentally friendly technology, discussions, and stories about the ways their human species entangles with the planet in their search for a life that is not ecologically devastating (Cajete, 2000). They call on all, whatever age, to acknowledge and act on the disruptions arising from our planet, the Earth.

Like Adreanne, we each engage work in our local communities, where we can hear the footsteps of ancestors, soft cries, whispers, the piercing of police bullets outside a family window, the rumbles of racial uprisings, watch the seashore erode, listen to a mother tucking her baby into bed with a story from a grandmother in another land. On these grounds we can still smell, see, feel, and touch, that is, sense the tremors, anxieties, traumas, and residue of colonialism, apartheid, carceral violence, or intimate violence even as we nourish the desire in ourselves and our children for a world not yet, a world that might be otherwise. On the ground is where we inquire with, alongside, or in ways that move through words and actions, silences and affects, relationships and social movements, embroidery, and poetry. We focus on praxis, where theory, methods, ethics, and practice entwine. As South African scholar Shose Kessi (2018) wrote,

> The focus on praxis translates into approaches to knowledge production that promote the participation of marginalized communities in research projects. Such orientations to research create meaningful conduits between the academy and lived experience and can mitigate the epistemic violence often produced and exercised against those who are researched. (p. 508)

In our very distinct settings, working with social movements and everyday people fighting and loving to survive, we all walk on that humble fragile bridge between academy and community, aware of our two-ness, feeling the heat of suspicion on both sides. For Maria and Michelle, these affects surface in our work in, through, with, and alongside women in prison. Surrounded by wisdoms borne in hell, notions of expertise explode and democratize.

Toward Radical Inclusivity in a Transnational Feminist Commons

We are moved by what happens when we hold space together, online, when we dedicate time and dare to listen to each other, across local spaces, contexts, and struggles. Here we draw on the writings of Miriam Ticktin (2020), naming the power of a transnational feminist commons that refuse enclosure. Ticktin warned that "the nation is not a harmless or protected space. . . . A focus on the nation as a space of supposedly nonviolent connection and care has already killed thousands and thousands of people" (p. 2). COVID-19 has invited us to ask "not how to isolate ourselves . . . but which forms of connection to attend to and cultivate and which ones to be careful of" (p. 3). She advances "new, horizontal forms of sociality . . . [as] the only way to survive . . . acknowledge our porousness . . . struggle against enclosures, against privatization of spaces of freedom [and] exclusions" (p.6).

Judith Butler (2011) joined the call for a transnational feminist commons when she wrote, "the Polis, properly speaking, is not the city-state in its physical location; it is the organization of the people as it arises out of acting and speaking together, and it's [*sic*] true space lies between people living together for this purpose, no matter where they happen to be." The "true" space then lies "between the people" and belongs properly to alliance itself. Butler called forth Hannah Arendt, for whom alliance is not tied to location but brings about its own location, highly transposable. In 1958 she wrote, "action and speech create a space between the participants which can find its proper location almost anywhere and anytime" (cited in Butler, 2011, p. 198). As Arendt imagined otherwise, we have built a home, together, online, rooted in the percussive winds that travel across, held in relationship and political desires for a world not yet.

How do we understand the mobility of transnational feministic connectivity that vibrates among us? This query was posed eloquently by Bhekizizwe Peterson (2021), brilliant scholar and filmmaker, recently deceased: "How do we maintain the ideas and live the forms of kinship and solidarities (ancestral, familial, communal, continental and global) that remain crucial even though they may be fragile, suffocating and even deemed retrograde and transgressive?" (p. 25).

We write as women rooted in decolonial feminist theory and a long thread of sisterhood, with toes buried in local grounds where we stand even as our heads and thoughts wander across, eager to lay down our epistemic blues and incites, and stitch a story not told, across, because we dare. We write from a loosely cobbled but loving transnational feminist commons, noting all the ways that power and hegemony, Whiteness and privilege flow across and through us, and thrilled by all the ways that our pores, frameworks, theoretical dissociations, our laughter, wisdoms, and our hearts open when we are together. We share sweet histories of trust and bare commitments to decolonizing praxis, with all our uncertainties and inequities made more vivid during COVID-19. We place stories of backlash in the yellow lines that connect our Zoom boxes, as Puleng did recently (July 2021) when a written snippet based on a radio interview focusing on the "fatherhood crisis" tied to apartheid which she did for one of the national radio stations was shared on social media. Puleng was attacked by letters from readers. "STOP!" they said, "do not connect the present to the past!" Yet she persisted. We dare to make public scholarship that historicizes current issues within the bloody past of White Supremacy—colonialism, apartheid, or U.S. White state violence. Yet we learn, quickly, that these are historic connections that many people do not want to hear, even as the coloniality of White supremacy carries forth, evident in another offering from Puleng:

> On the 31st of May 2021, pupils and their parents protested on the premises of one of the private schools in Pretoria because of the racism experienced by Black children at the school. One of the pupils addressed the school, saying that her first and most vivid memory of racism happened when she was in Grade 4 (she would have been 9 or 10 years old at the time). "I was happily on my way to break when a teacher stopped me," the pupil said. "She looked me dead in the eyes and said: Your hair's unpresentable, it is messy and it's not the Cornwall way. She also proceeded to tell me that I'd look better if I chemically straightened my hair," she said. "After that encounter, I believed there was something wrong with my natural, kinky hair and for a long time I was uncomfortable wearing my natural hair to school." It is in such moments where we are painfully reminded that the processes of decolonization and Africanization are necessary as coloniality continues to rear its head in the classrooms, during school breaks, always reminding us of the audacity of Whiteness as it pierces through people's sense of being in the world.

Like Puleng, as decolonizing scholars, we all have obligations to link the present conditions of coloniality and oppression to history and to radical imaginings of what else is possible. Like Puleng, we will confront backlash. If you are lucky, you will find colleagues, comrades, and sisters in struggle online, in the next office, in the restroom . . . someone or somewhere . . . to hold the pain and honor the courage.

To Be of Use

Our editors have invited us to offer you, our readers, provocations toward action, practice, and community engagement. In each space, these "moves" will vary, but on the ground, for instance at the Graduate Center, Michelle with colleague and critical neuropsychologist Desiree Byrd has launched a new course, Decolonizing Psychology. Cotaught by professors who are rooted in critical and neuropsychology, White and African American, senior and junior, students excavate collectively archives on the regressive history of psychology—testing, classification, criminalization, tracking or leveling in schools, pathologizing mental health struggles, "help" rather than liberation, conversion therapy, Guantanamo, institutionalization, and then deinstitutionalization. They find and resurrect sweet, buried radical possibilities launched by psychologists across the globe—and ignored by the canon—in prisons, in community mental health, across national borders, in movements and labor unions, in women's clinics, and at kitchen tables.

In Pretoria, Puleng has been teaching a module on community intervention strategies for students pursuing a master's in research psychology. One of the things the module focuses on is revisiting history as a way of getting deep understanding of how their various research topics cannot be understood outside colonial history and its impact on current challenges—we revisit history by spending time at the South African Freedom Park—(outside the classroom learning experience), which is a monument that serves as a space of remembrance that takes people on a historical journey of colonialism and apartheid. The exercise forces students to be outside their comfort zones and to think seriously about the intersectionality of their work and the politics of representation.

With the Public Science Project, María builds collective spaces annually at the Graduate Center during summer institutes where graduate students, professors, activists, and community workers come together for week-long intensives on critical participatory action research and reclaiming research as liberatory praxis. In the very halls in which people have previously dissected, diagnosed, predicted, and proclaimed, we challenge, reframe, and carve pathways for epistemic justice and research not on but by us that is of use for social movements. We spend time learning from and imagining engagements with research that goes beyond reporting back—that instead sparks conversation, becomes a presence to contend with, a recognition as well as a tool for creating sovereign spaces. Research findings take the form of zines, easily carried folded back-pocket reports, neighborhood chalking or wheat pastings, interactive theater pieces, community dinners, board games, policy talking points, and more (Cahill & Torre, 2008; Fox & Fine, 2012; Stoudt et al., 2019).

These, however, are just a few offerings. More importantly dear readers, is the reminder that living a decolonizing praxis means that our inquiries must be cultivated by and with communities under siege; that knowledges borne in struggle, survivance, resistance, and laughter must be honored—the knowledges of grandmothers and aunties, of published works and wisdom passed down kitchens, of stories shared at funerals and in organizing spaces where protests are planned. We each, and all, must refuse simple colonial frameworks for extractive inquiry. We each, and all, must continually question whether our inquiries are bold enough to address and dismantle the voracious appetite of global capitalism, the lingering wounds of colonialism, and the treacherous grips of patriarchy. We each, and all, should face the shadows of complicity and contradiction. And at the same time, we should relish the feeling of magic when our projects spark new ways of being. When we resist in our Zoom spaces, meeting across time and place; when we bring together activists, scholars, and community members to speak through what is, and what must be. And when the session ends and we text each other, hearts full, with emojis and "that was amazing," we must remember our long-gone friend, mom-tor, and brilliant feminist philosopher, Maxine Greene (1988) who wrote, "When freedom is the question, it is always time to begin" (p. 155). So, it is with this that we leave you. With a reminder and a call, for our discipline and all of us who are a part. For within psychology, decolonizing must begin, again.

RESOURCES

Barefoot Divas. (2012, January 26). *Festival TV: Barefoot Divas* [Video]. YouTube. https://www.youtube.com/watch?v=03OCVG9zBmQ

Bissel, E., Loyer, K., Orellana, T., Nowlain, L., & Begley, J. (n.d.). *The knotted line*. https://knottedline.com/

Canadian Museum for Human Rights. (2021, April 28). *The power of art: Artivism and witness blanket: Preserving a legacy* [Video]. YouTube. https://www.youtube.com/watch?v=2GOuiw4CjLg

Faculty of Humanities. (2019, November 1-9). *Intersecting violences exhibition* [Exhibit]. University of Cape Town. https://humanities.uct.ac.za/articles/2019-11-14-intersecting-violences-exhibition

Joseph, P. (Director). (2012). *Tatarakihi: The children of Parihaka* [Film]. NZ On Screen. https://www.nzonscreen.com/title/tatarakihi-the-children-of-parihaka-2012

Kessi, S. (2018). Photovoice as a narrative tool for decolonization: Black women and LGBT student experiences at UCT. *South African Journal of Higher Education, 32*(3), 101–117. https://doi.org/10.20853/32-3-2519

Kessi, S., Kaminer, D., Boonzaier, F., & Learmonth, D. (2019). Photovoice methodologies for social justice. In S. Laher, A. Fynn, & S. Kramer (Eds.), *Transforming research methods in the social sciences: Case studies from South Africa* (pp. 354–374). Wits University Press. https://doi.org/10.18772/22019032750.27

Luttrell, W. (2018). *Exhibitions* [Exhibit]. https://www.wendyluttrell.org/exhibitions

Masilela, P. (2020, June 9). Intuthuko Embroidery group band together to sew masks to put food on table amid the Covid-19 pandemic. *Benoni City Times*. https://benonicitytimes.co.za/392972/intuthuko-embroidery-group-band-together-to-sew-masks-to-put-food-on-table-amid-the-covid-19-pandemic/

The Public Science Project. https://publicscienceproject.org/

The Survivors Justice Project. https://www.sjpny.org/

Walker, S., Hall, R., Rika, M., & Kingi, T. (2014, July 25). *Stan Walker-Aotearoa ft. Ria Hall, Troy Kingi, Maisey Rika* [Video]. YouTube. https://www.youtube.com/watch?v=jWhAoZZh8fc

Zuholi, Z. (2019, September 20). *Zanele Muholi on "somnyama ngonyama, hail the dark lioness" at Seattle Art Museum* [Video]. YouTube. https://www.youtube.com/watch?v=fppJn5N2-Ks&t=2s

REFERENCES

Adichie, C. (2009). *The danger of a single story* [Video]. TED Conferences. https://www.ted.com/talks/chimamanda_adichie_the_danger_of_a_single_story

Alexandre, L. (2023). *For 200 years*. Center for Media Literacy. https://www.medialit.org/reading-room/200-years-alternative-press-voices-dissident-views

Anzaldúa, G. E. (1987). *Borderlands/La Frontera: The new mestiza*. Aunt Lute Books.

Anzaldúa, G. E. (2000). In A. Keating (Ed.), *Interviews/Entrevistas*. Routledge.

Arendt, H. (1958). *The human condition*. University of Chicago Press.

Arendt, H. (2006). The meaning of love in politics. A letter by Hannah Arendt to James Baldwin. *HannahArendt.net, 2(1)*. https://www.hannaharendt.net/index.php/han/article/view/95

Arvin, M., Tuck, E., & Morrill, A. (2013). Decolonizing feminism: Challenging connections between settler colonialism and hereropatriarchy. *Feminist Formations, 25*(1), 8–34. https://doi.org/10.1353/ff.2013.0006

Ayala, J., Cammarota, J., Berta-Ávila, M. I., Rivera, M., Rodríguez, L. F., & Torre, M. E. (Eds.). (2018). *PAR EntreMundos: A pedagogy for the Americas.* Peter Lang. https://doi.org/10.3726/b11303

Bandura, A., & Cherry, L. (2020). Enlisting the power of youth for climate change. *American Psychologist, 75*(7), 945–951. https://doi.org/10.1037/amp0000512

Barad, K. (2007). *Meeting the universe halfway: Quantum physics and the entanglement of matter.* Duke University Press. https://doi.org/10.2307/j.ctv12101zq

Barrett, P. (2006). Will unchecked global warming destroy civilization by century's end? What three degrees of global warming really means. *Policy Quarterly, 2*(1), 5–9. https://ojs.victoria.ac.nz/pq/article/view/4190/3696

Batabyal, S. (2014). *Environment, politics and activism: The role of media.* Routledge.

Bradbury, J. (2021). Narrative subjects: Tense, (in)tension and (im)possibilities for change. In C. Squire (Ed.), *Stories changing lives* (pp. 145–162). Cambridge University Press. https://doi.org/10.1093/oso/9780190864750.003.0008

Brodkin, K. (1998). *How Jews became White folks: And what that says about race in America.* Rutgers University Press.

Bryant-Davis, T., & Comas-Díaz, L. (Eds.). (2016). *Womanist and mujerista psychologies: Voices of fire, acts of courage.* American Psychological Association. https://doi.org/10.1037/14937-000

Buck, P. H. (1938). *Vikings of the sunrise.* Frederick A. Stokes Company.

Butler, J. (2011). *Bodies in alliance and the politics of the street.* European Institute for Progressive Cultural Policies. https://transversal.at/transversal/1011/butler/en

Cahill, C., & Torre, M. E. (2008). Beyond the journal article: Representations, audience, and products of research. In S. Kindon, R. Pain, & M. Kesby (Eds.), *Participatory action research approaches and methods: Connecting people, participation and place* (pp. 196–206). Routledge.

Cajete, G. (2000). *Native science: Natural laws of interdependence.* Clear Light Publishers.

Chuh, K. (2003). *Imagine otherwise.* Duke University Press.

Cole, E. R. (2009). Intersectionality and research in psychology. *American Psychologist, 64*(3), 170–180. https://doi.org/10.1037/a0014564

Comas-Díaz, L. (Ed.). (2020). *Liberation psychology.* American Psychological Association.

Crenshaw, K. (1991). Mapping the margins: Intersectionality, identity politics, and violence against women of color. *Stanford Law Review, 43*(6), 1241–1245. https://doi.org/10.2307/1229039

Davis, A. (1981). *Women, race and class.* Vintage Press.

de Sousa Santos, B. (2014). *Epistemologies of the south: Justice against epistemicide.* Routledge.

Du Bois, W. E. B. (1899). *The Philadelphia negro.* University of Pennsylvania Press.

Du Bois, W. E. B. (1903). *The souls of Black folk.* A. C. McClurg & Co.

Duffy, D. (2011). No room in the ark? Climate change and biodiversity in the Pacific Islands. *Pacific Conservation Biology, 17*(3), 192–200. https://doi.org/10.1071/PC110192

Duran-Becerra, B., Hillyer, G. C., Cosgrove, A., & Basch, C. H. (2020). Climate change on YouTube: A potential platform for youth learning. *Health Promotion Perspectives, 10*(3), 282–286. https://doi.org/10.34172/hpp.2020.42

Dutta, U., Sonn, C., & Lykes, M. (2016). Structural violence and community-based research and action. *Community Psychology in Global Perspectives, 2*(2), 1–20.

Fals-Borda, O. (1995, April 8). *Research for social justice: Some North–South convergences* [Plenary Address]. Southern Sociological Conference, Atlanta, GA, United States. https://www.scribd.com/document/453629125/Fals-Borda-Research-for-Social-Justice

Fanon, F. (1961). *Wretched of the earth*. François Maspero.

Fenton, L. K., Geissler, P. E., & Haberle, R. M. (2007). Global warming and climate forcing by recent albedo changes on Mars. *Nature, 446*(7136), 646–649. https://doi.org/10.1038/nature05718

Fernández, J. S., Sonn, C. C., Carolissen, R., & Stevens, G. (2021). Roots and routes toward decoloniality within and outside psychology praxis. *Review of General Psychology, 25*(4), 354–368. https://doi.org/10.1177/10892680211002437

Fine, M., & Torre, M. E. (2021). *Essentials of critical participatory action research*. American Psychological Association. https://doi.org/10.1037/0000241-000

Fox, M., & Fine, M. (2012). Circulating critical research: Reflections on performance and moving inquiry into action. In G. Cannella & S. Steinberg (Eds.), *Critical qualitative research reader* (pp. 153–165). Peter Lang.

Glaude, E. S. (2020). *Begin again: James Baldwin's America and its urgent lessons for our own*. Crown Publications.

Gqola, P. (2015). *Rape: A South African nightmare*. MF Books.

Gott, R. (2008, August 25). *Obituary: Orlando Fals Borda: Sociologist and activist who defined peasant politics in Colombia*. The Guardian.

Gray, N. F. (2015). *Facing up to global warming: What is going on and how you can make a difference?* Springer International. https://doi.org/10.1007/978-3-319-20146-7

Greene, M. (1988). *Dialectics of freedom*. Teachers College Press.

Guishard, M., Halkovic, A., Galletta, A., & Li, P. (2018). Toward epistemological ethics: Centering communities and social justice in qualitative research. *Forum Qualitative Sozialforschung/Forum: Qualitative Social Research, 19*(3). Advance online publication. https://doi.org/10.17169/fqs-19.3.3145

Kessi, S. (2018). Community social psychologies for decoloniality: An African perspective on epistemic justice in higher education. *South African Journal of Psychology. Suid-Afrikaanse Tydskrif vir Sielkunde, 47*(4), 506–516. https://doi.org/10.1177/0081246317737917

Kiddle, R., Elkington, B., Jackson, M., Ripeka Mercier, O., Ross, M., Smeaton, J., & Thomas, A. (Eds.). (2020). *Imagining decolonisation*. Bridget Williams Books. https://doi.org/10.7810/9781988545783

Klein, A. (2017, September 7). Eight low lying Pacific Islands swallowed whole by rising sea. *NewScientist*. https://www.newscientist.com/article/2146594-eight-low-lying-pacific-islands-swallowed-whole-by-rising-seas/

Lorde, A. (1978). *Uses of the erotic: The erotic as power*. Kore Press.

Lugones, M. (2007). Heterosexualism and the colonial/modern gender system. *Hypatia, 22*(1), 186–209.

Lugones, M. (2010). Toward a decolonial feminism. *Hypatia, 25*(4), 742–759. https://doi.org/10.1111/j.1527-2001.2010.01137.x

Manganyi, C. (2018). Making strange: Race science and ethnopsychiatric discourse. *Psychology in Society, 57*, 4–23.

Martín-Baró, I. (1994). *Writings for a liberation psychology*. Harvard University Press.

Mbiti, J. (1970). *African religions and philosophies*. Doubleday.

McCubbin, S., Smit, B., & Pearce, T. (2015). Where does climate fit? Vulnerability to climate changes in the context of multiple stressors in Funafuti, Tuvalu. *Global Environmental Change, 30* (January), 43–55. https://doi.org/10.1016/j.gloenvcha.2014.10.007

Mendoza, B. (2016). Coloniality of gender and power: From postcoloniality to decoloniality. In L. Disch & M. Hawkesworth (Eds.), *Oxford handbook of feminist theory* (pp. 100–121). Oxford Handbooks Online.

Mignolo, W. D. (2012). *The darker side of modernity: Global futures, decolonial options.* Duke University Press.

Mignolo, W. D. (2017). Coloniality is far from over, and so must be decoloniality. *Afterall: A Journal of Art, Context, and Enquiry, 43*(1), 39–45. https://doi.org/10.1086/692552

Mika, C. (2017). *Indigenous education and the metaphysics of presence: A worlded philosophy.* Taylor and Francis. https://doi.org/10.4324/9781315727547

Mkhize, N. (2018). Ubuntu-Botho approach to ethics: An invitation to dialogue. In N. Nortje, D. De-Jongh, & W. A. Hoffman (Eds.), *African perspectives on ethics for healthcare professionals* (pp. 25–48). Springer. https://doi.org/10.1007/978-3-319-93230-9_3

Montero, M., Sonn, C., & Burton, M. (2017). Community psychology and liberation psychology: A creative synergy for an ethical and transformative praxis. In M. A. Bond, I. Serrano-García, & C. B. Keys (Eds.), *Handbook of community psychology: Theoretical foundations, core concepts, and emerging challenges* (Vol. 1, pp. 149–167). American Psychological Association.

Moon, E. (2013). *Neoliberalism, political action on climate change and the youth of Aotearoa New Zealand. A space for radical activism?* [Unpublished master's thesis]. Victoria University Wellington.

Moraga, C., & Anzaldúa, G. (1981). *This bridge called my back: Writings by radical women of color.* Persephone Press.

Moreton-Robinson, A. (2017). Relationality: A key presupposition of an Indigenous social research paradigm. In J. M. O'Brien & C. Andersen (Eds.), *Sources and methods in Indigenous studies* (pp. 69–77). Routledge.

Mosley, D. V., Neville, H. A., Chavez-Dueñas, N. Y., Adames, H. Y., Lewis, J. A., & French, B. H. (2020). Radical hope in revolting times: Proposing a culturally relevant psychological framework. *Social and Personality Psychology Compass, 14*(1), e12512. https://doi.org/10.1111/spc3.12512

Nwoye, A. (2015). What is African Psychology the psychology of? *Theory & Psychology, 25*(1), 96–116. https://doi.org/10.1177/0959354314565116

Nwoye, A. (2017). A postcolonial theory of African Psychology: A reply to Kopano Ratele. *Theory & Psychology, 27*(3), 328–336. https://doi.org/10.1177/0959354317700000

Ormond, A., Kidman, J., & Tomlins-Jahnke, H. (2020). An indigenous Māori perspective of rangatahi personhood. In S. Swartz, A. Cooper, C. M. Batan, & L. Kropoff Causa (Eds.), *The Oxford handbook of Global South youth studies* (pp. 96–108). Oxford University Press.

Ormond, A., & Ormond, J. (2018). An iwi homeland: Country of the heart. *MAI Journal, 7*(1), 79–91. https://doi.org/10.20507/MAIJournal.2018.7.1.7

Panaligan, E. (2019, October 1). Youth and social media fuel movement demanding action to fight climate change. *Daily Bruin.* https://dailybruin.com/2019/10/01/youth-and-social-media-fuel-movement-demanding-action-to-fight-climate-change

Peña, D. G. (2011). Structural violence, historical trauma, and public health: The environmental justice critique of contemporary risk science and practice. In L. M. Burton, S. P. Kemp, M. Leung, S. A. Matthews, & D. Takeuchi (Eds.), *Communities, neighborhoods, and health: Expanding the boundaries of place* (pp. 203–218). Springer. https://doi.org/10.1007/978-1-4419-7482-2_11

Peterson, B. (2021). A love letter to those who passed on and those still tasked with creating a better future for all. *Safundi: The Journal of South African and American Studies, 22*(1), 23–25. https://doi.org/10.1080/17533171.2020.1823741

Piercy, M. (1982). *Circles on the water: Selected poems of Marge Piercy.* Knopf.

Pihama, L. (2010). Kaupapa Māori theory: Transforming theory in Aotearoa. *He Pukenga Kōrero, 9*(2), 5–14.

Pillay, S. (2020). The revolution will not be peer reviewed: (Creative) tensions between academic, social media and anti-racist activism. *South African Journal of Psychology. Suid-Afrikaanse Tydskrif vir Sielkunde, 50*(3), 308–311. https://doi.org/10.1177/0081246320948369

Pratt, M. L. (1991). Arts of the contact zone. *Profession*, 33–40. https://www.jstor.org/stable/25595469

Ramose, M. (1999). *African philosophy through Ubuntu.* Mond Books.

Rodriguez Castro, L. (2018). Feeling-thinking for a feminist participatory visual ethnography. In D. Kember & M. Corbett (Eds.), *Structuring the thesis—Matching method, paradigm, theory and findings* (pp. 319–328). Springer. https://doi.org/10.1007/978-981-13-0511-5_32

Runyan, A. S. (2018). Decolonizing knowledges in feminist world politics. *International Feminist Journal of Politics, 20*(1), 3–8. https://doi.org/10.1080/14616742.2018.1414403

Segalo, P. (2014). Embroidery as narrative: Black South African women's experiences of suffering and healing. *Agenda (Durban, South Africa), 28*(1), 44–53. https://doi.org/10.1080/10130950.2014.872831

Segalo, P. (2018). Women speaking through embroidery: Using visual methods and poetry to narrate lived experiences. *Qualitative Research in Psychology, 15*(2–3), 298–304. https://doi.org/10.1080/14780887.2018.1430013

Segalo, P. (2020). Poison in the bone marrow: Complexities of liberating and healing the nation. *Hervormde Teologiese Studies, 76*(3), 1–6. https://doi.org/10.4102/hts.v76i3.6047

Segalo, P., & Fine, M. (2017). Threading life stories. In M. Seedat., S. Suffla & D. J. Christie (Eds.), *Emancipatory and participatory methodologies in peace, critical and community psychology* (pp. 107–117). Springer.

Segalo, P., & Fine, M. (2020). Under lying conditions of gender-based violence—Decolonial feminism meets epistemic ignorance: Critical transnational conversations. *Social and Personality Psychology Compass, 14*(10), 1–10. https://doi.org/10.1111/spc3.12568

Segalo, P., Manoff, E., & Fine, M. (2015). Working with embroideries and counter-maps: Engaging memory and imagination within decolonizing frameworks. *Journal of Social and Political Psychology, 3*(1), 342–364. https://doi.org/10.5964/jspp.v3i1.145

Simmons, A. (2021). *Impacts of climate change on young people in small island communities.* Springer. https://doi.org/10.1007/978-3-030-50657-5

Smith, G. (2012). Interview: Kaupapa Māori: The dangers of domestication. *New Zealand Journal of Educational Studies, 47*(2), 10–20.

Smith, L. (2012). *Decolonizing methodologies: Research and Indigenous peoples* (2nd ed.). Zed Books.

Smith, L., Maxwell, T. K., Puke, H., & Temara, P. (2016). Indigenous knowledge methodology and mayhem: What is the role of methodology in producing indigenous insights? A discussion from mātauranga Māori. *Knowledge Cultures, 4*(3), 131–156.

Stoudt, B. G., Torre, M. E., Bartley, P., Bracy, F., Caldwell, H., Downs, A., Greene, C., Haldipur, J., Hassan, P., Manoff, E., Sheppard, N., & Yates, J. (2019). Researching at the community–university borderlands: Using public science to study policing in the South Bronx. *Education Policy Analysis Archives, 27*(May), 56. https://doi.org/10.14507/epaa.27.2623

Te Rangi Hiroa (Sir Peter Henry Buck). (1964). *Vikings of the sunrise.* Whitcombe and Tombs Limited.

Thunberg, G. (2019). *No one is too small to make a difference.* Penguin.

Ticktin, M. (2020). Building a feminist commons in the time of COVID-19: Feminists theorize COVID-19. *SIGNS Online Journal, 47*(1).

Torre, M., Fine, M., Stoudt, B., & Fox, M. (2012). Critical participatory action research as public science. In H. Cooper, P. M. Camic, D. L. Long, A. T. Panter, D. Rindskof, & K. J. Sher (Eds.), *Qualitative research in psychology: Expanding perspectives in methodology and design* (2nd ed., pp. 171–184). American Psychological Association. https://doi.org/10.1037/13620-011

Torre, M. E. (2009). Participatory action research and critical race theory: Fueling spaces for nos-otras to research. *The Urban Review, 41*(1), 106–120. https://doi.org/10.1007/s11256-008-0097-7

Torre, M. E., & Ayala, J. (2009). Envisioning participatory action research entremundos. *Feminism & Psychology, 19*(3), 387–393. https://doi.org/10.1177/0959353509105630

Torre, M. E., & Fine, M. (with Alexander, N., Billups, A., Blanding, Y., Genao, E., Marboe, M., & Salah, T.). (2008). Participatory action research in the contact zone. In J. Cammarota & M. Fine (Eds.), *Revolutionizing education: Youth participatory action research in motion* (pp. 23–43). Routledge.

United Nations Development Programme. (2019). *The heat is on: Taking stock of global climate ambition.* https://reliefweb.int/sites/reliefweb.int/files/resources/NDC_Outlook_Report_2019.pdf

Uzwiak, B. A., & Bowles, L. R. (2021). Epistolary storytelling: A feminist sensory orientation to ethnography. *The Senses and Society, 16*(2), 203–222. https://doi.org/10.1080/17458927.2020.1858656

Vizenor, G. (1999). *Manifest manners: Narratives on postindian survivance.* University of Nebraska Press.

wa Thiong'o, N. (2009). *Re-membering Africa.* East African Educational Publishers.

Weis, L., & Fine, M. (2012). Critical bifocality and circuits of privilege: Expanding critical ethnographic theory and design. *Harvard Educational Review, 82*(2), 173–201. https://doi.org/10.17763/haer.82.2.v1jx34n441532242

Wielk, E., & Standlee, A. (2021). Fighting for their future: An exploratory study of online community building in the youth climate change movement. *Qualitative Sociology Review*, *17*(2), 22–37. https://doi.org/10.18778/1733-8077.17.2.02

Williams, B. (2016). Radical honesty: Truth telling as pedagogy. In F. Tuitt, C. Haynes, & S. Steward (Eds.), *Race, equity and the learning environment: The global relevance of critical and inclusive pedagogies in higher education* (pp. 71–82). Stylus.

Wilson, S. (2008). *Research is ceremony: Indigenous research methods*. Fernwood Publishing.

PART **III** EDUCATION, PROFESSIONAL TRAINING, AND MENTORING

8

DECOLONIZING THE HIGH SCHOOL AND UNDERGRADUATE CURRICULUM

EDIL TORRES RIVERA AND IVELISSE TORRES FERNÁNDEZ

Decolonization is not new; however, the topic has gained increased attention over the last couple of decades, as evidenced by the number of presentations and publications (Goodman & Gorski, 2015; Moosavi, 2020; Trujillo-Pagan, 2013). Decolonization is a complex process. Considering the educational system's role in promoting critical thinking skills is therefore imperative (Moratilla, 2019; Stein & de Oliveireira Andreotti, 2016). This consideration is important given the current educational climate, when various U.S. states are politicizing elementary, middle, and high public schools' curricula. In addition, some state governments have pushed to prepare students to choose a career by the time they complete high school. This chapter focuses on decolonizing high school and undergraduate educational programs. It is important to underscore that no consensus on developing a decolonial curriculum has been reached given that many scholars see this process as a colonial artifact (Freire, 1996; Mena, 2021; Mignolo, 2017; Mignolo & Walsh, 2018). Decolonization is pluralistic: the concept is understood differently depending on the person's location, positionality, and political stance. This chapter conceptualizes decolonization as disrupting Western, educated, industrialized, rich, and democratic (or WEIRD)

https://doi.org/10.1037/0000376-009
Decolonial Psychology: Toward Anticolonial Theories, Research, Training, and Practice,
L. Comas-Díaz, H. Y. Adames, and N. Y. Chavez-Dueñas (Editors)

epistemologies. Decolonization also focuses on reclaiming and reframing what has been erased from history by adding knowledge reflected in the deconstruction of the colonial discourse (Sonn & Garth, 2021). The deconstruction of the colonial discourse represents the reintroduction of counternarratives to those that place colonized people as incapable, dependent, and needing rescue. To this end, we envision decolonization as the embodiment of diverse approaches to resist oppression and racialization while seeking to transform and rediscover Indigenous ways of knowing and being in the world (Mignolo & Walsh, 2018; Stein & de Olivereira Andreotti, 2016). Indigenous, Native, or other ways of knowing are the principal bases for the decolonization movement, indicating knowledge, culture, and civilization before the colonization took place.

Throughout history, educational settings have become the center stage of colonial reproduction and indoctrination. Academic institutions have thus relied on curriculum, accreditation standards, and other regulations to control knowledge production and determine the content of the curriculum, how it is delivered, and who can access formal education. Examples of these practices include (a) using the English language as the dominant language of instruction; (b) using texts and materials that depict primarily White, European American values; and (c) vilifying the cultures, languages, and values of ethnic minoritized groups (Lebeloane, 2017; Lumadi, 2021). Resistance to using critical pedagogies, models, and praxes that promote critical thinking, social awareness, and anti-oppressive education has highlighted the role of politics and power relations in the educational process (Moratilla, 2019). Critically examining how these practices continue perpetuating the colonial mentality and promoting the hidden curriculum is therefore imperative.

As stated, one of the major concerns of decolonizing education is our understanding of knowledge. What is often considered knowledge has been dictated by Western values, specifically from societies with economic power or what is described as the Global North. Many Native scholars argue that individuals with the power to define constructs of knowledge may distort, overlook, exaggerate, and extend ignorance to preserve their power at the expense of others. Meaning factual historical events are usually "whitewashed" or erased. An excellent example is the boarding schools during colonization, the use of English only, and the prohibition of Indigenous men from having long hair, among other restrictions imposed on colonized people (Duran et al., 2008; Moosa-Mitha, 2015; see also Films for Action, 2010).

In recent years, a strong movement has surfaced in the United States targeting public education curricula, particularly those that include critical race theory and a focus on diversity (George, 2021; Gholami, 2021). Other attempts to rewrite history using the curriculum have been made as well. For example, the Texas Board of Education has a long history of attempting to stop teaching slavery in the classroom (see Monroe, 2010; Romero, 2021). These actions underscore how colonized education is a tool to maintain power over others. Moane (2014) discusses how cultural control is exerted by determining the individuals, groups, and institutions that

- Have access to formal education
- Have the authority to make decisions about the curriculum
- Can have content intentionally removed from history books and archives
- Influence and control the media (e.g., the narrative presented in news outlets, online platforms, messages, and so on)

Furthermore, schools have served as "laboratories in which social injustices such as class, gender, language, and racial inequality were inculcated, tested, implemented, and perpetuated" (Lebeloane, 2017, p. 2). Thus decolonizing the curriculum requires examining which knowledge is being reproduced and denouncing the systems and mechanisms that historically have promoted the colonial ideology (Lumadi, 2021). Decolonization cannot occur without a clear understanding of the colonization process and the politics of power and control.

Two critical components are needed to disrupt and decolonize WEIRD epistemologies and curricula. First, promoting dialogue by connecting content with students' interests is pivotal. Decolonizing the curriculum involves increasing opportunities for students to connect with knowledge in meaningful and authentic ways (Freire, 1996). Second, dialogue usually leads to critical thinking; moving beyond teaching content and incorporating active learning strategies is equally important (Freire, 1996). For example, asking students to consider a possible solution to a community problem by incorporating the latest principle or theory covered in class. By combining these strategies, educators ensure that students develop meaningful connections with the content being taught, reflect critically on the information they are learning, including who is producing the knowledge, and create a new knowledge base that includes their meaning-making.

Decolonizing the curriculum requires actions that deconstruct reductionistic ideas. It also requires us to avoid presenting fragmented and incomplete aspects of history based on the idea that one group is superior to another. A decolonized curriculum also promotes the concept of the Other as a source of knowledge and liberation (Dusell, 1985). Last, while researching literature for this chapter, we noticed that only a few sources discussed the stages of colonization (Bulhan, 2015; Enriquez, 1994; Laenui, 2000; Thira, 1995). Developing an understanding of the process of colonization is essential for us to imagine, talk, and eventually engage in actions to deconstruct WEIRD epistemologies and curricula. To this end, the following section describes the stages of the colonization process outlined by Enriquez (1994) and later updated and clarified by Laenui (2000).

STAGES OF COLONIZATION

Scholars typically outline three to four stages of colonization to describe its systemic violence (Bulhan, 2015; Thira, 1995). We find that the stages of colonization described by Enriquez (1994) and Laenui (2000) are more helpful in both describing and understanding this process. The description and characteristics of each stage allow people to identify the tools utilized in the process (e.g., violence, erasure of history). We frame these stages as a form of indoctrination with a reeducation process by the colonizer. Denial and withdrawal characterize the first stage of colonization. In this stage, the colonizer encounters Native people and begins sending the message that Native people have nothing to offer, lack morals, and that their culture has no real value. In other words, this first stage creates doubt about people's values and humanity. In academic environments, this stage is reflected by minoritized ethnic groups experiencing racism, discrimination, and marginalization regarding how their groups are represented or invisible in the curriculum.

The second stage, focusing on destruction and eradication, is characterized by more substantial attempts to destroy and eradicate all physical representations of traditional Native cultures and symbols. Examples of eradication include banning books that center on Indigenous history and ways of knowing, omitting specific historical events from the curriculum, rewriting history to glorify the colonizer's history and knowledge, and attempting to block the inclusion of critical race theory and diversity as integral components of a curriculum. From an educational standpoint, erasing Indigenous history is easier if the elements that represent it have been destroyed or hidden.

In the third stage, denigration, belittlement, and insulting, history's actual erasure occurs. The colonizer meanwhile reconstructs the culture by creating new educational, health, legal systems, and religion by demonizing every aspect of the Native system (Enriquez, 1994; Laenui, 2000). During this stage, most of the formal education is substituted by the colonizer. An example of colonization in this stage refers to developing the common core curriculum and accreditation standards, which determines what subjects will be taught, the curricular content, and how the core competencies will be achieved. In the few instances that Native culture is represented in the curriculum, it is presented superficially and without context, leading to tokenism. A particular characteristic of this stage is the beginning of tolerance, also called the Christian syndrome, referring to the belief of many Christians that they are superior to those who do not share their religious faith (Sue et al., 2019). In academic settings, this stage is manifested by enacting policies that, on the surface, are geared toward "proving" that schools are inclusive and representative of diversity. For example, many scholars from the decolonization movement indicate that a fundamental piece of the Christian syndrome is the belief that creation and nature must be improved because the original sin and emotions show humanity's weakness. Therefore, only through Evangelical Christianity can we improve and become like the Christian God, which is also synonymous with the colonizer, that is, White, Christian, and English-speaking (Blume, 2020; Morales, 2018). Thus, the erasure of history and contribution to society from other cultures as well as the tokenism in the form of affirmative action.

The final stage is the transformation and exploitation stage, characterized by the colonizer's appropriating Native customs and traditions, erasing and whitewashing Native culture. In educational spaces, we see this stage via the romanticization of Native cultures, where most cultural appropriation occurs.

As illustrated in these stages, the indoctrination and recreation of a new reality occur throughout the colonization process, which begins with devaluing Native cultures and continues with the commercialization and cultural appropriation of Native traditions. Hence colonization can be visualized as progressing across several stages in the curricula. Although the illustrations of these stages suggest a linear sequence, this is not always the case. Colonization is not linear and neither is decolonization. We recommend that a curriculum be living and dynamic, acknowledging that knowledge is not always discovered. Instead, it could be created and discovered simultaneously; one aspect is not more important than the other. In the next section, we describe different approaches to decolonizing the curriculum and propose a model.

APPROACHES TO DECOLONIZE THE CURRICULUM

Decolonizing the curriculum is a multipronged process. A curriculum has been decolonized when reviewed, improved, and confronted with its epistemic violence. Lebeloane (2017) recommended seven domains to decolonize the curriculum and promote equity and social justice, including deconstruction and reconstruction, self-determination, ethics, language, internationalization of Indigenous experiences, history, and critique. Last, the author stressed that promoting critical thinking and reflection are key elements to fostering equity and social justice in educational systems.

In addition to these elements, Lumadi (2021, p. 2) asserted that a decolonizing curriculum should address several questions: Who is teaching? Who is being taught? What is the learning content? How is it being taught? These questions are particularly relevant considering the complexities involved in this process. Thus Lumadi challenges us to reflect on our understanding of how mainstream pedagogy contributes to the reproduction of oppressive practices and how best to move toward an education that is liberating and transformative. This task requires us to name, confront, and dismantle the structures perpetuating and reproducing colonial knowledge. Decolonizing the curriculum involves shifting the current narrative by ensuring that diverse perspectives are centered. In other words, developing an inclusive curriculum that celebrates diversity and inclusivity and promotes non-Western ways of knowing.

Decolonizing the curriculum within the high school and undergraduate context also suggests rethinking current educational practices and creating spaces for critical dialogue, problem-solving, and reclaiming the silenced voices (Moratilla, 2019). In this regard, Tejeda et al. (2003) advocated for anticolonial and decolonizing pedagogical praxis that promote the development of critical consciousness and work toward ending the "mutually constitutive forms of violence that characterize our internal neocolonial condition" (p. 14). Therefore, decolonizing the curriculum requires examining which knowledge is being reproduced and denouncing the systems and mechanisms that have historically promoted the colonial ideology (Lumadi, 2021).

A Model to Decolonize the High School and Undergraduate Curriculum

In the framework we propose to decolonize the curriculum, we use the questions proposed by Lumadi (2021), the work of Tate et al. (2015), and elements of Martín Baro's (1998) principles of liberation psychology as theoretical foundations. Integrating these bodies of work presents valuable points we can use to decolonize our approach to formal education and curriculum development. Although it is essential to recognize that it might be difficult to present a discourse that challenges the status quo given the high politicization of the environment in education, we also believe that using universal dialogue principles could result in a positive outcome. We recommend using language of equals, curiosity, creativity, humility, respect, and humor. It could also be beneficial to find allies who understand the need for such work in advancing education in general and not only concerning minorities.

Stage I: Reframing the Discussion, Searching for Erased History

Living in a colonized society is a constant reminder of the oppression and the brutal control it bestows on the colonized. The first stage of the framework focuses on teaching the history of people and groups who have experienced colonization (Riggs & Badgley, 1995). During the rediscovery process, the fundamental principle is that colonized peoples learn about their entire history and can recover their culture, language, and identity (Lebeloane, 2017). Reclaiming their lost history creates the basis for the following stages.

History is written from the oppressor's perspective for many oppressed populations, particularly those colonized by foreign societies and cultures. A critical component of liberation psychology is that, in the absence of understanding the actual etiology of the oppression and the conditions that subjugation caused, authentic understandings from the perspective of the oppressed are not possible. Thus, for high school and undergraduate students, a course in global history or ethnic studies grounded heavily in the history of racial and ethnic minoritized groups could be the basis to accomplish this first stage. Three resources with ideas and methods for decolonizing the curriculum are a starting point. The Zinn Education project provides good examples of decolonizing the syllabus and selecting inclusive content (see Zinn Education Project, 2023). The University of Waterloo, School of Public Health Sciences, provides educators with steps to create more equitable and inclusive classrooms, courses, and learning experiences. This document includes additional resources, including websites and recommended books (see University of Waterloo, n.d.). The Kidsbridge Tolerance Center provides resources to decolonize the classroom. Resources include videos, websites, links, and children's resources (see Kidsbridge Center, n.d.).

Stage II: De-Ideologization, Reflecting on Erased History

This second stage centers on people lamenting their victimization and beginning processing that painful part of their lives. This stage is crucial for healing. The late bell hooks posited that no decolonization process is complete without the ex-colonized subjects experiencing deep emotions, including sadness, pain, and loss (bell hooks, cited in Riggs & Badgley, 1995). For high school and undergraduate students, a course in early critical thinking is one way to reflect on erased history. Such classes combine and describe how marginalized communities learn to analyze their social conditions critically. This process will support individuals liberating themselves from oppression rooted in the educational theory of Freire with real-life experiences, a call echoed by Martín-Baró (see Freire, 2000; Martín-Baró, 1998).

In this de-ideologization state, students are guided and supported as they deconstruct, reconstruct, and critique the curriculum they have experienced

(Lebeloane, 2017). The following two resources support the goal of stage two and can be helpful in other stages as well.

The National Council of Teachers of English (NCTE) guides strategies educators can implement to decolonize their classrooms (see NCTE, 2019). Recommendations include but are not limited to the following:

- diversify materials and content
- teach to learning outcomes that address power and social justice
- design assessments that allow diverse students to demonstrate mastery in various ways
- involve students in the creation of knowledge, content, and curriculum
- embrace diverse language usage in interactions, writing, and tests
- apply oneself at the institutional, local, state, and national levels to advocate for equity

The PBS Teachers' Lounge is an excellent resource for educators wanting to learn more about decolonizing their classroom, particularly the importance of examining one's biases and beliefs. It includes PBS in the Classroom, Technology Tools, Virtual Professional Learning, and Voices in Education (see PBS Education, 2020).

Stage III: The Strength of the People, an Essential Component of Liberation

The third stage centers on the crucial role of decolonial action. During this stage, colonized people can explore their cultures and envision their future in more detail. Thinking and working toward possibilities are encouraged and expressed through debate, dialogue, and discussions, eventually creating the basis for new beginnings. Martín Baró (1998) pointed out that it is crucial to utilize the virtues of oppressed people when working to improve their lives. He described the virtues of the oppressed people of his own country. The strengths-based approach highlighted by Martín-Baró allows social scientists to depend on oppressed people to produce the tools and energy that may lead them to liberation.

Further, utilizing the virtues of oppressed peoples takes the tools used to cope with oppressive circumstances for generations and transforms them into indispensable instruments or bridges for liberation (see Adames & Chavez-Dueñas, 2017). In the third stage, high school and college students may benefit from learning about the strengths of their ancestors. For example, *cuentos* (folktales) from Latin cultures can be used to present adaptive behavior models tailored to bridge Latin cultures' bicultural conflict, such as Juan Bobo. Additionally, the use of other historical events or books like "La visión Indigena de la conquista" and "Mitos del pueblo Taíno" (differing accounts of the history of Latin American colonization from the Indigenous perspective), to mention a few resources as well some other pre-Colombian resources to emphasize the value of previous cultures (Adames & Chavez-Dueñas, 2017; Akkeren, 2007; Dominguez, 2021).

Stage IV: Conscientization by Integrating Stages I Through III

The path to decolonizing educational spaces necessitates the development of critical consciousness. That is, individuals need to understand how colonized views and perspectives have dominated the academic discourse so that they can begin questioning the structures that have perpetuated such colonization. In addition, individuals may create opportunities for reclaiming their erased history, discuss the impact of colonization, and begin the healing process. The healing process entails including antioppressive education, creating spaces for critical dialogues about issues of diversity and inclusion and of revamping curriculum and accreditation standards, among others. This process is dynamic and circular; therefore, similar characteristics will overlap with each other and appear in different stages.

Critical collaboration inquiry is the use of problematization—the act of questioning and, in that process, eroding the foundations of some beliefs and habits (Montero, 2009), in particular the de-ideologized understanding of the erased history, in conjunction with the people's strengths, to understand and work on the problems that oppressed groups face. As mentioned earlier, the goal of liberation, according to Freire, is the creation of critical thinking. That could be illustrated as problematization will lead to reflection. Reflection will lead to critical consciousness. Critical consciousness will lead to change (action). The illustration of the model looks like this: problematization > reflection > critical consciousness > action > reflection dynamics. This suggested model has based on the premise that transitions between stages follow a natural progression and that creating critical thinking will lead to action. The liberation psychology literature supports this approach (see Comas-Díaz & Torres Rivera, 2020; Sharma & Hipolito-Delgado, 2021).

One resource to consider is the Council of International Schools, which provides a blog on strategies to decolonize the curriculum. The site offers five questions that guide educators and leaders committed to decolonizing the curriculum and specific actions, including incorporating project-based learning (for more, see CIS 2021). The particular action items discussed include the need to examine the course syllabus and curriculum sequence documentation. As part of the process, educators are invited to reflect on the following questions:

1. What is being noticed about the content?

2. What would it look like from a postcolonial perspective?

3. Regarding the content of the readings and materials presented in class, to what extent are cultural references, historical facts, authors, and discoveries presented as Western, male dominated, and European?

4. To what extent does the content offer students diverse views and stories from First Peoples, Africa, Asia, pre-Columbian civilizations, the Middle East, and Oceanic regions?

5. What, if any, critical discussions are happening in the classroom to ensure deep reflection on the power of representation in how textbooks present materials to learners?

CONCLUSION

Striving for equity, inclusion, social justice, and anti-oppressive education within the U.S. educational system is important. However, decolonizing the curriculum and integrating practices that disrupt and challenge the systems perpetuating oppression, discrimination, and marginalization of minoritized and racialized groups continues to be complicated. The challenge is primarily associated with the dominant discourse of imposing Eurocentric values at the expense of demonizing and devaluing Indigenous ways of knowing. As mentioned earlier, at every step, the colonization process tries to degrade and dehumanize Native cultures by controlling their authority, economics, knowledge, subjectivity (education), and gender and sexuality, which Quijano (2000) identified as the matrix of power. The colonizer uses the tools of violence, political exclusion, economic exploitation, control of sexuality and culture (education), and fragmentation to gain power (Moane, 2014). Decolonizing educational spaces requires a deep understanding of colonization and integrating a liberatory praxis, including critical reflexivity, problematization, and social transformation. We hope this chapter motivates educators and academics to engage in critical dialogues regarding what is being taught, how information is presented, which groups are included and excluded, and what traditional values are being promoted. We assert that even though decolonizing academic spaces is a complex and challenging process, it is imperative if we strive to achieve equity and promote antioppressive education.

RESOURCES

Carson, Q. (2017, August 25). *Pedagogy of the decolonizing* [Video]. TEDxUAlberta. https://www.youtube.com/watch?v=lN17Os8JAr8
Diaz, P. (Director). (2010). *The end of poverty?* [Film]. https://cinemalibrestudio.com/theendofpoverty/

REFERENCES

Adames, H. Y., & Chavez-Dueñas, N. Y. (2017). *Cultural foundations and interventions in Latino/a mental health: History, theory and within group differences*. Routledge.

Akkeren, R. V. (2007). *La visión Indígena de la conquista* [The Indigenous view of conquest]. Fundación del Centro de Investigaciones Regionales de Mesoamérica.

Blume, A. (2020). *A new psychology based on community, equality, and care of the earth: An Indigenous American perspective*. Praeger.

Bulhan, H. A. (2015). Stages of colonialism in Africa: From occupation of land to occupation of being. *Journal of Social and Political Psychology, 3*(1), 239–256. https://doi.org/10.5964/jspp.v3i1.143

Comas-Díaz, L., & Torres Rivera, E. (Eds.). (2020). *Liberation psychology: Theory, method, practice, and social justice*. America Psychological Association. https://doi.org/10.1037/0000198-000

Council of International Schools (CIS). (2021). Decolonising the curriculum. https://www.cois.org/about-cis/news/post/~board/perspectives-blog/post/decolonising-the-curriculum

Dominguez, R. A. (2021). *Juan Bobo: Cuentos insólitos*. ibukku, LLC.

Duran, E., Firehammer, J., & Gonzalez, J. (2008). Liberation psychology as the path toward healing cultural soul wounds. *Journal of Counseling and Development, 86*(3), 288–295. https://doi.org/10.1002/j.1556-6678.2008.tb00511.x

Dusell, E. (1985). *Philosophy of liberation*. Orbis Books.

Enriquez, V. G. (1994). *From colonial to liberation psychology: The Philippine experience*. De La Salle University Press.

Films for Action. (2010). *Schooling the world* [Film]. https://www.filmsforaction.org/watch/schooling-the-world-2010/

Freire, P. (1996). *Pedagogy of the oppressed* (Rev. ed.). Penguin Group.

Freire, P. (2000). *Cultural action for freedom*. Harvard Educational Review.

George, J. (2021). A lesson on critical race theory. *The American Bar Association*, 1–9. https://www.americanbar.org/groups/crsj/publications/human_rights_magazine_home/civil-rights-reimagining-policing/a-lesson-on-critical-race-theory/

Gholami, R. (2021). Critical race theory and Islamophobia: Challenging inequity in higher education. *Race, Ethnicity and Education, 24*(3), 319–337. Advance online publication. https://doi.org/10.1080/13613324.2021.1879770

Goodman, R. D., & Gorski, P. C. (Eds.). (2015). *Decolonizing "multicultural" counseling through social justice*. Springer. https://doi.org/10.1007/978-1-4939-1283-4

Kidsbridge Center. (n.d.). *Decolonization of the classroom resources*. https://www.kidsbridgecenter.org/resources-for-decolonizing-the-classroom/

Laenui, P. (2000). Processes of decolonization. In M. A. Battiste (Ed.), *Reclaiming Indigenous voice and vision* (pp. 150–160). The University of British Columbia Press.

Lebeloane, L. D. M. (2017). Decolonizing the school curriculum for equity and social justice in South Africa. *Koers, 82*(3), 1–10. https://doi.org/10.19108/KOERS.82.3.2333

Lumadi, M. W. (2021). The pursuit of decolonising and transforming curriculum in higher education. *South African Journal of Higher Education, 35*(1), 1–3. https://doi.org/10.20853/35-1-4527

Martín Baró, I. (1998). *Psicología de la liberación*. Editorial Trotta.

Mena, J. (2021). *Decolonizing curriculum*. https://www.tc.columbia.edu/decolonizing-psychology-conference/

Mignolo, W. (2017). Coloniality is far from over, and so must be decoloniality. *Afterall: A Journal of Art, Context and Enquiry, 43*(Spring/Summer), 38–45. https://doi.org/10.1086/692552

Mignolo, W., & Walsh, C. E. (2018). *On decoloniality: Concepts, analytics, praxis*. Duke University Press.

Moane, G. (2014). Liberation psychology, feminism, and social justice psychology. In J. Diaz, Z. Franco, & K. Nastasi, Bonnie (Eds.), *The Praeger handbook of social justice and psychology: Vol. 1. Fundamental issues and special populations* (pp. 115–132). Praeger.

Monroe, B. (2010, May 24). How Texas' school board tried to pretend slavery never happened and why your kid's school may be next. *HuffPost*. https://www.huffpost.com/entry/how-texas-school-board-tr_b_586633

Montero, M. (2009). Methods for liberation: Critical consciousness in action. In M. Montero & C. Sonn (Eds.), *Psychology of liberation: Theory and applications* (pp. 73–91). Springer.

Moosa-Mitha, M. (2015). Situating anti-oppression theories within critical and difference-centred perspectives. In S. Strega & L. Brown (Eds.), *Research as resistance: Revisiting critical, indigenous, and anti-oppressive approaches* (2nd ed., pp. 65–96). Canadian Scholars' Press: Women's Press.

Moosavi, L. (2020). The decolonial bandwagon and the dangers of intellectual decolonisation. *International Review of Sociology, 30*(2), 332–354. https://doi.org/10.1080/03906701.2020.1776919

Morales, E. (2018). *Latinx: The new force in American politics and culture*. Verso.

Moratilla, N. C. A. (2019). Revisiting Paulo: Critical pedagogy and testimonial narratives as liberative spaces in the Philippines' K–12 curriculum. *The Journal for Critical Education Policy Studies, 17*(2), 246–278.

National Council of Teachers of English. (2019, April 11). *Decolonizing the classroom: Step 1*. https://ncte.org/blog/2019/04/decolonizing-the-classroom/

PBS Education. (2020, August 3). *Decolonizing our classrooms starts with us*. https://www.pbs.org/education/blog/decolonizing-our-classrooms-starts-with-us

Quijano, A. (2000). Coloniality of power and Eurocentrism in Latin America. *International Sociology, 15*(2), 215–232. https://doi.org/10.1177/0268580900015002005

Riggs, M., & Badgley, C. (1995). *Black is . . . Black ain't*. Newsreel.

Romero, S. (2021, May 20). Texas pushes to obscure the state's history of slavery and racism. *The New York Times.* https://www.nytimes.com/2021/05/20/us/texas-history-1836-project.html

Sharma, J., & Hipolito-Delgado, C. P. (2021). Promoting anti-racism and critical consciousness through a critical counseling theories course. *Teaching and Supervision in Counseling, 3*(2), 15–25. https://doi.org/10.7290/tsc030203

Sonn, C. C., & Garth, S. (2021). Tracking the decolonial turn in contemporary community psychology: Expanding socially just knowledge archives, ways of being and modes of praxis. In S. Garth & C. C. Sonn (Eds.), *Decoloniality and epistemic justice in contemporary community psychology* (pp. 1–19). Springer. https://doi.org/10.1007/978-3-030-72220-3_1

Stein, S., & de Olivereira Andreotti, V. (2016). Historicizing decolonization and higher education. In M. Peters (Ed.), *Encyclopedia of educational philosophy and theory* (pp. 370–375). Springer. https://doi.org/10.1007/978-981-287-532-7_479-1

Sue, D. W., Sue, D., Neville, H. A., & Smith, L. (2019). *Counseling the culturally diverse: Theory and practice* (8th ed.). Wiley.

Tate, K. A., Torres Rivera, E., & Edwards, L. M. (2015). Colonialism and multicultural counseling competence research: A liberatory analysis. In R. D. Goodman & P. C. Gorski (Eds.), *Decolonizing "multicultural" counseling through social justice* (pp. 41–54). Springer. https://doi.org/10.1007/978-1-4939-1283-4_4

Tejeda, C., Espinoza, M., & Gutierrez, K. (2003). Toward a decolonizing pedagogy: Social justice reconsidered. In P. P. Trifonas (Ed.), *Pedagogies of difference: Rethinking education for social change* (pp. 9–38). Routledge.

Thira, D. (1995). Beyond the four waves of colonization. *Centre for Native Policy and Research Collection.* https://chodarr.org/sites/default/files/chodarr0255.pdf

Trujillo-Pagan, N. (2013). *Modern colonization by medical intervention: U.S. medicine in Puerto Rico.* Brill. https://doi.org/10.1163/9789004243712

University of Waterloo. (n. d.). *Resources for instructors to decolonize and indigenize teaching and learning.* https://uwaterloo.ca/public-health-sciences/resources-instructors-decolonize-and-indigenize-teaching

Zinn Education Project. (2023, January 1). *#Teachtruth syllabus.* https://www.zinnedproject.org/news/teachtruth-syllabus/

9 UNLEARNING COLONIAL PRACTICES AND (RE)ENVISIONING GRADUATE EDUCATION IN PSYCHOLOGY

CARRIE L. CASTAÑEDA-SOUND, MIGUEL GALLARDO, AND SUSANA O. SALGADO

We have come to realize that we are not alone in our struggles nor separate nor autonomous but that we . . . are connected and inter-dependent. We are each accountable for what is happening down the street, south of the border, or across the sea.

—Gloria Anzaldúa (Anzaldúa & Keating, 2002, p. 19)

Professional training for aspiring licensed psychotherapists within the United States requires an individual to complete rigorous curricular and clinical training requirements. These requirements are codified, standardized, and monitored by state licensing boards, professional organizations, accrediting organizations, ethics boards, and higher education institutions. This approach is intended to protect the public from harm and stems from a medical education and training model. Unfortunately, with this protection come colonizing pedagogical viewpoints and practices that sometimes can ultimately harm the communities that they intend to serve. Communities that traditionally have been underserved or pathologized by the mental health system pay the price for

https://doi.org/10.1037/0000376-010
Decolonial Psychology: Toward Anticolonial Theories, Research, Training, and Practice,
L. Comas-Díaz, H. Y. Adames, and N. Y. Chavez-Dueñas (Editors)

a one-size-fits-all approach to education and training in psychology. Drawing from scholarly work from critical pedagogical studies, cultural studies, and liberation psychology, this chapter illustrates the importance of training masters and doctoral students with an ecologically attuned curriculum. Decolonization involves questioning, identifying, and disrupting the processes and effects of colonization within systems and structures that maintain power and control. We embrace, center, and elevate approaches that reclaim Indigenous ways of knowing, being, and healing. Indigenous ways of knowing embody a deep respect for and reciprocal relationship with the land and the elements as well as the unseen spiritual world. Knowledge is informed by experiences with community and the natural elements, and this knowledge is often shared via oral tradition across generations.

We are mindful of the limitations of a prescriptive approach to defining the decolonization of graduate education and training. Fellner (2018) viewed decolonization as "tricky concept" to define and experiences some of these limitations as deriving from the English language. She explained:

> I have heard countless definitions and varied understandings of what deco-loniality means and what it entails. I have also heard numerous Indigenous people criticize these terms and concepts, with some asserting that they should not be used at all primarily due to their vague nature and the impossibility and, often, undesirability, of an absolute decolonization. For me, this is always the catch with the English language. (p. 284)

As a result, Fellner wrote about "embody[ing] decoloniality" to defray these limitations by "walking the talk—living decolonizing and Indigenizing both inside and outside of the classroom" (p. 284).

Aligned with a decolonized approach, we include our voices at different points throughout this chapter to contextualize our experiences and share our positionality in our journey to decolonize our teaching and practice. We engage in *testimonio*, a form of storytelling grounded in resistance, solidarity, and empowerment with roots in Chicanx studies, liberation psychology, and mujerista liberation psychology. Testimonio is a method employed by educators, researchers, mental health professionals, and healers (Cienfuegos & Monelli, 1983; Comas-Díaz, 2020a; Comas-Díaz 2020b; Delgado Bernal et al., 2012). Reyes and Curry Rodríguez (2012) explained, "What is certain is that testimonio is not meant to be hidden, made intimate, nor kept secret. The objective of the testimonio is to bring to light a wrong, a point of view, or an urgent call for action" (p. 525). In addition to our testimonios, we synthesize the areas of graduate training that we believe need to be decolonized. We also share challenges and strategies for navigating the process of decolonization. We provide examples of conceptual and structural concerns for developing a specialty track at the doctoral level, as well as Aliento (breath), a Latinx master's program where decolonizing practices, such as liberation psychology, are central to the training and education students receive. Finally, we discuss the praxis of decolonization in the clinical supervision of graduate students.

EMBRACING CRITICAL CONSCIOUSNESS AND A SOCIAL JUSTICE ETHIC

> Our profession calls on us to 'do no harm', but it also sits in a place of inaction while societal abuse is being perpetuated. (Lewis, 2020, para. 6)

Lewis's statement about do no harm was written to raise consciousness about the lack of antiracist efforts within the medical and health care systems. It also reflects the realities of our discipline in psychology. What role should psychology have in addressing the structural violence and systems of oppression that impact the daily lives of many devalued communities? What standards and expectations should be in place to ensure that our graduate training frameworks do a better job in revisiting theories and intervention models that may have limited applicability with many Black, Indigenous, People of Color (BIPOC) communities? As some debate these questions, pushback and critique from some in White communities continues, and some folks of color (it has always been about one's level of consciousness over the color of one's skin), within psychology about what our role should be. The Universal Declaration of Ethical Principles for Psychologists (International Union of Psychological Science, 2008) is one example that outlines four principles that provide the backdrop by which we should consider our role and function in creating a more peaceful society. The preamble to the declaration states that

> Psychologists recognize that they carry out their activities within a larger social context. They recognize that the lives and identities of human beings both individually and collectively are connected across generations, and that there is a reciprocal relationship between human beings and their natural and social environments. Psychologists are committed to placing the welfare of society and its members above the self-interest of the discipline and its members. (p. 1)

The preamble goes on to state that the declaration provides a moral framework by which organizations "(a) evaluate the ethical and moral relevance of their ethics codes; (b) . . . use as a template to guide the development or evolution of their codes of ethics; (c) . . . encourage global thinking about ethics, while also encouraging action that is sensitive and responsive to local needs and values; and (d) . . . speak with a collective voice on matters of ethical concern" (p. 1). What we value and appreciate about the declaration is the focus on shared human values and a commitment from psychology communities to build a better world where peace, freedom, justice, humanity, and moral values succeed. Suppose this truly is our goal within the various psychological communities. In that case, it raises the question for us as psychologists and the organizations that govern the discipline of what it means to do no harm.

Unfortunately, definitions of what doing no harm means vary. Does it imply meeting the minimal standards and requirements in the American Psychological Association (APA) Ethical Principles of Psychologists and Code of Conduct (2017a), primarily rooted in White Euro-settler values? Or does it imply revisiting and reimagining what our work can and should look like? We would argue the latter. Several versions of ethical codes and guidelines have been developed— by the Association of Black Psychologists (2019), the Society of Indian Psychologists (García & Tehee, 2014), and, more recently, the National Latinx Psychological Association (NLPA, 2020)—that demonstrate what a moral, ethical compass might look like if we were truly placing the interests of those that we serve before our own. I (Miguel Gallardo) learned long ago that the path to hell is paved with good intentions. Our good intentions are simply not enough. More recent efforts have developed synchronicity between the APA Ethics Code and those of the various multicultural communities within psychology (Domenech Rodríguez et al., 2020). These efforts continue, but the challenges of centering our work within culturally embedded frames remain.

Wendt and her colleagues (2015) wrote, "The history of modern medicine suggests that 'harm' does not have a straightforward, objective, or obvious meaning. Rather, harm is a social construct that is interpreted and negotiated, however informally, in relation to norms about well-being, clinical treatment, and social relations" (p. 346). The concept of harm is distorted by dynamics such as concerns about litigation, the financial status of the client, and mental health legislation (Wendt et al., 2015, pp. 346–347). Systemic racism, sexism, classism, heteronormative values, and the concept of what constitutes a family from Euro-settler viewpoints, to name a few, were developed to rationalize the justification of unjust and inhumane treatment of many BIPOC communities, including the systemwide support of organizational policies over people, wealth over health, and laws that continue to sustain and support the status quo. The fields of psychology are not immune to the influences and impact of these various systems of oppression. The "isms" of the world are in the air we breathe. If we as individuals and organizations are not intentionally filtering the air, we will violate our moral and ethical compass, maybe without even realizing it at times. The power of colonialism runs deep, and the will to unlearn colonialist values and attitudes runs shallow. The profession developed and was designed to assist people with the pain and challenges they may experience can also reinforce harmful and oppressive practices at times. As a result, good, well-intentioned psychologists may be faced with the dilemma of investing in their self-protection over engaging in what they deem the most effective and culturally congruent interventions necessary to create a healing space for their clients (Gallardo et al., 2009). However, we cannot blame the individual psychologist who relies on the system to fulfill societal and professional expectations. We should hold these systems—which placed psychologists and trainees in unrealistic and unethical situations—accountable.

Why Western Euro-Settler Perspectives Should Be Deconstructed

The psychology profession continues to attempt to integrate multicultural and social justice principles in ethics codes, the *Diagnostic and Statistical Manual of Mental Disorders* (American Psychiatric Association, 2022), guidelines, and training programs, to name a few. However, these principles are often placed alongside mainstream notions of what psychology should look like but without any analysis of how the two merge and diverge from one another. Without an analysis and the intentional deconstruction of these two often opposing forces, competence, as defined by White Euro-settler values, will often displace multicultural and social justice competencies (APA, 2017b) for many. We argue that multicultural principles, social justice ethics, and human rights for all are necessary essentials to address in psychology graduate education programs to minimize the harm that some Eurocentric psychological perspectives, theories, interventions, and overall values can have in the lives of those most vulnerable. If we do not address these issues with some level of intentionality, we will continue to ill equip our students in addressing underserved and unserved communities' needs. We argue that the discrepancies between most current curriculum standards and the work demanded of students when they graduate are both a disservice to the students and unethical. This is one of those moments when good well-intentioned providers, might be unintentionally violating those they are attempting to serve.

A BRIEF EXCERPT IN A LIFELONG JOURNEY OF UNLEARNING AND RELEARNING: MIGUEL'S TESTIMONIO

As the program director of Aliento, I (Miguel Gallardo), and our faculty, work to create the space for our students to develop their voices and address unjust circumstances, both within the university setting, and outside. This is not always an easy process, and the process itself reinforces our decolonial and liberatory approaches. As a result, our students are vocal, which I hope is an affirmation that we have created the space for them to express what matters most to them, and more importantly, to listen to them. One of the most difficult outcomes of our efforts is to hear comments directed at our program, and at times, to me, particularly critical feedback about how decisions have been made, how a class may be unfolding, or negotiating the challenges of being in colonial system that assume all students know exactly how to benefit most from it. As the program director, I have struggled at times with my own colonial approaches to issues arising in our program and within the larger university system. I have long said that I work as hard as anyone else at remaining conscious and intentional in all that I do, but like all others, I stumble and fall. It is part of the work. I am often reminded of being inculcated in traditional academic settings that did not always do a good job decolonizing the curriculum and training experiences. I have learned that movement is not the same thing as progress. The movement must be intentional and meaningful and followed with intentional and meaningful actions and behaviors. I have existed within systems for many years that have long operated within the confines of Euro-settler values and ideas, and getting tangled within those bounds is easy. After all, I reap the benefits of the great oppressive force known as colonialism. I am paid to teach, mentor, supervise, direct, research, and consult because my university has given me the space to do so. In fact, if you are reading this chapter, you will likely also benefit from the systems we are attempting to deconstruct and hoping to reconstruct. This book is being published by the American Psychological Association, the gatekeeper of psychological knowledge, including whether something can and should be disseminated and validated as credible information with strong evidence to support it. Many within the APA will balk at a book on decolonial approaches and do not like it when we speak about the deconstruction of anything. However, as I sit and write this chapter out of interest and to collaborate with great colleagues, I know that it will benefit me in my academic institution. As I constantly negotiate between doing what I think is right and just for the students and program, meanwhile attempting to manage traditional academic and colonial systems, I have felt hypocritical, as if I were speaking out of both sides of my mouth at times. Trying to find the rhythm keeps me up at night. I remember hearing Dr. Cornell West speak at the University of California, Irvine, close to 18 to 19 years ago, when I worked there; when he was asked why he does not occupy more administrative positions within academic settings, he responded that the higher one goes up within most, if not all, systems, the more one loses their voice. His words resonated with me at the time, and I am constantly reminded of them as I think of my work of more than 21 years in the field of psychology. Developing and overseeing the Aliento program is like being in a constant battle to honor the work and to continue to find ways to be creative and imaginative in ensuring meaningful action behind the words and language we use, all within systems created to support limited ideas of the world and those of us in it. One of the greatest calamities of colonialism is the loss of creativity and imagination. We try to teach our students these critical values. No one does anything alone or in isolation. I have had help all along the way. I have had other BIPOC colleagues in the system and allies who have supported my and our efforts in the program. Two of them are my coauthors for this chapter. Both have challenged me in different ways for different reasons, and both have been instrumental in sustaining the Aliento program. We also have incredible faculty and supervisors dedicated to the program and the students. Without them, we have no program.

The Aliento Program

Prilleltensky (1997) wrote, "Discourse without action is dangerous because it creates the impression that progress is taking place when in fact, only the words have changed" (p. 530). This remains central in all that we do in the Aliento program and also represents one of our greatest challenges as a program. The Aliento, the Center for Latinx Communities at Pepperdine University, is a terminal master's degree program that attempts to decolonize more traditional methodologies within a colonized university system. Housing three interrelated spaces, including a terminal master's degree program, a research institute, and community outreach, it was launched in 2012. These three spaces all work in sync with one another by providing opportunities for master's level students to gain research experience with BIPOC communities through our research institute and by providing students with opportunities to deliver psychoeducational workshops and training that have a direct impact on Latinx communities. One year later, in 2013, we admitted our first cohort of students invested in serving Latinx communities. Brown (2009) stated that the dominant culture always writes history. When two cultures clash, the dominant culture becomes the historian, the keeper and disseminator of all knowledge and how history is recorded, how ethnocultural communities are then vilified, and how the rights and privileges of the majority are raised. Award-winning journalist Maria Hinojosa explained: "My stories didn't appear. We were invisible. I was invisible from the media narrative. No one in the reporting that I saw looked like me [and] looked like my family, so I began to think that maybe somehow my life—my story—was less valuable" (TEDx, 2015, 1:11). The sentiments Brown and Hinojosa expressed reflect what we hope to undo and teach our students to unlearn with the Aliento program. We have learned that decolonizing anything in words and language is much easier than taking action and instituting meaningful change. The goals of the program include training students to work with Latinx communities from strength-based perspectives. Our hope is to prepare students to integrate a community-based, liberatory lens in their conceptualization and therapeutic approaches when working with underserved and unserved Latinx communities. The program is also committed to developing students' cultural and linguistic responsiveness by training bilingual (English and Spanish) speakers in working with monolingual Spanish communities in more linguistically congruent ways. We offer two semesters of mental health Spanish-language classes for bilingual students who enter our program. These classes are taught entirely in Spanish and students read, write, and present all class content in Spanish. During the second semester of Spanish-language classes, we offer students an opportunity to travel for an immersion program where they learn about mental health systems, practices, and cultural practices of diverse Latinx communities. Thus far, the immersion trip has been to Buenos Aires, Argentina (Pepperdine campus), and to Lima and Cusco, Peru.

An essential component of a decolonial Latinx training program is ensuring that we are not silencing the students' voices. Most students in the program are bilingual Latinas, the first generation in college in their families. They have endured an educational system that has invalidated and devalued the authenticity of their and our stories. As a result, our curriculum was cocreated with community feedback, including lay community members and professionals in the field. The feedback formed approximately half of the entire curriculum, which includes about 30 units of Latinx-specific course content, including the two semesters of Spanish mental health classes.

The program's foundations are rooted in the teachings of liberation psychology (Martín-Baró, 1994) and *Pedagogy of the Oppressed* (Freire, 1970). In our efforts to implement a program that is decolonial, we invite students to help cocreate the content of our classes. The classroom is built heavily on discourse and challenges the notion of the banking system of education (Freire, 1970). Freire's banking system of education highlights the professor or teacher as the primary active participant in the learning process, and the students as passive recipients of the information communicated by the professor or teacher. Freire stated that the professor or teacher communicates what is important (i.e., making deposits), which students passively receive, only to try to memorize and repeat the information later. The banking system, where deposits are made into the students' fund of knowledge, assumes that the professor or teacher is the holder of all knowledge and information that is important and relevant, and that the students are mere recipients of our knowledge, meanwhile minimizing what they know, their lived experiences, and their contributions in cocreating knowledge in the classroom. If we want our students to walk with Latinx communities in an effort toward liberation, we need to walk with our students to assist them in unlearning and liberating the colonial ideologies and values they unconsciously bring to our program (i.e., that their experiences are not valid, legitimate, or as important as others). Additionally, we teach about Indigenous healing practices, which are central in our work toward reconnecting with ancestral wisdom, traditions, and practices. Indigenous healing practices have their origins with a specific culture and are accepted within that culture to heal and treat any needs that may arise within that culture. The practices are intended to oftentimes treat the whole person, mind, body, spirit, and emotions. An imbalance in these areas of our wholeness are thought to be the cause of physical and emotional challenges we may experience. Indigenous healing practices have existed for centuries and yet their validity in healing continues to be questioned by many in Western psychology, including by their omission in many graduate training programs. Only when Western culture appropriates these practices do they become "legitimate" forms of healing. In the Aliento program, these practices remain central both to uplifting what our students have been exposed to in their lives and to ensuring that they receive the message that Indigenous practices are culturally valid, relevant, and necessary for healing to occur for many Latinx communities.

Each Aliento-specific class is an exercise in critically examining Euro-settler perspectives about what psychology historically has indicated what our work should look like from more traditional viewpoints. From the *Diagnostic and Statistical Manual of Mental Disorders* (American Psychiatric Association, 2022) to psychological theories and interventions to the family life cycle, each class examines the historical underpinnings of colonial knowledge, with an intentional reenvisioning of Western ideologies in ways that are more reflective and liberating for Latinx communities. The program's decolonial practices begin with our syllabi, which include antiracist intersectional, territorial or land, pronoun, and family or community statements. The family or community statement is particularly important for our students in that it creates the space where our students can bring family and loved ones to our classroom community. The statement reads as follows:

> The Aliento Program believes that if we want more BIPOC communities and women in academia, that we should expect children/loved ones to be present in some form, at some point in our class. Currently, the university does not have a formal policy on children/loved ones in the classroom. The policy described here is a reflection of the Aliento programs beliefs, values, and commitments to student, staff and faculty parents/caregivers.

Many challenges are associated with operating a decolonial program in a colonial system, too many to name here. However, the Aliento program hopes to challenge how mainstream psychology continues to colonize. Goodman and Gorski (2015) identified ways in which psychology is still colonizing through its efforts to deny and destroy culture, minimize and dehumanize cultural values and practices, and control how cultural values are expressed within the already existing infrastructure built and maintained by the colonizer.

When we launched the Aliento program, other professionals in the field struggled with what we required them to do if they wanted our Aliento students at their practicum sites. As our students were placed in community agencies to fulfill their practicum placements, we required sites to provide supervision in Spanish if they were asked to provide services in Spanish. We got pushback: people were unhappy and did not understand why this mattered. It mattered because we needed to ensure that our Spanish-English bilingual students received the support they needed and were not being further oppressed as laborers within systems where they were trying to liberate their communities while being paid nothing for their labor. The lack of compensation also keeps me up at night. For years, trying to educate other mental health professionals and agencies about why this mattered was one of my and our greatest fights. Although the pushback on ensuring that students have adequate support while providing services in Spanish has lessened significantly over the last decade, the question of why this is really necessary remains in the air in psychology and mental health more generally. Agencies and providers still perpetuate lessons learned through colonialist values without the explicit awareness of their oppression and devaluing of the work our Spanish- and English-speaking students provide. The need for services is considerable; if agencies or other entities want to provide those services to marginalized communities, resources need to be there. Otherwise, these entities will attempt to provide services to Latinx and other BIPOC communities in a way that may further increase disparities, create unnecessary barriers, and decrease access to services intended to heal and not further harm. The path to hell can be paved with good intentions.

Viray and Nash (2014) stated that to experience the suffering of others and then try hard to lessen that suffering is the most salient social justice action of all. I do not know whether this captures the essence of what social justice actions mean, but it resonates with me and with the work of the Aliento program. Most of our students are of the community and have experienced the pain and suffering they see in those they serve. One way that decolonial work shows up in the Aliento program is in affirming and validating the students' lived experiences while assisting them in unlearning unhelpful ways of understanding themselves and others. In essence, liberation and radical healing, and self-love start with oneself. We hope that their liberation as Latinx individuals trying to reconcile the legacies of colonialism within themselves, at times, leads to the liberation of those they serve.

TEACHING WITH SPIRIT AND CORAZÓN: CARRIE'S TESTIMONIO

> By approaching the discussion and enacting a borderlands experience, I am situating my pedagogy in an untraversed process where traditional pedagogy becomes linear and spiritual pedagogy becomes serpentine. (Figueroa, 2014, p. 35)

Maria Figueroa (2014) wrote about spiritual pedagogy and how she infuses a holistic approach into her work. She explained how her spiritual pedagogy integrates subjective, emotional, and intuitive elements of her student's lives and the objective and cognitive components. This approach resonates with my experience as a teacher and learner throughout my life. Teaching has been a spiritual journey that began when I was a child standing in front of a class pretending to teach a lesson to my younger cousin. My grandmother, a custodian at an elementary school, let us play in the classrooms while she worked. The lesson I was teaching my cousin escapes my memory, but I can still feel the excitement of being in the front of a classroom, and that feeling has never left me. Yet I was also afraid I would be caught in this pretend play by the "real teachers." Unfortunately, this feeling and belief also stayed with me. Part of unlearning this internalized fear of being caught pretending involved finding my voice and experience in the scholarship I read and wrote, the colleagues I worked with, and in the communities where I lived and worked. I found answers within ethnic and gender studies, social psychology, and critical educational studies. This was when I was exposed to the work of Paulo Friere, Ignacio Martín-Baró, bell hooks, Gloria Anzaldúa, and scholars in critical race theory. These scholars spoke to my mind, emotions, and soul. Their work reflected the lived experiences of my family members and generational challenges with institutions of power.

The Mayan wisdom "In Lak'ech Ala K'in [I am you, and you are me]" has influenced my life (Valdez, 1973). As a midcareer faculty member teaching from a liberation psychology framework in a clinical psychology doctorate program, I experience teaching as a relationship between all who step into the classroom. Teaching and learning have always been relational, spiritual, storied, and more than a transaction for me. I am changed by every class I facilitate and the community the students and I cocreate.

Cada Cabeza es un Mundo (Each Person Is Their Own World)

One of the approaches to decolonization of the curriculum that I (Carrie Castañeda-Sound) incorporate is to introduce and enact frameworks such as liberation psychology, Mujerista psychology, and womanism. Embedded in these frameworks are critical consciousness, and a relational consciousness. The relationship I have with my students is comparable to the elements of liberation psychotherapy presented by Comas-Díaz (2020b) but adapted for the classroom. They are radical humility, radical empathy, *acompañamiento*, creativity, spirituality, and social justice. These elements overlap, are simultaneously embedded throughout the class, and show up in our dialogues, assignments, and readings.

Radical humility deconstructs the notion that the instructor holds all the knowledge and is the expert. The reality, even though I have more years of lived experience as a psychologist, is that students come to the classroom with knowledge and wisdom. Asking students to tap into their knowledge and wisdom is often challenging because they are conditioned to be receivers of knowledge and forget, or are afraid, to listen to their intuition. This forgetting can have different etiologies. Although not every student can engage in the process of connecting with their inner wisdom, I model this through *acompañamiento* and radical empathy. *Acompañamiento* allows me as an instructor to witness and join my students in our collective journey of critical consciousness. I ask them to identify how coloniality has affected their lives specifically (e.g., benefits, detriments, or both) and those of their clients' lives. Moreover, we interrogate how we may have caused harm by actions or inaction in our roles as therapists and trainees. These dialogues sometimes include students' sharing instances when they or loved ones have been the target of harm by the mental health profession.

This process of *acompañamiento* is complemented by radical empathy. In psychotherapy, radical empathy requires that the therapist be able to "intuitively feel their [client's] pain" (Comas-Díaz, 2020b p. 176). We begin and end every class with a check-in, and I often will use prompts that require "sensorial modes of connection and other nonrational kinds of knowledge" (p. 176). Sometimes this entails using music, poetry, spoken word, literature, films, podcasts, and imagination. I often envision their clients in the classroom with us and ask each student in the class to think of a client and imagine what they would want us to know about their life experiences. I also ask students to look around and name the "voices" not present in the classroom. These voices reflect people with marginalized identities or people who have experiences that place them on the fringes of society. This helps graduate students learn to attune to what is not only visible but also invisible (or erased).

Creativity, spirituality, and social justice are core elements of my classes. I have guest speakers in my class who are traditional healers and activists to talk about forms of spiritual healing that happen in culturally specific ways and often are tied to social justice movements. Getting students to think about liberatory frameworks outside our classroom's four walls is important to me. Using activities such as Theatre of the Oppressed (Boal, 1979) in the local community, we embody a decolonized approach to learning and being in the community. Theater of the Oppressed is a method that takes social issues "into the street" to engage in dialogue with people and to raise awareness and consciousness. In my class, students formed three to four groups to address different mental health issues (e.g., isolation and depression, microaggressions based on gender and race, and issues of classism). We then went into the court-yard near the campus and created scenes that people who walked by could react to. A few students stood outside the scene and engaged in dialogue with passersby. A few people were angry at some of the scenes depicting racism and sexism and asked that it be changed to be more just and empowering. For a more in-depth discussion of this theatrical form in teaching, read the work of Jason Platt (2016).

Another example of my attempts to bring the outside world into the class-room includes asking students to share photos taken outside the classroom representing their reality and those of communities where they live and work. This typically leads to discussions about positionality and how the environment shapes our daily lives. Of all these elements, radical humility and radical empathy are two processes that evolve slowly over the course of the semester and I often initiate. They entail vulnerability and intuition on my part that is often not found in academia.

Just as I invite the student to examine the threads of connection between their lives and their clients, I identify my points of connection and disconnection between the students and myself. Differences in age, gender, ethnicity, and education are the most visible in the classroom, but this becomes a way to model conceptualizing one's positionality in relation to others. After sharing my own, I give examples of my intersectional identities as a cisgender, heterosexual, Latina mother working in academia and clinical practice and how that dynamically affects my teaching and clinical work. Sharing these details about my identity made me feel vulnerable at the beginning of my career. However, over time I realized that it was hypocritical to ask students to do this self-reflexive work while I withheld my transparency. I assign a book chapter I wrote that includes my testimonio as a Latina psychologist (Castañeda-Sound, 2018). This sparks a discussion about various topics using a lens of critical consciousness: ethnic and racial identities and development, destigmatizing mental health, and intergenerational trauma.

Challenges of Decolonizing Doctoral Training

Writing about decolonizing graduate-level training is challenging not only for the reasons Miguel already identified, but also because many voices could be included. The perspectives of instructors, trainees, supervisors, and clients are examples. Yet I could also include the epistemologies from research within psychology and the journals that choose what is published in the field and constitutes evidence-based practice.

A powerful narrative within graduate training in psychology is the power and value of accreditation by the American Psychological Association. A doctoral program's status of APA accreditation has an impact on many professional milestones in the student's career. For example, graduating from an accredited graduate program will help students be competitive when applying for a clinical internship, seeking postdoctoral training, and pursuing licensure. With this accreditation status at the doctoral level come requirements and guidelines that make teaching from a decolonized approach difficult. Unfortunately, I do not have all the answers. I am also still evolving as an unapologetic instructor in the service of communities where students do their clinical training. A meaningful discussion and assignment in my multicultural track class (for a description, see Castañeda-Sound, 2020) is to ask students to identify the different voices in professional psychology about multiculturalism, decolonization, diversity, social justice, antiracism, liberation psychology, and so on. I call this the diversity of standpoints paper; it broadens the lens for them to see how these visions and tensions in the field are not new but have instead evolved over time. After presenting two to three theories or frameworks, I ask the following questions: Are your voices, experiences, community, or ancestors present in these theories? Are your clients' voices, experiences, communities, or ancestors present in these theories? If not, what is missing? Further, how does this influence your theoretical approach? How would you integrate this into your clinical work? This paper and subsequent discussion allow them to identify their positionality in relation to the field of professional psychology.

My goal is to demonstrate that a decolonized approach to teaching involves much more than scholarly readings and assignments listed in a syllabus. No matter how much planning goes into the design of a course, flexibility is critical. As Medina (2014) so beautifully wrote, "We must be able to adapt when necessary, to flow like the wind, to be open to change, to be flexible with our plans, to be able to cleanse and renew ourselves" (p. 167). This was evident when COVID-19 caused campuses worldwide to shut down and compelled instructors to provide classes remotely. Our students and we were tasked with flexibility amid uncertainty. Moreover, it is incomprehensible that an instructor would teach a class about psychology during George Floyd's murder without acknowledging racial inequality and police violence. Approaching a classroom as a decontextualized, sterile environment is antithetical to decolonized teaching. We must hold discussions about current events, identify the structural and historical connections and precursors, and share how these events affect the communities and us where we work and live.

SUSANA'S TESTIMONIO

Mi Apa (my father) inculcated the idea of questioning norms; he taught me to question the pervasive narrative being pushed down our throats by the Mexican and White American media. He implored me to question the underlying sexist, racist, and colorist messages that were the underpinnings for the portrayal of the mujer Indigena with darker skin in a subservient role, and the villainized women who displayed anger, ambition, and confidence. My mother's lessons were beautifully, and at times unintentionally, modeled. My mother, a Mexican woman de piel morena, like myself, was determined to have her voice and opinions heard without fear of being labeled a mujer que no sabe su lugar. In fact, I think she likes to defy that stereotype and taught me how to advocate for myself in a world that constantly tries to silence me. Intellectually, my clinical self was birthed into existence and supported by liberation psychologies, womanist-mujerista-feminist epistemologies, and multicultural frameworks. I did not however, always give myself permission to dismantle my clinical and supervisory work from a decolonial perspective. The sterilized air of academia propagated inherent colonized, White supremacist ideologies as ethical and professional standards making it so that I thought I was "refining" myself when in reality I was being stripped away from my cultural ways, socialized to exercise professionalism in manners that perpetuated White supremacist values.

I was younger than 30 when I began my supervision journey. My age, coupled with being a first-generation professional and an early career psychologist drew me into the "safety" of behaving as professional as I could and to not blur the boundaries between supervisor or mentor, let alone friend or therapist.

I tried to be serious, more objective, limited my emotional support of my supervisee's personal life; I "toned down" my personality and even dressed in professional attire that did not reflect my personality. Like many Latinx professionals, I was afraid of not "being enough." Not serious enough, not academic enough, not trained enough, not professional enough. . . . The list goes on. Little by little I remembered my truth—my values—and started unlearning and regrounded myself by no longer complying with respectability politics that at times seemed to only apply to Black, Indigenous, Women of Color (BIWOC). I called back my spirit and remembered why I pursued the field of psychology in the first place. It was never about the profession; it was always about serving my community and I needed to be my authentic self to do this work. I reintroduced makeup and attire that reflected my personality and I began the process of questioning, unlearning, and using my voice. Throughout the years, BIWOC supervisees, especially those who were indoctrinated longer through doctoral training would say things like "I didn't know you could wear red lipstick" or "I always thought that displaying emotion at work was unprofessional" often followed by a sigh of relief that they could be themselves as professionals. During this time, I also delved into understanding in depth my Mexican Indigenous values, healing practices, and theories that actively dismantle ideologies that are in place to protect the status quo, rather than my supervisee or the client they are serving.

Serving as a group supervisor in the Aliento program, I have witnessed many stories of breaking generational cycles through questioning and dismantling their familial or cultural norms. Yet many of our students are grappling with unlearning perspectives entrenched in colonization while relearning and contextualizing Indigenous approaches. Like many beginning therapists, they often want a road map on how to do this work. My approach to decolonizing supervision is one based on holding space for the interconnectedness between us, intentionally honoring all of us as whole and centering their and our cultural wisdom.

The next section addresses decolonized supervision with trainees from the Aliento program. My methodology is storytelling through testimonios and is rooted in mujerista literature and liberation theories (Comas-Díaz, 2020a; Comas-Díaz, 2020b). My words in Spanish are deliberately not italicized here as an expression of resistance in particular, as I delve into what it means to decolonize supervision. It is also congruent with many bilingual literary authors who have chosen not to italicize Spanish and other non-English languages. Similarly, I want to highlight that (a) I am intentionally centering the in-between space and the complexity of bilingual BIPOC perspectives starting with the use of our languages, (b) the majority of this section is my voice and

Spanish words are not foreign to me, and (c) I do not stop to differentiate my Spanish words from my English words when I speak.

I acknowledge that Spanish, much like English, is a colonizing language. The complexity of decolonizing is that we no longer have access to the rich and diverse Indigenous languages that afford us the depth and breadth of our pre-Colombian value systems, our rich and interconnected spirituality and our vast medicinas and healing systems. Instead, we are left with decoding, translating, remembering, and piecing together fragments of our collective memories from this in-between space of knowing. The colonization of our languages relegates us to a simplified and at times monolithic interpretation of our Indigenous lineages. Yet for many of us, Spanish is our mother tongue, el idioma, and feels the closest to home. As I attempt to decolonize and have a deeper understanding of what this means, I hold two important and contradicting truths: first, my brain was colonized before I was born; and, second, my body, spirit and heart are imprinted with ancestral wisdom beyond my brain's comprehension. Decolonization is an action, a conscious practice of questioning where our truths come from. As I delve into this work, I often use words in Náhuatl (the Indigenous legacy closest to my roots) as portals to a worldview that is past and present in many of us today. Although some argue that discussions about colonization are moot and that they rehash history that perpetuates hatred and divisiveness, we should recognize that Indigenous and BIPOC communities' mental health continue to suffer the effects of colonization (Dupuis-Rossi, 2021). At the root of decolonizing mental health, we need to start with our trainees. It needs to be deeper than how we talk about decolonizing therapy; we need to lead by example by decolonizing the supervision process and how we discuss and conceptualize clients in supervision. The majority of our socialization and training in doing therapy happens in supervision, and yet research on the impact of supervision on trainees, particularly as it pertains to training BIPOC clinicians, remains limited. Therefore, the supervision process, the relationship between supervisors and supervisees, and understanding of the client should center on the impact colonization has had and continues to have on communities and the trickle-down effects on the client (e.g., individual, couple, or family).

Supervision Rooted in Decolonial Perspectives

My supervision style and clinical work go hand in hand. Yes, I am aware of the different schools of thought on this issue but my guides remain the same. A fundamental tenet of liberation psychology is bringing to awareness that everything is value-laden, and therefore to pretend that who I am as a person or clinician does not enter the supervisory relationship is not only inauthentic but oppressive (Martín-Baró, 1994; Prilleltensky, 1997). I am transparent about my identities and my values when I enter the supervisory relationship, and I do not ask anything of my supervisees that I am not willing to do myself.

As mentioned earlier, my approach to therapy is grounded in liberation psychologies and is guided by holistic mujerista influenced by womanist and social justice frameworks. I actively work toward decolonizing myself and the mental health frameworks in the various roles I occupy. I use a trauma-informed lens to address the underlying impact of personal and historical and race-based trauma. I weave Indigenous ancestral wisdom (e.g., the use of the natural elements such as earth, water, air and fire or the invitation of ancestors and prayer), energy work (e.g., emotional freedom techniques also known as tapping, and reiki, the Japanese energy healing system, and somatic interventions (e.g., movement combined with breathwork and body sensory awareness) to complement talk therapy and engage the whole person in their healing process. I see the therapeutic relationship as a vehicle for change that allows me to be an obsidian mirror, in other words, a truth teller, someone who will reflect the complexity of the person in front of me, their unspoken yet palpable shadow and what they are presenting to the work. My hope is that I do this in an affirming and compassionate way, which in turn facilitates healing, acceptance, and change for clients.

Supervision Process and Decolonial Intentions

The context for decolonizing supervision has been heavily influenced by my journey of remembering my Indigenous Mexican cultural worldviews and unlearning an entire worldview grounded in White supremacy. These colonial messages were not actively taught in my training program yet were everywhere around me. I was indoctrinated with them in the halls of academia and the trenches of clinical supervision. Much of this transformation of unlearning and relearning has been through pláticas with cultural keepers and cultural spiritual healers who have been influenced by Mexican Indigenous traditions and those of Indigenous communities across Turtle Island, which represents North America for many Indigenous peoples. Pláticas could be summed up as a conversation however it is much more synergistic. Pláticas are our oral tradition of passing down cultural wisdom, storytelling encoded with life lessons, cultural traditions, our cosmology, and creation stories. They are often informal, yet at other times within a educational or ceremonial context.

Consistent with my Mexican American upbringing, I do not think in linear terms and I no longer try to do so. I now understand that learning, like healing, is circular, each time understanding the lesson in more profound ways. In writing this chapter, I am tasked with trying to capture a synchronous process that ensues within the interconnectedness of my supervisees, the client who is metaphorically or spiritually in the room and myself. In my mind, decolonial approaches are not so much what one says or does but rather how one conceptualizes the process of supervision, our roles as supervisors, and how and what we choose to give space. Like the cosmos, it is a constellation of energy in constant movement. The areas I highlight as part of decolonizing supervision are not meant to be prescriptive, nor is there only one approach. The aspects of my Indigenous Mexican cultural worldviews most relevant to this chapter are those of interconnectedness, conceptualization of self-care that encompasses spiritual and communal care, a deeper understanding of our bodies as sacred, and the role of ancestral stories and ceremonies in learning, teaching and healing. I highlight (a) eliciting feedback from the beginning of supervision, (b) self-care for therapists, (c) that we grow, heal, and transform in community, and (d) decolonial interventions.

Eliciting Feedback From the Beginning

Supervision is a dynamic cocreated space in which I invite trainees to be active in making it what they want, including determining the order in which things should happen. I am one person and do not assume to have all the answers, particularly given that I am also in this journey of decolonizing myself and will make mistakes. I set the tone for eliciting feedback from the beginning. One important aspect to this approach is being flexible and eliciting feedback that has the potential to alter the process of supervision. This may be a given, but I think most of us can relate to the exercise of providing feedback and feeling that it was just an exercise that did not have the option of eliciting change. I do not think we as supervisors set out to not incorporate supervisees' feedback as much as our colonized minds fool us into believing that we know better because we are familiar with the literature or are the more seasoned supervisor and sometimes unconsciously ignore feedback.

Trainees are invited to cocreate a group supervision process that best meets their needs for a period of time with an understanding that we must have a check-in, make space for self-care within the group, discuss clients (e.g., conceptualization, interventions, and process) or a clinical issue and we must all participate in meaningful discourse. The process has allowed trainees to share difficult feedback to us as a program and has shifted as our group members change to meet their needs, but the main ingredients remain.

Self-Care for Therapists

I lay the foundation for self-care as an act of resistance from the very first supervision meeting. I echo the lessons of Audre Lorde (1988) and the work of so many Black activists such as Tricia Hersey (2016), founder of the Nap Ministry, who reminded us that "rest is resistance." We start to lay a foundation by sharing perspectives, mini-testimonios, and brief overviews of the impact of colonization compounded by immigration, on our lack of value for self-care as Latinx in the United States. We joke about our parents saying things like "descanso cuando me muera" (I will rest when I die) and then we get serious and emotional as we engage in discourse about the roots and implications of these messages. We make connections to productivity as a source of self-worth and how this mindset sustains capitalism. We share feelings that we are not enough when we are not of use, not producing, or our productivity does not meet standards grounded in White supremacy. We also go back, way back, and create hope by reminding each other that we engage in self-care and rest for us and for our ancestors.

In addition, it is imperative that trainees understand that we are not colluding with colonized perspectives of treating our bodies as objects and that our worth and value are not based on how much we suffer or sacrifice ourselves for others. When trainees join group supervision, we set the foundation that who they are matters and that their well-being matters. I often have to hold the paradox of the trainees being members of Latinx communities who suffer the pain of colonization and who at times struggle with issues similar to those their clients struggle with, even as they are tasked to support their communities with little or no monetary compensation. These are practicum trainees. They too have financial struggles, have to make decisions about work versus advancing their education, feel pulled in multiple directions, and have little to no time for self-care. I attempt to dismantle the pervasive narratives in our profession that perpetuate the notion that our emotional labor should be free and that they need to be selfless as clinicians or invisible in the room. I invite them to be intentional about bringing themselves in the therapeutic process and modeling self-care during the therapy hour with their clients. Focus is on the collective.

We practice self-care and tending to our bodies in group supervision. We start all group supervision meetings with a general check-in. Supervisees are invited to share how they are doing and feeling whether it be about their personal-emotional well-being or their practicum-academic experience. We give as much space to this as needed before we move on to a grounding or self-care practice (e.g., breathwork, meditation or visualization) guided by one of the trainees or myself. We take turns guiding the practice followed by a short debrief on anything that came up for folxs during this practice and provide feedback to the facilitator.

We Grow, Heal, and Transform in Community

In theory, group supervision offers a plethora of opportunities for growth and healing in community, which is at the corazón of decolonial perspectives that strive to move away from an individualized, expert, top-down discourse. A fundamental tenant in liberation psychologies is that there is not any single expert and that the field is one of many approaches to healing and transformation. Most of us were trained to relate to countertransference as an undesirable experience and were taught that if your supervisee has countertransference with a client it was something to keep an eye on. As with anything in our field, it depends. For this chapter, I highlight that not all countertransference will necessarily interfere with the therapeutic process. From a decolonial perspective, countertransference and genuine reactions are reframed from the perspective of interconnectedness. The idea that we create meaning, grow, heal, and transform in relationship to others is explored with the intention of facilitating trainees to notice how they can cocreate meaning with their clients, simultaneously engage in their healing journey, and as a result be transformed through the process of working with their clients. From this perspective, it is important that we as professionals and trainees acknowledge the notion of sacred reciprocity, that our clients play a pivotal role in our clinical and personal development. When relevant, we make a direct link between trainee's decolonization process and their clients' healing through decolonizing and liberating themselves. We acknowledge these gifts aloud and remind each other of our interconnectedness. Cultural countertransference is also common with our trainees because, as mentioned earlier, the majority of the trainees are Latinas and have experienced many of the same hardships as our Latinx clients. I also want to be clear that exploration of countertransference also includes increasing awareness of self as therapist, developing boundaries between the trainee and the client while keeping the focus of the clinical work on the client.

In supervision, we understand that change comes from within the community. At times, it is a bottom-up approach in our group, sometimes I am sharing knowledge and other times we are working from a true collaborative approach. I am transparent about how I work, my areas of specialty, and what I believe I bring to the table even as I am also intentional about my areas of growth, particularly as it pertains to decolonial work, how they have changed me, and what I have learned from them. I try to share my process with them throughout supervision rather than only at the end of that relationship.

Decolonizing Interventions

From my decolonial lens, I see my role of group supervisor as a maestra, one who teaches interventions by sharing my medicina, my approach to facilitating healing, reminding them of their medicina, their gifts and cultural wisdom from their lived experiences, by guiding them back to themselves, and modeling being inquisitive and not always knowing the answer. I also see my role as a cultural reactivator by reminding them of who they are through the use of Spanish and, primarily, Spanglish, sharing and eliciting family and cultural stories, testimonios, Indigenous legends, the use of Náhuatl, and being transparent about my use of Indigenous healing practices. I actively engage the group in critical thinking and cofoster creativity in developing interventions that are congruent with liberation psychologies and decolonial practices. Trainees and I take turns discussing cases from a decolonial perspective; when we get stuck, we go back to basics, a decolonial framework. I remind them to connect with what they know based on their cultural and ancestral knowledge and what strength-based means in the context of their Latinx clients, then we all engage in discourse about the various interventions or approaches we can take with a particular client. We normalize the idea that the client can be the medicina or the vessel for their medicina and expand or contract what their role as a clinician sitting with their client could be.

When a trainee discusses a case, I often ask how they feel in their heart and their bodies when they sit with their clients. I ask them to tune into their intuition and use it as a guide to engage in exploratory work with their client. If it is not relevant to the client, I sometimes challenge them, and other times I gently encourage them to explore what comes up for themselves.

As a group supervisor within a colonial system in a litigious world, I am cognizant that I am part of a team in supporting trainees. Therefore I do not act alone; I challenge trainees to expand and be inclusive of non-Western interventions, particularly those congruent with their cultural worldviews or that of their clients. Similarly, I ask that they talk with their primary supervisor about the use of non-Western interventions. I invite trainees to expand their therapeutic frameworks by gaining concrete knowledge of Indigenous and other cultural interventions, and to respectfully engage with those healing systems. When trainees have a familiarity with cultural interventions, whether it is through lived cultural experiences or previous training, I guide students in how to incorporate these interventions in their therapeutic work. The integration of cultural interventions is a collaborative and intentional decision involving the trainee, client, and supervisor and is given the same clinical consideration we would give when incorporating any other type of intervention. An integral aspect of decolonial work is to treat this knowledge with respect and to be careful to not commodify these modalities given that they are part of a much larger healing system that we are barely beginning to relearn. Last, I ask trainees to reconceptualize therapy as a sacred process that truly tries to address the whole person in mind, body, and spirit. A full discussion on decolonizing interventions is beyond the scope of this chapter, but I hope this paints a broad picture.

Unique Considerations in Supervising From Decolonial Perspectives

As Hernández-Wolfe (2011) asserted, a decolonial framework asks that we place ourselves in the colonial history of the Americas and that we construct knowledge from the borderlands. In this case, borderlands, a concept birthed by Gloria Anzaldúa (1999) encompasses a psychological and social location representing the margins, a place where those with intersecting identities whose voices are rendered to the margins are centered. As a first-generation Latinx professional, I live in nepantla—that in-between space that those of us who have power have to navigate, where we honor the knowledge that we have worked so hard to attain while cultivating humility by remembering that we still have a lot to learn from those that came before and after us. Staying grounded in humility without minimizing my or others' knowledge or accomplishments in supervision is key. As a professional, I am keenly aware of how much my professional upbringing is embedded in colonial and White supremacist values, yet I still see value in my training. My goal in supervision is to continue the thread of liberation theories that are taught in the program and give it aliento by critically thinking through cases from this perspective and applying decolonial interventions. I remind them that decolonial perspectives are not meant to be binary but instead can coexist with other models. I am intentional about questioning and challenging concepts that we have learned as facts, even as they pertain to our Latinx cultures, because I remind them, and myself, that our Latinx mindset has been colonized.

A challenge in decolonizing supervision, which many of us doing this work are apprehensive in addressing, is that supervisors have a responsibility to protect. We need to have considerable clarity when encountering challenges in supervision that we are using our power to protect people and not systems of oppression or, simply put, White supremacy. As a group supervisor, I am part of a larger training team that includes Dr. Gallardo as the director of the program and a number of supervisors who provide group supervision. Although I have used APA's competency benchmarks in previous settings, my process for evaluation is oral and ongoing. I have the flexibility in this context to work collaboratively with my colleagues and share ongoing feedback and concerns about all trainees.

In sum, in writing this chapter, I found myself feeling that what I do in supervision is common sense, but I also want to validate supervisors who are actively decolonizing their supervision methods by not confusing their ascribed power (based on our role) with omniscience and superiority, and instead fully show up for themselves and trainees.

CONCLUSION

Throughout this chapter, we have weaved our testimonios and perspectives with scholarly literature to demonstrate our approaches to decolonizing clinical training for masters and doctoral students who aspire to be counselors and psychologists. Decolonizing our teaching and supervision compels us to question the practices and values that have dominated teaching and supervision and instead center and destigmatize ancestral ways of knowing. In addition, we include hopeful resistance (Villanueva, 2013) and learn from Norte (2011, cited by Villanueva, 2013), who reminds us that in addition to critical awareness, we must also create spaces for collective healing, imaging a new reality, and then the commitment and action to realize these dreams.

We end with part of a collective poem developed by students in one of Carrie's doctoral classes. It was inspired by a workshop titled "Poetry as data, data as poetry: Prosas de Resistencia," held at the National Latinx Psychological Association's 2021 conference. Ellen McWhirter and Brian Rojas-Arauz shared how poetry can be used in data collection for research. Adapting their approach for use in a classroom, Carrie gave each student prompts to complete, and then they shared their responses in class. Carrie collected these responses and combined them to create two collective poems she shared on the last day of class to represent the community they created in the classroom.

¿Quién eres, quienes somos? (Who are you, who are we?)
I am because we/they are
My name is not regret
I am spirit
My name is a song and is blessed
I am Choctaw
My name is stolen, but not forgotten
My community is perseverance
I am gay
My name is not f-g.
I am loved by God.
My community is important to me.
People who like me do not judge me.

Mi hogar, mi lugar (My home, My place)
The wind and mulberry smells like home.
Chimes and leaves dancing sound like home.
Scented candles smell like home and
Loud laughter sounds like home.
Ocean waves crashing on the sand sound like home.
My community is polishing its crown.
I am home, we are home.

RESOURCES

Amplify Restorative Justice. (2021). *Decolonize your classroom.* https://www.amplifyrj.com/decolonize-your-classroom

Asian American Justice + Innovation Lab. https://www.aajil.org/

Community-Based Global Learning Collaborative. (n.d.). *Decolonizing thought and action—and higher education.* https://www.cbglcollab.org/decolonizing-thought-and-action

CRESTS. (2021, June 21). *Decolonizing mental health training: Using a culture-centered approach to working with Black youth* [Video]. YouTube. https://youtu.be/caxNKHuU-rQ

de Oliveira Andreotti, V., Stein, S., Susa, R., Ahenakew, C., Caikova, T., Pitaguary, R., & Pitaguary, B. (2021). *Calibrating our vital compass: Unlearning colonial habits of being in everyday life.* Instituto Paulo Freire de España. https://www.rizoma-freireano.org/articles-3030/calibrating-our-vital

Lehman, K. (2016). *Unlearning colonial and nation-state history in documentary film by and about Indigenous peoples. alter/nativas, spring 6.* https://alternativas.osu.edu/en/issues/spring-6-2016/essays3/lehman.html

Manathunga, C., Davidow, S., Williams, P., Willis, A., Raciti, M., Gilbey, K., Stanton, S., O'Chin, H., & Chan, A. (2022). Decolonising the school experience through poetry to foreground truth-telling and cognitive justice. *London Review of Education, 20*(1). https://doi.org/10.14324/LRE.20.1.06

Owusu, M. (2017, April 14). *Decolonising the curriculum* [Video]. TEDx: University of Leeds. YouTube. https://www.youtube.com/watch?v=zeKHOTDwZxU

Sanchez, N. (2019, March 12). *Decolonization is for everyone* [Video]. TEDxSFU. YouTube. https://youtu.be/QP9x1NnCWNY

Sharpe, J. (2013). *Unlearning colonialism: Storytelling and the accord* [Paper]. Adult Education Research Conference, St. Louis, MO, United States. https://newprairiepress.org/aerc/2013/papers/43/

Stein, S. (2017, December 5). *So you want to decolonize higher education? Necessary conversations for non-Indigenous people* [Podcast/Article]. https://medium.com/@educationotherwise/https-medium-com-education-otherwise-so-you-want-to-decolonize-higher-education-4a7370d64955

Students and faculty of the Community Psychology, Liberation Psychology, and Ecopsychology MA/PHD program. *Hearing voices 2018-2019.* Pacifica Graduate Institute. https://www.pacifica.edu/wp-content/uploads/2018/10/hearing_voices_2018-web.pdf

REFERENCES

American Psychiatric Association. (2022). *Diagnostic and statistical manual of mental disorders* (5th ed., text rev.). https://doi.org/10.1176/appi.books.9780890425787

American Psychological Association. (2017a). *Ethical principles of psychologists and code of conduct* (2002, amended effective June 1, 2010, and January 1, 2017). https://www.apa.org/ethics/code/index.aspx

American Psychological Association. (2017b). *Multicultural guidelines: An ecological approach to context, identity, and intersectionality.* https://www.apa.org/about/policy/multicultural-guidelines.pdf

Anzaldúa, G. (1999). *Borderlands/La frontera* (2nd ed.). Aunt Lute Books.

Anzaldúa, G., & Keating, A. (2002). *This bridge we call home: Radical visions for transformation.* Psychology Press.

Association of Black Psychologists (ABPsi). (2019). *Ethical standards of Black psychologists.* https://www.abpsi.org/pdf/EthicalStandardsAssociationofBlackPsychologists.pdf

Boal, A. (1979). *The theatre of the oppressed.* Pluto Press.

Brown, D. (2009). *The DaVinci code.* Anchor Books.

Castañeda-Sound, C. L. (2018). Weaving identities and theoretical perspectives of cultural competency in *Nepantla.* In L. Comas-Díaz & C. Vasquez (Eds.), *Latina psychologists: Thriving in the cultural borderlands* (pp. 146–157). Routledge. https://doi.org/10.4324/9781315175706-9

Castañeda-Sound, C. L. (2020). Liberation, inspiration, and critical consciousness: Preparing the next generation of practitioners. In L. Comas-Díaz & E. Torres Rivera (Eds.), *Liberation psychology: Theory, method, practice, and social justice* (pp. 265–282). American Psychological Association. https://doi.org/10.1037/0000198-015

Cienfuegos, A. J., & Monelli, C. (1983). The testimony of political repression as a therapeutic instrument. *American Journal of Orthopsychiatry, 53*(1), 43–51. https://doi.org/10.1111/j.1939-0025.1983.tb03348.x

Comas-Díaz, L. (2020a). Journey to psychology: A mujerista testimonio. *Women & Therapy, 43*(1–2), 157–169. https://doi.org/10.1080/02703149.2019.1684676

Comas-Díaz, L. (2020b). Liberation psychotherapy. In L. Comas-Díaz & E. Torres Rivera (Eds.), *Liberation psychology: Theory, method, practice, and social justice* (pp. 169–185). American Psychological Association. https://doi.org/10.1037/0000198-010

Delgado Bernal, D., Burciaga, R., & Flores Carmona, J. (2012). Chicana/Latina *testimonios*: Mapping the methodological, pedagogical, and political. *Equity & Excellence in Education, 45*(3), 363–372. https://doi.org/10.1080/10665684.2012.698149

Domenech Rodríguez, M. M., Gallardo, M. E., Rosario, C. C., Delgado-Romero, E. A., & Field, L. D. (2020). Ethical guidelines of the National Latinx Psychological Association: Background. *Journal of Latina/o Psychology, 8*(2), 95–100. https://doi.org/10.1037/lat0000150

Dupuis-Rossi, R. (2021). The violence of colonization and the importance of decolonizing therapeutic relationship: The role of helper in centering Indigenous wisdom. *International Journal of Indigenous Health, 16*(1), 108–117. https://doi.org/10.32799/ijih.v16i1.33223

Fellner, K. D. (2018). Embodying decoloniality: Indigenizing curriculum and pedagogy. *American Journal of Community Psychology, 62*(3–4), 283–293. https://doi.org/10.1002/ajcp.12286

Figueroa, M. (2014). Toward a spiritual pedagogy along the borderlands. In E. Facio & I. Lara (Eds.), *Fleshing the spirit: Spirituality and activism in Chicana, Latina, and Indigenous women's lives* (pp. 34–42). The University of Arizona Press.

Freire, P. (1970). *Pedagogy of the oppressed.* Continuum.

Gallardo, M. E., Johnson, J., Parham, T. A., & Carter, J. A. (2009). Ethics and multiculturalism: Advancing cultural and clinical responsiveness. *Professional Psychology, Research and Practice, 40*(5), 425–435. https://doi.org/10.1037/a0016871

García, M. A., & Tehee, M. (2014). *Society of Indian Psychologists commentary on the American Psychological Association's (APA) Ethical Principles of Psychologists and Code of Conduct.* Society of Indian Psychologists. https://www.nativepsychs.org/_files/ugd/0ab9f1_176486908e7d43c2b559fb046b46b6d7.pdf

Goodman, R. D., & Gorski, P. C. (Eds.). (2015). *Decolonizing "multicultural" counseling through social justice.* Springer. https://doi.org/10.1007/978-1-4939-1283-4

Hernández-Wolfe, P. (2011). Decolonization and "mental" health: A Mestiza's journey in the borderlands. *Women & Therapy, 34*(3), 293–306. https://doi.org/10.1080/02703149.2011.580687

Hersey, T. (2016). The Nap Ministry. https://thenapministry.wordpress.com/

International Union of Psychological Science. (2008). Universal declaration of ethical principles for psychologists. https://www.iupsys.net/about/declarations/universal-declaration-of-ethical-principles-for-psychologists/

Lewis, T. (2020, June 25). How to make healthcare anti-racist. The Paper Gown. https://thepapergown.zocdoc.com/how-to-make-healthcare-anti-racist/

Lorde, A. (1988). *A burst of light: Essays.* Firebrand Books.

Martín-Baró, I. (1994). *Writings for a liberation psychology* (A. Aron & S. Corne, Eds.). Harvard University Press.

Medina, L. (2014). Nepantla spirituality: My path to the sources of healing. In E. Facio & I. Lara (Eds.), *Fleshing the spirit: Spirituality and activism in Chicana, Latina, and Indigenous women's lives* (pp. 167–185). The University of Arizona Press.

National Latinx Psychological Association (NLPA). (2020). Ethical guidelines of the National Latinx Psychological Association. *Journal of Latina/o Psychology, 8*(2), 101–111. https://doi.org/10.1037/lat0000151

Platt, J. (2016, September). Pedestrians as professors: Theatre of the Oppressed in Mexico City. *Psychology International Newsletter.* APA Office of International Affairs. https://www.apa.org/international/pi/2016/09/pedestrians-professors

Prilleltensky, I. (1997). Values, assumptions, and practices: Assessing the moral implications of psychological discourse and action. *American Psychologist, 52*(5), 517–535. https://doi.org/10.1037/0003-066X.52.5.517

Reyes, K., & Curry Rodríguez, J. (2012). Testimonio: Origins, terms, and resources. *Equity & Excellence in Education, 45*(3), 525–538. https://doi.org/10.1080/10665684.2012.698571

TEDx. (2015, July 14). From invisible to visible | Maria Hinojosa [Video]. YouTube. https://www.youtube.com/watch?v=mAucrEPi4sM

Valdez, L. (1973). *Pensamiento serpintino*: The law of in Lak'Ech Ala K'in. *Chicano Theater One, 1*, 7–19.

Villanueva, T. S. (2013). Teaching as a healing craft: Decolonizing the classroom and creating a space of hopeful resistance through Chicano-Indigenous pedagogy praxis. *The Urban Review, 45*(1), 23–40. https://doi.org/10.1007/s11256-012-0222-5

Viray, S., & Nash, R. J. (2014). Taming the madvocate within: Social justice meets social compassion. *About Campus: Enriching the Student Learning Experience, 19*(5), 20–27. https://doi.org/10.1002/abc.21170

Wendt, D. C., Gone, J. P., & Nagata, D. K. (2015). Potentially harmful therapy and multicultural counseling: Bridging two disciplinary discourses. *The Counseling Psychologist, 43*(3), 334–358. https://doi.org/10.1177/0011000014548280

10 THE DECOLONIAL MENTORING FRAMEWORK

Advancing an Anticolonial Future in Psychology and Beyond

MACKENZIE T. GOERTZ, HECTOR Y. ADAMES,
CHELSEA PARKER, NAYELI Y. CHAVEZ-DUEÑAS,
RADIA DELUNA, AND JESSICA G. PEREZ-CHAVEZ

*We must decolonize our minds and redefine ourselves . . . in all respects,
culturally, politically, socially.*

—Roach, n.d.

The life and well-being of humankind has been denigrated by a ravaging legacy of colonization. Coloniality is an enduring pattern of abuse of power that emerged from colonization and permeates virtually all aspects of humanity through a system of domination and exploitation created and perpetrated by White European Americans (Maldonado-Torres, 2007; Quijano & Therborn, 2007). Coloniality is the foundation of White supremacy culture, which is built on a system of racial classification. Manifesting through insidious power structures and socialization practices, White supremacy culture promotes dominance of people who are racially White and has deleterious consequences for those who are Black, Indigenous, and People of Color (BIPOC; Adames et al., 2021; Grzanka et al., 2019; Helms, 2019). Under coloniality, racism remains one of the most general forms of domination in the world (Quijano & Therborn, 2007).

https://doi.org/10.1037/0000376-011
Decolonial Psychology: Toward Anticolonial Theories, Research, Training, and Practice,
L. Comas-Díaz, H. Y. Adames, and N. Y. Chavez-Dueñas (Editors)

To resist colonialism and advance an anticolonial future, this chapter reimagines professional mentorship in psychology through the decolonial mentoring framework (DMF). We define decolonial mentoring as a racially conscious, growth fostering relationship that seeks to promote critical consciousness, self-acceptance, and transformative action for an anticolonial world. In the field of psychology, mentoring commonly occurs within the context of training relationships that aim to support holistic development, such as academic advisor or research mentor (Schlosser & Foley, 2008). Mentorship has been referred to as the archetype of graduate training because it is the process by which trainees are socialized to uphold the profession's values, practices, and ethical standards (American Psychological Association, 2006; Lunsford et al., 2017). In practice, traditional approaches to mentorship socialize mentees to uphold Eurocentric values of individualism, competition, and meritocracy. Thus, as trainees are mentored into the profession, they are directly and indirectly taught to reproduce a science that is fundamentally oppressive (Miller & Miller, 2020; Teo & Afşin, 2020).

The DMF intends to interrupt this long-standing tradition of mentorship in psychology that reinforces a status quo of coloniality. In tandem, the framework seeks to reorient mentees to decolonial praxis in psychology while recognizing the interplay of racial identity and power in the mentoring relationship. The enduring aim of decolonial mentoring is to advance an anticolonial future in psychology and beyond. This chapter introduces and describes the four pillars of the DMF (4Rs): resisting psycolonization, reorienting to a decolonial psychology, recognizing racial Identity and power, and rebuilding for an anticolonial future. The framework applies guiding principles from liberation psychology (Comas-Díaz & Torres Rivera, 2020; Martín-Baró, 1994; Torres Rivera, 2020) and addresses the explicit influence of race and relational power on mentorship through the racial identity social interaction model (RISIM), developed by Helms (1990; Helms & Cook, 1999). We conclude with a discussion of how to apply the DMF in everyday practice.

THE DECOLONIAL MENTORING FRAMEWORK

The DMF, as noted, is constructed of four primary pillars that capture the theory and action of decolonial mentorship (see Figure 10.1). Each pillar connotes an integral, necessary component of the total framework. Combined, the pillars provide a comprehensive approach to decolonial mentorship that is both practical and aspirational. The following section describes the four pillars (4Rs).

FIGURE 10.1. The Decolonial Mentoring Framework

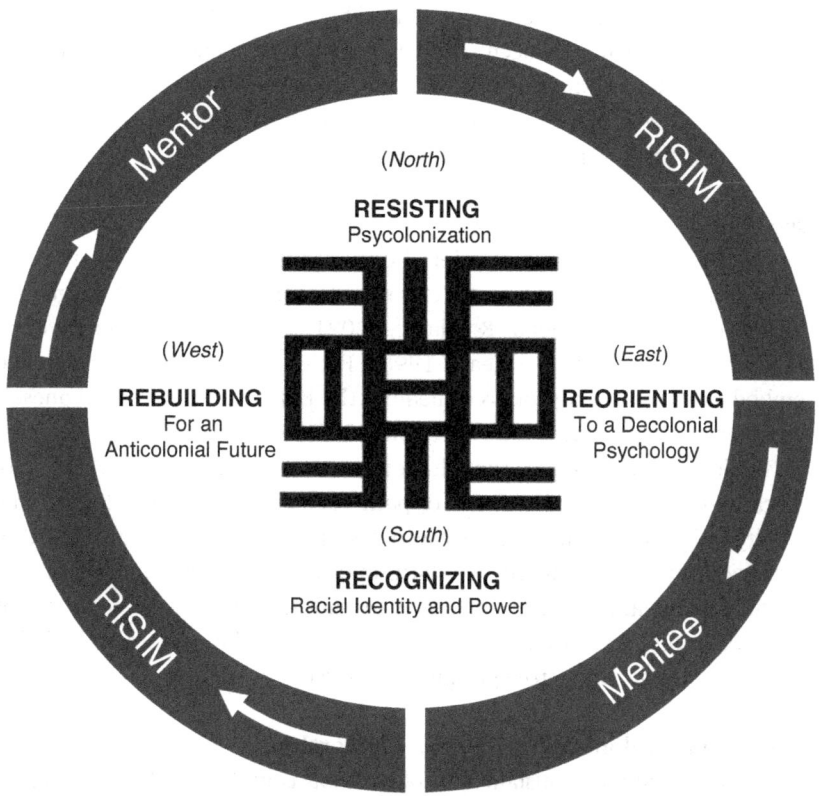

Note. Represented by four pillars (4Rs), the decolonial mentoring framework is characterized by its enduring aim of resisting psycolonization (North), reorienting to a decolonial psychology (East), recognizing racial identity and power (South), and ultimately rebuilding for an anticolonial future (West). The framework is visualized via the African Adinkra symbol of "Nea Onnim No Sua a, Ohu" [The one who does not know], representing lifelong education and the continued quest for knowledge (Kojo Arthur, 2017, p. 276). The arrows in the figure represent the reflexive and recursive nature of decolonial mentoring, whereby engagement with one pillar informs subsequent pillars in an ongoing, repeated fashion. RISIM = racial identity social interaction model. © Goertz, Adames, Parker, Chavez-Dueñas, DeLuna, Perez-Chavez. Reprinted with permission.

Pillar 1: Resisting Psycolonization

As a global discipline, psychology is guilty of reproducing and reinforcing coloniality. Since its inception, psychology has propagated universalist assumptions of mental health based on a hegemonic Western Eurocentric framework (Adames et al., 2023; American Psychological Association, 2021; Sonn & Stevens, 2021). This process is described by Teo and Afşin (2020) as psycolonization, in which a Eurocentric psychology is forced upon communities for which it has no relevance. Psycolonization pathologizes the Global Majority and propagates White supremacy culture. Thus the task of resisting psycolonization is the first pillar of decolonial mentoring.

Resisting psycolonization requires an understanding of how BIPOC perspectives on illness and healing are painfully relegated to the margins in the global mental health field. Rendered invisible are the cultural knowledge, therapeutic skills, and healing remedies that stem from centuries of Indigenous experience (Chavez-Dueñas & Adames, 2021; Waziyatawin & Yellow Bird, 2012; Yellow Horse Brave Heart, 1998). For example, Indigenous science embodies a reciprocal process of healing the Earth in order to heal oneself and community (Chavez-Dueñas et al., 2022; Hernandez, 2022). Yet such psychological perspectives that challenge Eurocentric norms are routinely discarded as mere pseudoscience or pathologized (Hernandez, 2022). This loyalty to Eurocentrism positions psychology as a tireless agent of coloniality working to sustain the oppressive status quo. To this end, a foundational task of the decolonial mentoring process is to understand these wrongdoings of the profession and learn how to resist them. Mentorship sustains coloniality, yet it can also provide fertile ground to do the opposite.

Resisting Psycolonization Through Mentorship

A primary avenue that sustains psycolonization is professional mentorship of emerging trainees in the field. Traditional mentorship models typically fail to critically engage the role of identity, power, and oppression, even while ignoring the saliency of race and racism. In practice, traditional mentoring models primarily use color-blind racial ideologies (see Neville et al., 2000) and emphasize Eurocentric values of individualism, competition, and meritocracy. Decolonial mentoring can resist these norms by explicitly attending to the influence of race, culture, and socialization. For instance, naming and critically evaluating race and culture across each environment and mentoring exchange can disrupt the avoidance behaviors that underpin psycolonization.

Mentors can challenge mentees to question how knowledge is produced and consider the role of racism in determining what knowledge is considered valid (i.e., White Eurocentric perspectives). A key component of resisting psycolonization also includes fostering a sense of willingness and genuine commitment to decolonial practice in the mentee. Mentors can encourage mentees to identify their role in perpetuating oppressive norms as well as their responsibility to fight for a better world. Developing the capacity for self-reflection while empowering a sense of self-agency are essential. Ultimately, these practices should aim to interrupt the Eurocentric socialization of the mentee to instead focus on developing an anticolonial orientation. Whereas traditional mentorship is a messenger of coloniality, decolonial mentorship offers the advent of an anticolonial future.

Pillar 2: Reorienting to a Decolonial Psychology

Moving beyond resisting psycolonization, the second pillar of the DMF embodies reorienting to a decolonial psychology. Decoloniality centers a return to Indigenous wisdom, science and worldviews to advance strategies for liberation (Chavez-Dueñas et al., 2022; La Torre, 2016; Tuck & Yang, 2012; Waziyatawin & Yellow Bird, 2012; Yellow Horse Brave Heart, 1998). As Maldonado-Torres (2011 stated, decolonization is a "necessary task that remains unfinished" and that requires us to critically analyze existing ideas and theories (p. 2). Many scholars have aimed to define decolonization and yet their definitions remain largely open to context and interpretation. This difficulty in operationalizing decolonization may speak to the nuanced, intimate, and complex nature of decolonization as a theory and praxis. For instance, Tuck and Yang (2012) warned against the equivocation of naming other forms of resistance against oppression as decolonization because it may serve in shifting blame and evading accountability for our own parts in colonization. In this chapter, we describe decoloniality as the ongoing process of abandoning colonial socialization through critical transformation of one's attitudes, beliefs, and behaviors.

In our reorientation of psychology, we hope to emphasize the purposeful action of return to Indigenous ways of thinking but also the repatriation of Indigenous land and life. Still, the symbiotic nature of the relationship between White supremacy culture and colonization is ever present. Comas-Díaz (2021), adding to the work of Indigenous scholar Villanueva (2018), proposed racial equity as a step toward healing and working toward decolonization. Given the salience of race in both coloniality and White supremacy culture, we argue that decoloniality requires that individuals develop a healthy racial identity. This process includes garnering an appreciation for the complexity of race in one's life and the lives of others while maintaining an active commitment to ending a system of racial oppression (Helms, 1990, 2019).

Movements of resistance throughout history have embraced decoloniality to seek liberation from White hegemony. In psychology, several distinct yet overlapping approaches engage a decolonial paradigm. Examples include Black psychology (Cross, 1971; White, 1984), community psychology (Nelson & Prilleltensky, 2010), ethnopolitical psychology (Comas-Díaz, 2000), liberation psychology (Comas-Díaz & Torres Rivera, 2020; Martín-Baró, 1994; Torres Rivera, 2020), psychology of radical healing (Adames et al., 2023; French et al., 2020), and decolonial psychology (Comas-Díaz, 2021; Sonn & Stevens, 2021). Collectively, these critical approaches aim to advance an anticolonial future in which all people, regardless of social group belonging, have equal access to a life of dignity, belonging, and well-being.

Liberation psychology offers core principles that can reorient the mentee and mentor toward a decolonial psychology. This approach stems from a global movement of theology, philosophy, and critical pedagogy that seeks liberation for all people from the oppression of a ruling class. Liberation theory was developed by independent actors across the Americas, Africa, and Europe during the second half of the 20th century (for a full history, see Burton & Guzzo, 2020). A core tenet of is belief that people are active agents of social change and capable of facilitating collective transformation (Comas-Díaz & Torres Rivera, 2020; Torres Rivera, 2020). Philosopher and psychologist Martín-Baró (1986) was the first to apply liberation theory to construct a new psychology. At the time, psychology had become a widespread discipline with little relevance to the Global Majority, propagating Eurocentric presumptions of universal norms and scientific neutrality. Martín-Baró observed the field as essentially irrelevant and unable to produce practical knowledge to effect social change (Burton & Guzzo, 2020; Martín-Baró, 1986, 1994). In describing liberation psychology, Martín-Baró (1986, 1994) proposed three essential elements: (a) shifting focus of psychology away from defining itself as a scientific discipline toward instead providing effective interventions in service to the majority, (b) pursuing knowledge from the perspective of those who are directly affected most by oppressive structures, and (c) emphasizing the need for action of the researcher and practitioner alongside the oppressed. As a discipline, liberation psychology recognizes psychological distress as a direct consequence of the social conditions of oppression and marginalization. In turn, psychological wellness can only be achieved through active resistance and transformation of our social conditioning.

Reorienting With Principles of Liberation Psychology

Scholars of liberation psychology have articulated core principles to ground everyday practice toward liberation (Comas-Díaz & Torres Rivera, 2020; Martín-Baró, 1994; Torres Rivera, 2020). These principles provide a road map that enables unlearning the knowledge, theories, and epistemologies of psycolonization while reorienting to a decolonial psychology. Given the centrality of race in coloniality, the process of reorienting is intimately connected to deconstructing racial socialization. In this section, we apply principles of liberation psychology as a way to foster a healthy racial identity development. We emphasize six liberation psychology principles necessary for decolonial mentoring: recovering historical memory, honoring people's strengths, de-ideologization and denaturalization of everyday experience, problematization, conscientization, and praxis (see Table 10.1).

Recovering historical memory. Recovering historical memory demands that history must be reclaimed from the perspective of those who have been oppressed and whose voices have been silenced (Martín-Baró, 1994). In decolonial mentoring, this principle aims to provide mentees with factual knowledge that captures the true narratives of oppression and resistance throughout history (Chavez-Dueñas & Adames, 2021). For BIPOC mentees, recovering accurate and full history is necessary to externalize oppression and identify strategies communities use across time to resist and heal. Following this principle, mentors can task BIPOC mentees with studying historical narratives that provide alternatives to the limited, White Eurocentric history taught in the United States. Alternatives can include oral, written, musical, artistic media that highlight strengths and contributions of BIPOC people. Learning the stories of their ancestors can help BIPOC mentees celebrate the ingenuity,

TABLE 10.1. Six Selected Principles of Liberation Psychology

Core principle	Description
Recovering Historical Memory	Developing an accurate understanding of history that includes the role of oppression and critical resistance in the lives of our ancestors.
Honoring People's Strengths	Recognizing and uplifting the psychological strengths of marginalized peoples who have resisted oppression for centuries.
De-Ideologization and Denaturalization of Everyday Experience	Deconstructing the dominant ideologies we have been taught to accept unconditionally while recognizing these norms as abnormal and unnatural.
Problematization	Developing a clear understanding of the problems inherent in coloniality; recognizing the system of domination as problematic and not the individual.
Conscientization	Developing critical knowledge and awareness of oppressive social conditions and one's capacity to transform them.
Praxis	Exercising theory and practice simultaneously, understanding that knowledge must be accompanied with action.

creativity, and enduring spirit of those who have come before them. Knowing the many contributions and talents of their ancestors can help BIPOC mentees locate their inner resources to thrive in today's world.

For White mentees, exposure to the reality of their ancestor's oppressive legacy is necessary for reckoning with their role in perpetuating coloniality today. Developing an understanding of the history of colonization, including mass genocide and enslavement of BIPOC, is a critical aspect of confronting modern-day racism. Mentors may assign mentees readings of BIPOC accounts of historical events, with the task of critically engaging with the role their ancestors played in perpetuating colonization. Ultimately, acknowledging history can challenge White mentee's socialized tendencies to avoid, deny, or minimize the reality of White supremacy. Further, learning about the strengths and accomplishments of BIPOC throughout history can help challenge and correct pathologizing biases of Communities of Color. Engaging with their history of colonization and racial oppression may provoke critical racial awareness in White mentees for the first time. Mentors may ask White mentees to examine their defenses and emotions that arise as a result, and sit with the discomfort, rather than engage in avoidance of the realities of White supremacy. By recovering historical memory, decolonial mentoring can help mentees critically examine what they have been socialized to believe about themselves and others.

Honoring people's strengths. Honoring people's strengths emphasizes the identification of positive skills, attributes, talents, and knowledge that have allowed individuals and groups to survive and thrive in the face of coloniality (Adames & Chavez-Dueñas, 2017). Within decolonial mentoring, this principle encourages mentees to acknowledge their strengths and inner resources, as well as to recognize and center the virtues of others. This principle aims to shift the mentee's perspective away from pathologizing BIPOC values and toward highlighting them as tools "to cope with impossible circumstances for generations" (Torres Rivera, 2020, p. 46). For BIPOC mentees, this includes highlighting the strengths of the group that the BIPOC mentee belongs to and identifying figures who embody such strengths (e.g., historical figures, community leaders, artists, writers, public figures). Further, mentors can remind BIPOC mentees to use their inner strengths when faced with systemic challenges. Mentors may ask BIPOC mentees to identify personal, professional and political examples where cultural strengths were used to combat systemic racism (e.g., Latinx immigrant women in detention centers writing letters to advocate for themselves and their children's humanity, Indigenous people maintaining their culture and oral traditions despite colonization, the Black Lives Matter movement started by Black mothers whose children's lives were lost at the hands of policing). White mentees can be guided to recognize and prioritize the historical and ongoing strengths and contributions of BIPOC communities and conversely, resist pathologizing colonial beliefs that frequently frame such strengths as unhealthy. For instance, White mentees might learn that BIPOC's distrust in health providers is a healthy and normal reaction rather than an indicator of psychopathology. Further, mentors may connect mentees with literature that highlights the psychological strengths and contributions of Communities of Color (e.g., Adames & Chavez-Dueñas, 2017; White, 1984). Finally, within the mentoring relationship, the mentees (and mentors) life experiences, knowledge, and skills can be honored as strengths, an element that is sometimes lacking within traditional mentorship. A spotlight on strengths provides contrasting paradigms to colonial practices that have pathologized BIPOC communities and failed to recognize their incredible strengths.

De-ideologization and denaturalization of everyday experience. *De-ideologization* captures the journey of deconstructing the inhumane ideologies of coloniality that many of us have learned to accept unconditionally. In tandem, *denaturalization* is the process of uncovering the complete abnormality of these ideologies while rejecting the assumptions and beliefs we have taken for granted as being "natural" (Torres Rivera, 2020). The goal is to identify and reject those aspects of coloniality we have been taught to believe are normative and natural. In other words, for both BIPOC and White mentees, this principle represents the process of questioning everything that we think we know. For BIPOC mentees, de-ideologization and denaturalization are necessary to practice de-pathologizing normal reactions to abnormal situations and identify that coloniality and White supremacy culture are abnormal situations. For White people, this principle can help guide their critical examination of socialized thoughts, beliefs, and actions that are harmful toward BIPOC and that perpetuate coloniality and their sense of racialized superiority. Within the mentorship relationship, mentors can offer examples of how they question and challenge their training, education, and ideas about their personal and professional responsibilities (e.g., what is right, best, or the truth). They can also role model critical analysis of the information and knowledge we consume by asking certain questions: Who produced this piece of knowledge? What is their understanding of systems of oppression? What information was left out? What other context is necessary to consider? Only through critically examining our imposed reality can we begin to rebuild anew.

Problematization. Liberation psychology seeks to externalize the problem from the person or community while recognizing troubles as a manifestation of coloniality; this is known as *problematization*. Shifting our perspective toward examining how the environment recreates colonial norms can help us understand context over personal characteristics. The goal is to process, discuss, question intentionally, and identify what systems are the "problem." For BIPOC mentees, problematization is necessary to avoid internalizing blame for the remnants of the colonial system. Identification of the root causes of suffering (i.e., systemic, cultural, and institutional racism) for BIPOC communities can open avenues for healing as well as for resistance. A mentor can draw attention to when BIPOC mentees express thoughts and feelings of self-doubt, low worth, shame, and not being good enough, and help them understand that these are a by-product of living in a oppressive environment that reinforces White supremacist ideologies, and not a measure of their inherent value or potential. For White mentees, problematization is necessary to continuously challenge and unlearn the denigrating and pathologizing beliefs from which they benefit. Mentors can encourage White mentees to engage in deliberate self-reflection of inherent biases, ways of benefiting (i.e., racial privilege), and identifying how their beliefs and actions perpetuate systems of coloniality. Furthermore, mentors can role model this principle by naming and calling out existing deficit narratives of BIPOC communities and placing responsibility where it belongs, that is, on the colonial machine's reproduction of White supremacy.

Conscientization. *Conscientization* was first termed by Freire (1970) and involves the active process of "continual discovery and action related to the 'truth'" (Torres Rivera, 2020, p. 46). This discovery process includes a critical analysis of one's collective history (Watts et al., 2011) and subsequent action to apply the consciousness to daily interaction. This principle aims to develop an awareness of one's historical, sociocultural, and political reality while engaging in actions to transform a new reality. For BIPOC mentees, this process is necessary to facilitate reflection on how they may continuously and indirectly internalize systems of oppression and actively build collective agency. For White mentees, conscientization is necessary to develop critical racial awareness, engage in actions that make the world a more just place, and challenge oneself and other White people to be accountable to coloniality. Mentors can help raise critical consciousness by engaging in dialogue and reflection with mentees about material (e.g., workshops, lectures, podcasts, documentaries, chapters) that focuses on subjects such as the history of colonization, critical race theory, racial identity theory, and BIPOC resistance movements. Mentors can help mentees reflect, process, and make sense of the material by asking open-ended questions. What are your reactions to the material? What surprised you? How is this different or similar to what you knew before? How have you been hurt by systems of oppression? How have you benefited from systems of oppression? How does this material affect your worldview and behaviors? Critical consciousness is an active and reiterative process that necessitates not one but ongoing reflection and questioning.

Praxis. The final guiding principle is *praxis,* which describes the combination of theory and practice or the action necessary for changing the circumstances that create suffering. The goal of praxis in decolonial mentoring is to communicate to mentees that the world will change through deliberate action. This principle challenges mentees to enact decolonial praxis in their lifetime while passing this responsibility of unlearning, relearning, and rebuilding on to others. For BIPOC mentees, the praxis principle includes fostering their commitment to imagining; voicing and connecting; empathizing; and celebrating the self and others within the community.

As Chavez-Dueñas et al. (2022) discussed, mentors can assist BIPOC mentees to "envision a future of liberation and self-determination" that reflects their culture and not the oppressor's (p. 12). This could include encouraging BIPOC mentees engage in self-care practices that promote well-being or role modeling collective action. Further, mentors may ask BIPOC students to mentor other BIPOC mentees as a way to continue the legacy of mentorship and commitment to an anticolonial future.

Praxis is necessary to keep passing the responsibility forward and act in direct opposition to what coloniality reinforces. For White mentees, praxis is essential to guide accountability for their oppressive legacy, which requires not only simple reflection but also striving to internalize and practice knowledge. This demands several actions, including challenging racism at all times, modeling deliberate action, and demonstrating a commitment to continued effort through antioppressive engagement with other White people.

As White people are socially rewarded for regression to the colonial mean, maintaining action is especially important. Informed, engaged, and consistent action with a continuous commitment to unlearning and relearning remains a primary goal for White people with decolonial mentorship. Additional application of the praxis principle is explored in the fourth pillar, rebuilding for an anticolonial future.

The six principles from liberation psychology provide guideposts for developing a decolonial orientation in psychology and beyond. Although these guiding principles are critical, they are theoretical and challenging to transform into action. To translate theory into action, the decolonial mentoring relationship must be attuned to issues of race and power. The third pillar considers how these factors (i.e., racial identity, social power) influence the ability of mentorship to be growth fostering or growth hindering.

Pillar 3: Recognizing Racial Identity and Power

The third pillar of the DMF captures the essential requirement of recognizing racial identity and power within the mentoring relationship. As with all social interactions, mentorship is affected by the interplay of racial identity and relational power dynamics. Racial identity is shaped by a process of racial socialization wherein individuals internalize messages about race and racism. These messages are a reflection of dominant ideologies that exist across personal, institutional, and systemic levels (Harro, 2000). Racial messages are internalized in the form of schemas, described as cognitive and affective filters that affect how we perceive and respond to racialized content (Helms, 1990). Essentially, schemas help organize incoming stimuli and allow for a sense of prediction and control in our social environments. Thus racial identity schemas dictate how one approaches topics related to race and culture.

The process of racial socialization is both insidious and life long. Because they are a reflection of dominant ideology (i.e., White supremacy culture), racial identity schemas are the mechanism by which the individual internalizes power and violence. Although racial socialization is collective, racial identity itself is expressed at the individual level. Because one of the primary aims of decolonial mentoring is to foster healthy racial identity development, explicit recognition of the individual mentor and mentee's racial identity schemas is paramount. The degree to which mentoring can facilitate growth depends on, first, the maturity of one's racial identity schemas, and, second, the relational dynamics that manifest in response to social power or status.

To illustrate this dynamic interplay, we apply Helms's (1990; Helms & Cook, 1999) racial identity social interaction model as a tool to advance decolonial mentoring. The model considers racial identity and social power or status, and how these two factors interact to affect the alliance. The RISIM is broadly applicable to relationships in which power relations are unequal, such as where one person has more social power than the other (e.g., mentor–mentee, teacher–student, supervisor–supervisee, parent–child; Helms, 1990; Helms & Cook, 1999). In the next section, we briefly describe these RISIM components and describe their application to decolonial mentorship.

Racial Identity

Racial identity theory provides a foundation for examining the salience of racial dynamics in mentorship. Pioneered by the work of Helms (1990, 1995, 2019), racial identity theory captures the cognitive, behavioral, and affective processes that occur as an individual comes to understand the role of race in their lives and the lives of others. Establishing a healthy racial identity requires a person to develop an accurate sense of who they are in a racialized society while actively deconstructing dominant narratives that sustain White supremacy culture. Individuals will vacillate through different ego statuses as they progress (or regress) in their racial identity development. Each such status is characterized by a predominant racial schema that illustrates how the individual interprets and responds to racial stimuli.

The process of racial identity development for BIPOC and White people is characteristically different due to a pervasive culture of White supremacy. For BIPOC, racial identity development underscores the need to actively resist the internalization of racism while developing coping strategies to combat racism and committing to a lifelong effort to resist and dismantle oppression in its varying forms (Helms, 2019). The model describes five identity ego statuses that BIPOC may experience and move between conformity, dissonance, immersion or emersion, internalization, and finally integrative awareness. BIPOC's identity status may shift from internalizing racist ideologies (e.g., denial, ambivalence) to externalizing racism and working toward community liberation (e.g., hyperawareness, intellectualization of racism, flexibility). The final status, integrative awareness, highlights the ability to remain aware of and act against racial inequity as well as other forms of oppression (Helms, 1990; Jernigan et al., 2010). This ability to conceptualize oppression existing in groups other than one's own and to understand the strengths and challenges of different groups makes this status optimal for sustained decolonial praxis.

For White people, racial identity development describes the lifelong process by which White people must deliberately work to overcome their personal, cultural, and institutional racist socialization and ideologies in favor of building an antiracist identity (Helms, 2019). The model delineates two multidimensional phases of identity: the abandonment of racism (i.e., contact, disintegration, reintegration), and the development of a nonracist identity (i.e., pseudoindependence, immersion or emersion, autonomy). Whereas phase 1 maintains a status quo of White superiority and includes efforts to avoid, deny, and reinforce racism, phase 2 includes efforts to challenge White racial socialization norms (Helms, 2019). Because both BIPOC and White individuals vacillate between racial identity schemas in the unrelenting storm of coloniality, the RISIM specifically considers the schemas held most primarily and consistently by the mentee and mentor.

Relational Power

Traditional mentorship in psychology is hierarchical, with relational power disproportionality afforded to the mentor. The RISIM considers relational power dynamics that occur when one individual in a dyad is ascribed greater social power or status on the basis of expectations of their given role. With this relational power differential, the role afforded the most power (e.g., mentor) has a greater responsibility to facilitate the development of the role with lesser power (e.g., mentee). By definition, mentors are likely to be more advanced in their career or be in a position where they are teaching, guiding, evaluating, or generally facilitating growth within the mentee (American Psychological Association, 2006). Given that the mentor holds a power-over stance in the relationship, the RISIM postulates that they are likely to have a greater ability to steer the relationship toward or away from engagement with issues of race and culture.

Interaction of Racial Identity and Relational Power Dynamics

The interaction of racial identity and power within a social dyad influences how individuals can engage with one another on issues of race and culture—the RISIM considers these complexities. In doing so, the RISIM highlights varying mentoring alliances that range from dysfunctional to growth promoting (Helms, 1990; Helms & Cook, 1999). According to the RISIM, the mentor may promote, inhibit, or stall the mentee's racial identity development by way of three types of alliances: parallel, regressive, and progressive.

Parallel. Parallel dyads are present when both the mentor and mentee have a similar predominant racial identity schema, even though they may also have different racial identities (e.g., a Black mentor who is in the conformity schema interacting with a White mentee who is in the contact schema). The mentor and mentee have similar views on racism (e.g., color-blind ideologies). Thus they are both prone to deny or ignore the salience of race and will fail to challenge one another's worldview. This type of alliance is most likely to stagnate growth for both the mentor and mentee. Pillars of decolonial mentoring may be challenging to enact within this type of dyad.

Regressive. Regressive dyads occur when the individual in the role with the most social power has a less developed identity schema than their counterpart (e.g., a mentor in immersion-emersion and a mentee in internalization). This relationship may range from stagnant to dysfunctional and long-lasting conflicts may be present. When a mentor assumes a dramatically less advanced identity schema, the relationship may be incredibly counterproductive, and they may avoid discussions of race altogether. The mentee's efforts to grow will be stifled and inhibited by the mentor with less advanced viewpoints. In this interaction, the mentor will continue to attempt to regress to the mean of White supremacy and coloniality.

Progressive dyads. Progressive dyads, the ideal relationship dynamic for decolonial mentorship, occur when the individual with more role power has a more advanced identity schema than the individual with less. An example would be a mentor using an integrative awareness schema and a mentee using an immersion-emersion schema. Progressive relationships are growth promoting because the mentor is more attuned to issues of race and able to encourage the mentee's advancement toward decolonial praxis. The tension by the mentor being more knowledgeable in their racial identity and having greater role power provokes growth and encourages attunement to issues of race and culture in meaningful and transformative ways (Helms & Cook, 1999; Jernigan et al., 2010). The progressive relationship dyad ensures that the mentor and the mentee continually engage in learning to advance their identity schemas and racial worldview. The mentor can support and challenge the mentee in their identity development and decolonial praxis while continuing to further grow to remain more advanced than their mentee.

Using the RISIM in Practice

The RISIM has previously been applied to counseling and supervision dyads (e.g., Helms & Cook, 1999; Jernigan et al., 2010; Thrower, Helms, & Manosalvas, 2020; Thrower, Helms, & Price, 2020); here we apply the model to mentorship. Although mentorship and supervision overlap in their aim to support trainee development, they are not synonymous. For instance, even though supervisors may assume a mentoring stance, not all supervision evolves to mentorship (Morgan & Sprenkle, 2007). Instead, mentorship aims to support the trainee's holistic development beyond a singular training experience or position (Atkinson et al., 1994; Schlosser & Foley, 2008).

Only by attending to issues of race and power in the relationship can mentoring be decolonial. The RISIM is a tool for critical analysis of racial identity and power between mentor and mentee. Mentors and mentees can use it to examine how identity and power interact within the relationship and use this understanding to inform both relational and individual growth. Mentees and mentors may use the RISIM to facilitate decolonial mentoring in various ways to

- identify the prominent racial identity status or schema both mentors and mentees are operating from at any moment;

- generate ongoing discussion of how racial identity and power promote, stifle, or hinder development;

- create an open and ongoing dialogue to examine how racial identity and power affect mentoring processes (e.g., professional guidance, psychosocial support);

- facilitate self-reflection for the mentor and mentee regarding their identity development while highlighting growth areas;

- help the mentee recognize when they are in a regressive dyad (e.g., when a mentor has a less developed racial identity) and resist internalizing harmful interactions of the relationship; or

- help the mentor acknowledge when the mentee is more advanced in their racial identity development and help connect the mentee with someone with a healthier identity.

Pillar 4: Rebuilding for an Anticolonial Future

The fourth pillar of the DMF intended to emphasize the lifelong, committed action necessary to advance an anticolonial future. Complementing the work of resisting psycolonization, reorienting to decolonial psychology, and recognizing the interplay of race and power, this final pillar asks what you are going to do about it. Providing mentees with the knowledge to develop a decolonial orientation is necessary, yet knowledge without action is futile. Rebuilding an anticolonial future requires mentees to engage in daily action. This pillar seeks to make the principle of praxis (i.e., theory plus action) explicit while helping the mentee assume an enduring commitment to rebuilding a more just world.

Developing a practice for daily anticolonial action requires thoughtful commitment from both mentor and mentee. Mentors can encourage direct action by providing guidance, critical feedback, and fostering mentees' sense of agency in challenging injustice. Mentors can model in their lives and facilitate in mentees in numerous ways.

- Be attentive to racism and oppressive behaviors in yourself and those around you. Build and execute skills for interrupting coloniality in your daily social interactions.

- Maintain a reflective practice of economic activity while moving toward supporting BIPOC owned and operated businesses. Keep score of where you are spending money, who you are investing in, and where you can divest from (see Movement for Black Lives, 2021).

- Develop skills to identify and resist institutional policies and practices reinforcing a colonial status quo. For example, ensure that BIPOC voices are recognized, taught, and cited across theoretical and clinical courses, in addition to one's research. The Psychology of Radical Healing Syllabus (French et al., 2019) is an excellent starting resource.

- Respect and value Indigenous peoples, their histories, land, and traditions. Begin by learning about the Native land you inhabit and its history by using the map developed by the Indigenous-led nonprofit Native Land Digital (2019).

- Grow your understanding of the impact of psycolonization in the teaching and practice of psychology. For instance, study texts such as *Even the Rat Was White* (Guthrie, 2003) and the *Apology to People of Color* (American Psychological Association, 2021).

- Learn about critical psychological approaches and frameworks developed by BIPOC and for BIPOC communities to engage with decolonial paradigms. Consider learning about psychological frameworks such as radical healing (Adames et al., 2023; French et al., 2019) and intersectionality awakening model of womanista (Chavez-Dueñas & Adames, 2021), intersectionality in psychotherapy (Adames et al., 2018), or listening to podcasts such as *Liberation Now*, which explores the healing and liberation of BIPOC (Liberation Lab, 2020).

- Engage in consistent, intentional conversation with peers, colleagues, and loved ones to examine your socialized biases and internal reactions to the world around you.

- Question what you think you know, often and with others.

THE DECOLONIAL MENTORING FRAMEWORK IN EVERYDAY PRACTICE

Rather than a prescriptive step-by-step model, the DMF is a reflective, action-driven tool that can be used to inform decolonial mentoring. The 4Rs of the framework are described in the active form of a verb: resisting, reorienting, recognizing, rebuilding. Action-oriented language is intended to capture the behavioral dimension of practicing decolonial mentoring. As a tool for daily practice, the DMF can help generate critical self-reflection, shared discussion, and collaborative action in mentoring dyads. Reflection prompts to consider include, how am I (are we) exercising each of the 4Rs, how are racial identity and power interacting to affect the quality of our mentorship, and what anti-colonial actions am I (are we) engaging in as a result of mentoring.

In everyday practice, it is helpful to consider the DMF as a reflexive and recursive tool: information generated through analysis of one pillar helps inform engagement with subsequent pillars (i.e., reflexive) in a repeated and ongoing fashion (i.e., recursive). For example, knowledge developed through conscientization (pillar 2) can guide individuals to exercise their voice in speaking out about injustice (pillar 4) while providing insight into how one's racial socialization is influencing the relational dynamics of mentoring (pillar 3).

Notably, optimal dynamics for decolonial mentoring occur in progressive dyads (Helms & Cook, 1999), wherein the mentor holds a more advanced racial identity schema relative to the mentee. Research indicates that mentoring relationships are most often initiated by the mentee (Forehand, 2008; Lundgren & Orsillo, 2012). Thus the reality remains that the burden of locating decolonial mentors is likely to fall on the mentee. When seeking out decolonial mentors, mentees may look for the following characteristics:

- Behavioral indicators of the mentor's commitment to racial equity and social justice (e.g., participation in protests and political demonstrations, speaking out in professional spaces or listservs).

- Evidence of the mentor's willingness to give and receive critical feedback (e.g., feedback shared in coursework, via social networking platforms, in personal exchanges).

- Engagement beyond academia and the professional realm, including their commitment and contributions to diverse communities.

- Ability to reflect on their racial identity schemas and development (e.g., endorsement of antiracist attitudes versus color-blind ideologies).

- Ability to talk openly about race and the role that race plays in the setting, as well as in the mentorship relationship itself.

- Ability to identify their internalized oppression surrounding BIPOC abilities and skills and its impact on their relationship with BIPOC students and mentees.

- Acknowledgment and understanding of the reality of the experiences of BIPOC.

Last, the DMF is intended to inform a broad approach to mentorship. Rather than restricting its application to a single mentoring experience, readers should consider how the DMF can inform their general orientation to mentoring praxis. As discussed at the beginning of this chapter, mentorship in psychology typically sustains a colonial ethos and reinforces White supremacy culture. Given this reality, the reader is likely to have had mentoring experiences or be actively involved in mentoring relationships that stifle growth or are regressive. By using the DMF to reimagine mentoring, readers may develop new insight and skills for fostering racially conscious, growth-promoting mentoring relationships toward an anticolonial future.

CONCLUSION

Our collective action is urgently needed to dismantle White supremacy culture and rebuild an anticolonial future. Psycolonization is a weapon of White supremacy that should be resisted and radically transformed. Current approaches to professional mentorship in psychology perpetuate this ethos of psycolonization, under which the livelihood and well-being of BIPOC are systematically denigrated (American Psychological Association, 2021; Sonn & Stevens, 2021). Given this reality, we must critically transform our approach to mentoring in psychology. The DMF offers an immediate vision of racially conscious mentorship that is growth fostering. Through decolonial mentoring, we can socialize a new generation of professionals to resist psycolonization while rebuilding for an equitable world. Given the immeasurable and everlasting destruction of coloniality, to decolonize is an aspirational act. Thus we will never truly decolonize this world, yet we can and must always strive for an anticolonial future. "The world we want to transform has already been worked on by history and is largely hollow. We must nevertheless be inventive enough to change it and build a new world . . . Remember that ideas are also weapons" (Marcos, n.d.).

RESOURCES

Castellanos, J., White, J. L., & Franco, V. (2022). *Riding the academic freedom train: A culturally responsive, multigenerational mentoring model*. Stylus Publishing.

Neville, H. (Host). (2020–present). *Liberation now* [Audio podcast]. Liberation Lab. https://illinoisliberationlab.libsyn.com/

Our Home on Native Land [Digital Tool]. https://native-land.ca/

Psychology of Radical Healing Collective. (2019). *Psychology of Radical Healing syllabus*. https://psychologyofradicalhealingdotcom.files.wordpress.com/2021/06/radical-healing-syllabus.pdf

UCI Libraries. (2016, February 24). *Dr. Joseph L White and Dr. Thomas Parham White's mentoring approach* [Video]. YouTube. https://www.youtube.com/watch?v=v22P9gW1uJ8

REFERENCES

Adames, H. Y., & Chavez-Dueñas, N. Y. (2017). *Cultural foundations and interventions in Latino/a mental health: History, theory, and within group differences.* Routledge Press.

Adames, H. Y., Chavez-Dueñas, N. Y., & Jernigan, M. M. (2021). The fallacy of a raceless Latinidad: Action guidelines for centering Blackness in Latinx psychology. *Journal of Latina/o Psychology, 9*(1), 26–44. https://doi.org/10.1037/lat0000179

Adames, H. Y., Chavez-Dueñas, N. Y., Lewis, J. A., Neville, H. A., French, B. H., Chen, G. A., & Mosley, D. V. (2023). Radical healing in psychotherapy: Addressing the wounds of racism-related stress and trauma. *Psychotherapy, 60*(1), 39–50. https://doi.org/10.1037/pst0000435

Adames, H. Y., Chavez-Dueñas, N. Y., Sharma, S., & La Roche, M. J. (2018). Intersectionality in psychotherapy: The experiences of an AfroLatinx queer immigrant. *Psychotherapy, 55*(1), 73–79. https://doi.org/10.1037/pst0000152

American Psychological Association. (2006). *Centering on mentoring.* https://www.apa.org/education/grad/mentor-task-force

American Psychological Association. (2021). *Apology to People of Color for APA's role in promoting, perpetuating, and failing to challenge racism, racial discrimination, and human hierarchy in U.S.* Resolution adopted by the APA Council of Representatives. https://www.apa.org/about/policy/resolution-racism-apology.pdf

Atkinson, D. R., Casas, A., & Neville, H. (1994). Ethnic minority psychologists: Whom they mentor and benefits they derive from the process. *Journal of Multicultural Counseling and Development, 22*(1), 37–48. https://doi.org/10.1002/j.2161-1912.1994.tb00241.x

Burton, M., & Guzzo, R. (2020). Liberation psychology: Origins and development. In L. Comas-Díaz & E. Torres Rivera (Eds.), *Liberation psychology: Theory, method, practice, and social justice* (pp. 17–40). American Psychological Association. https://doi.org/10.1037/0000198-002

Chavez-Dueñas, N. Y., & Adames, H. Y. (2021). Intersectionality awakening model of womanista: A transnational treatment approach for Latinx women. *Women & Therapy, 44*(1–2), 83–100. https://doi.org/10.1080/02703149.2020.1775022

Chavez-Dueñas, N. Y., Adames, H. Y., & Perez-Chavez, J. G. (2022). Anti-colonial futures: Indigenous Latinx women healing from the wounds of racial-gendered colonialism. *Women & Therapy, 45*(2–3), 191–206. https://doi.org/10.1080/02703149.2022.2097593

Comas-Díaz, L. (2000). An ethnopolitical approach to working with people of color. *American Psychologist, 55*(11), 1319–1325. https://doi.org/10.1037/0003-066X.55.11.1319

Comas-Díaz, L. (2021). Afro-Latinxs: Decolonization, healing, and liberation. *Journal of Latina/o Psychology, 9*(1), 65–75. https://doi.org/10.1037/lat0000164

Comas-Díaz, L., & Torres Rivera, E. (Eds.). (2020). *Liberation psychology: Theory, method, practice, and social justice.* American Psychological Association. https://doi.org/10.1037/0000198-000

Cross, W. E. (1971). The Negro to Black conversion experience: Towards a psychology of Black liberation. *Black World, 20*(9), 13–27.

Forehand, R. L. (2008). The art and science of mentoring in psychology: A necessary practice to ensure our future. *American Psychologist, 63*(8), 744–755. https://doi.org/10.1037/0003-066X.63.8.744

Freire, P. (1970). *Pedagogy of the oppressed.* Continuum.

French, B. H., Lewis, J. A., Mosley, D. V., Adames, H. Y., Chavez-Dueñas, N. Y., Chen, G. A., Neville, H. A., & Adam, A. (2019). Psychology of radical healing syllabus. https://psychologyofradicalhealingdotcom.files.wordpress.com/2021/06/radical-healing-syllabus.pdf

French, B. H., Lewis, J. A., Mosley, D. V., Adames, H. Y., Chavez-Dueñas, N. Y., Chen, G. A., & Neville, H. A. (2020). Toward a psychological framework of radical healing in communities of color. *The Counseling Psychologist, 48*(1), 14–46. https://doi.org/10.1177/0011000019843506

Grzanka, P. R., Gonzalez, K. A., & Spanierman, L. B. (2019). White supremacy and counseling psychology: A critical–conceptual framework. *The Counseling Psychologist, 47*(4), 478–529. https://doi.org/10.1177/0011000019880843

Guthrie, R. (2003). *Even the rat was white: A historical view of psychology* (2nd ed.). Pearson.

Harro, B. (2000). The cycle of socialization. In M. Adams, W. J. Blumenfeld, R. Casteñeda, H. Hackman, M. Peters, & X. Zúñiga (Eds.), *Reading for diversity and social justice* (pp. 16–21). Routledge.

Helms, J. E. (Ed.). (1990). *Black and White racial identity.* Praeger.

Helms, J. E. (2019). *A race is a nice thing to have: A guide to being a White person or understanding the White persons in your life* (3rd ed.). Microtraining Associates.

Helms, J. E. (1995). An update of Helm's White and people of color racial identity models. In J. G. Ponterotto, J. M. Casas, L. A. Suzuki, & C. M. Alexander (Eds.), *Handbook of multicultural counseling* (pp. 181–198). Sage Publications.

Helms, J. E., & Cook, D. A. (1999). *Using race and culture in counseling and psychotherapy: Theory and process.* Allyn & Bacon.

Hernandez, J. B. (2022). *Fresh banana leaves: Healing Indigenous landscapes through Indigenous science.* North Atlantic Books.

Jernigan, M. M., Green, C. E., Helms, J. E., Perez-Gualdron, L., & Henze, K. (2010). An examination of people of color supervision dyads: Racial identity matters as much as race. *Training and Education in Professional Psychology, 4*(1), 62–73. https://doi.org/10.1037/a0018110

Kojo Arthur, G. F. (2017). *Cloth as a metaphor: (Re)reading the Adinkra cloth: Symbols of the Akan of Ghana* (2nd ed.). iUniverse.

La Torre, J. C. (2016). *Decolonizing and re-/Indigenizing Filipinos in diaspora* [Master's thesis, California State University].

Liberation Lab. (2020). *Liberation Now Podcast.* https://illinoisliberationlab.libsyn.com/

Lundgren, J. D., & Orsillo, S. M. (2012). The science and practice of mentoring in psychology doctoral training. *Journal of Cognitive Psychotherapy, 26*(3), 196–209. https://doi.org/10.1891/0889-8391.26.3.196

Lunsford, L. G., Crisp, G., Dolan, E. L., & Wuetherick, B. (2017). Mentoring in higher education. In D. A. Clutterbuck, F. K. Kochan, L. G. Lunsford, N. Domniquez, & J. Haddock-Miller (Eds.), *The SAGE handbook of mentoring* (pp. 316–332). SAGE Publishing. https://doi.org/10.4135/9781526402011.n20

Maldonado-Torres, N. (2007). On the coloniality of being. *Cultural Studies, 21*(2–3), 240–270. https://doi.org/10.1080/09502380601162548

Maldonado-Torres, N. (2011). Thinking through the decolonial turn: Post-continental interventions in theory, philosophy, and critique: An introduction. *Transmodernity: Journal of Peripheral Cultural Production of the Luso-Hispanic World, 1*(2), 1–15.

Marcos, S. (n.d.). Subcomandante Marcos quotes. *AZ Quotes.* https://www.azquotes.com/quote/803718

Martín-Baró, I. (1986). Hacia una psicología de la liberación [Toward a psychology of liberation]. *Boletín de Psicología, 22*(1), 1–11.

Martín-Baró, I. (1994). *Writings for a liberation psychology* (A. Aron & S. Corne, Eds.). Harvard University Press.

Miller, L. L., & Miller, M. J. (2020). Praxivist imaginaries of decolonization: Can the psy be decolonized in the world as we *know* it? *Feminism & Psychology, 30*(3), 381–390. https://doi.org/10.1177/0959353519900220

Morgan, M. M., & Sprenkle, D. H. (2007). Toward a common-factors approach to supervision. *Journal of Marital and Family Therapy, 33*(1), 1–17. https://doi.org/10.1111/j.1752-0606.2007.00001.x

Movement for Black Lives. (2021). *Vision for Black lives.* https://m4bl.org/policy-platforms/

Native Land Digital. (2019). Our Home on Native Land. https://native-land.ca/

Nelson, G., & Prilleltensky, I. (Eds.). (2010). *Community psychology: In pursuit of liberation and well-being* (2nd ed.). Palgrave Macmillan. https://doi.org/10.1007/978-0-230-37008-1

Neville, H. A., Lilly, R. L., Duran, G., Lee, R. M., & Browne, L. (2000). Construction and initial validation of the Color-Blind Racial Attitudes Scale (CoBRAS). *Journal of Counseling Psychology, 47*(1), 59–70. https://doi.org/10.1037/0022-0167.47.1.59

Quijano, A., & Therborn, S. (2007). Coloniality and Modernity/Rationality. *Cultural Studies, 21*(2–3), 168–178. https://doi.org/10.1080/09502380601164353

Roach, M. (n.d.). Max Roach Quotes. *AZ Quotes.* https://www.azquotes.com/quote/1241888

Schlosser, L. Z., & Foley, P. F. (2008). Ethical issues in multicultural student–faculty mentoring relationships in higher education. *Mentoring & Tutoring, 16*(1), 63–75. https://doi.org/10.1080/13611260701801015

Sonn, C. C., & Stevens, G. (2021). Tracking the decolonial turn in contemporary community psychology: Expanding socially just knowledge archives, ways of being and modes of praxis. In G. Stevens & C. C. Sonn (Eds.), *Decoloniality and epistemic justice in contemporary community psychology* (pp. 1–19). Springer International. https://doi.org/10.1007/978-3-030-72220-3_1

Teo, T., & Afşin, B. (2020). The impossible conditions of the possibility of an alter-global psychology. In L. Sundararajan, K.-K. Hwang, & K.-H. Yeh (Eds.), *Global psychology from Indigenous perspectives* (pp. 159–174). Springer International. https://doi.org/10.1007/978-3-030-35125-0_10

Thrower, S. J., Helms, J. E., & Manosalvas, K. (2020). Exploring the role of context on racially responsive supervision: The racial identity social interaction model. *Training and Education in Professional Psychology, 14*(2), 116–125. https://doi.org/10.1037/tep0000271

Thrower, S. J., Helms, J. E., & Price, M. (2020). Racial dynamics in counselor training: The racial identity social interaction model. *The Journal of Counselor Preparation and Supervisor, 13*(1), 1–35. https://doi.org/10.7729/131.1313

Torres Rivera, E. (2020). Concepts of liberation psychology. In L. Comas-Díaz & E. Torres Rivera (Eds.), *Liberation psychology: Theory, method, practice, and social justice* (pp. 41–51). American Psychological Association. https://doi.org/10.1037/0000198-003

Tuck, E., & Yang, K. W. (2012). Decolonization is not a metaphor. *Decolonization*, *1*(1), 1–40.

Villanueva, E. (2018). *Decolonial wealth: Indigenous wisdom to health divides and restore balance.* Berret-Koehler.

Watts, R. J., Diemer, M. A., & Voight, A. M. (2011). Critical consciousness: Current status and future directions. *New Directions for Child and Adolescent Development*, *2011*(134), 43–57. https://doi.org/10.1002/cd.310

Waziyatawin & Yellow Bird, M. (Eds.). (2012). *For Indigenous minds only: A decolonization handbook.* SAR Press.

White, J. (1984). *The psychology of Blacks: An Afro-American perspective.* Prentice Hall.

Yellow Horse Brave Heart, M. (1998). The return to the sacred path: Healing the historical trauma and the unresolved grief response among the Lakota through psychoeducational group intervention. *Smith College Studies in Social Work*, *68*(3), 287–305. https://doi.org/10.1080/00377319809517532

11

WISE FACE, FIRM HEART
Ethics and Decolonial Psychology

MELINDA A. GARCÍA

In the current psychology training and practice environment in the United States, psychologists are typically not encouraged to be a vital part of the community in which they live and work. They are often trained to see themselves as independent observers of people and encourage individuals to be independent and self-reliant. Many psychology researchers, particularly applied scholars, spend considerable effort trying to study smaller units of behavior and causality to discover nuggets that might be universal to people worldwide. They often study behavior independent of context and history, and the widely accepted generalizability of those results has been questioned with good reason (Henrich et al., 2010).

In this context, the Ethical Principles of Psychologists and Code of Conduct of the American Psychological Association (APA; 2017) provide minimal guidelines for practice, teaching, and research. Even as basic as the guidelines are, they are aspirational. They do not guide psychologists' development individually or within their communities. They are too general and depend on each

Correspondence concerning this chapter should be addressed to Melinda A. García at melinda@highestpath.org, or 2918 Mountain Rd. NW, Albuquerque, NM 87104.

https://doi.org/10.1037/0000376-012
Decolonial Psychology: Toward Anticolonial Theories, Research, Training, and Practice,
L. Comas-Díaz, H. Y. Adames, and N. Y. Chavez-Dueñas (Editors)

psychologist to interpret concepts such as "maintaining competence" (APA, 2017, Standard 2.03) or "respect for people's rights and dignity" (APA, 2017, Principle E) as they see fit. Ethnic minoritized psychologists have described how the APA Ethics Code can harm when applied to Communities of Color (see Association of Black Psychologists, 2021; M. A. García & Tehee, 2014).

In 2018, the APA Ethics Code Task Force (ECTF) began a rigorous, thorough, and transformational revision of the Ethics Code more in line with the humanistic values of the 21st century. The Ethics Code, which is still under development at the time of writing, is planned to be based on eight principles, including (a) beneficence and nonmaleficence; (b) human and civil rights; (c) integrity; (d) interrelatedness of people, systems, and environment; (e) professionalism and responsibility; (f) respect for the welfare of persons; (g) peoples' scientific mindedness; and (h) social justice (Campbell, 2021a, 2021b). Each of the ten standards will explicitly be linked to the corresponding principles, and plans are to include a decision-making model. The goal is for the new Ethics Code to be more relevant and complete than the current code and to infuse content related to diversity and social justice. Like the current codes, the new code will also be aspirational given that the APA has no enforcement mechanisms. Individual states and countries may adopt all or simply parts of it. As improved as we hope the new code will be, it is unlikely to be decolonial because that would require a decentering of settler colonial perspectives (Tuck & Yang, 2012), nor has any announcement been made that this stance is being considered. Because this is a code of ethics for members of the APA, a solidly capitalist institution, a decolonial perspective is unlikely to be adopted and centered by the ECTF.

In the face of a profession that gives only lip service to the ethical treatment of marginalized and colonized populations, it is no wonder that few publications in either liberation psychology or decolonizing approaches to psychology have included a section on ethics. Nonetheless, having a frame of reference for what constitutes integrity from a decolonial or Indigenous point of view is constructive. Although many authors have written about the need to rediscover traditional wisdom from colonized peoples, fewer have explicitly integrated those wisdom teachings into their scholarly writings— a goal of this chapter.

To this end, the chapter focuses on and describes the contributions of three wisdom traditions that provide ancient, well-established road maps to the healthy development of anyone who works as a psychologist, researcher, or practitioner. I turn toward ancient wisdom traditions from the Global South, the first wisdom tradition is the Náhuatl culture of Mexico as recorded almost 500 years ago by Fray Bernardino de Sahagún and his Indigenous collaborators (de Sahagún et al., 1969, 1981, 1982) to describe the role of the *tlamatini*, the wise ones who both taught in the schools and whom the people consulted (González, 2019). The research on Náhuatl culture has been undertaken by anthropologists or cultural studies scholars unfamiliar with decolonial psychology. The Spaniards burned many, if not all, of the original Náhuatl texts. What survives are 16th-century works recorded by Indigenous scribes from cultural informants who were educated before the arrival of the Spaniards. Franciscan friars had educated the scribes to write in Latin and Náhuatl but with a Latin alphabet, as opposed to the preconquest pictographic style of writing. These texts were translated into Spanish and German before there was interest or funding to translate them into English (de Sahagún et al., 1982). Colonial attitudes in the United States about the value of Mexican culture have kept U.S. students of ancient Indigenous cultures ignorant of its treasures. Some sources used for this chapter was translated from Náhuatl directly to English between 1940 and 1981 (de Sahagún et al., 1982).

The second wisdom tradition is contemporary Indigenous teachings. Psychological understanding of the current Indigenous cultures of North America is receiving more attention than ever (see M. A. García et al., 2020). Although many U.S. and Canadian tribes do not have a writing tradition, they do have oral history traditions. Current Indigenous scholars from multiple disciplines are working diligently to document and preserve Indigenous knowledge. Two psychological resources are presented as examples of such Indigenous documentation: the current ethical frameworks from Indigenous traditions in North America as described in the *Guiding Principles for Engaging in Research With Native American Communities* (Straits et al., 2012), and the *Society of Indian Psychologists Commentary on the American Psychological Association's (APA) Ethical Principles of Psychologists and Code of Conduct* (M. A. García & Tehee, 2014).

The third area is Buddhist philosophy, specifically the Noble Eightfold Path and the role of the Bodhisattva. Many books have been written about Buddhist philosophy and how it relates to Western psychology (see Hanh, 2004; Kabat-Zinn, 2013; Kornfield, 2008); however, most books in English use a settler-colonial framework. A current wave of texts are by African American Buddhist teachers (see Johnson, 2014; King, 2018; Manuel, 2015; Owens, 2020; Williams et al., 2016). Although many of these do not connect the practice of Buddhism to decolonial frameworks, some have discussed the importance of Buddhist practice as a way to survive and live a healthy life while encountering oppression (Manuel, 2015; Owens, 2020).

Far more information is available for each area than can be reviewed in one chapter. Thus this chapter concentrates on concepts most relevant to a decolonial ethics in psychology and discusses how these can contribute to meaningful, relevant, and healthy ways of being and working as psychologists.

WHY DOES A DECOLONIALIZED PSYCHOLOGY NEED ETHICS?

Although many books on decolonial psychology often describe critical ways to decolonize ourselves and the practice of a discipline that has harmed many people, the noble cause does not mean that we will automatically behave in noble ways all the time. If we do not outline what we mean by ethical decolonial behavior, many different ideas of what that could mean will likely follow. As Pope et al. (2021) posited, "Our ethics acknowledge and affirm our profession's responsibilities" (p. 3). Similarly, the practice of decolonial psychology needs to examine the qualities and skills necessary to be a decolonial psychologist. Fortunately, most psychologists know how to find and read histories that were glossed over or ignored in training. Doing that, though, should be basic education for decolonial psychologists. We can also take courses in power, privilege, and oppression. But how do we put that theoretical, book-based learning into practice? What skill level do we need? Is it possible to engage in this without embarrassing ourselves? My answer to the last question is no. But with practice, I believe we can learn to recover gracefully.

Do we learn the colonizer's language to transform colonial psychology? Or do we declare colonial psychology bankrupt for us and present dynamic and relevant psychologies that have been used for centuries? Many argue for a middle position, to take the best of both. But without an in-depth education about what has been available to northern Indigenous and Global South people for several thousands of years, we have no idea what choosing the best of each would look like. Are we talking about a 50:50 split or perhaps 30% European colonial and 70% Indigenous and Global South? Some other proportion? And to what end? Undoing colonialism implies orienting oneself toward colonialism first. This saps energy by ruminating on what is wrong. I propose that we engage in strength-based growth and healing first by learning and mastering ways that are centuries old. We can then look at Western psychology with "a wise countenance and a firm heart" that does not waver.

Cultural Wisdom and Historical Memory

For many years before writing the commentary on the American Psychological Association's (APA's) Ethics Code (M. A. García & Tehee, 2014), the Society of Indian Psychologists shared frustrations at their annual conference about European-based psychology that permeated almost all our academic and workplace settings. Specifically, we found that culturally based colonial assumptions permeated American society and that American psychology absorbed those assumptions wholesale. These include the ideas that behavior can be best studied as discrete units to understand the whole, compartmentalizing helps promote the understanding of how humans function, and individuals should be autonomous and self-reliant. As Adames and Chavez-Dueñas have noted, these assumptions have directly contributed to a reductionistic psychology that is (a) devoid of context; (b) fails to consider racial, gender, or caste issues; (c) fails to consider history; and (d) implies that all knowledge can be measured and discovered instead of cocreated (2021).

In 2012, a consortium of Indigenous and White researchers in New Mexico published the *Guiding Principles for Engaging in Research With Native American Communities* (Straits et al., 2012), a best-practices manual describing methods that yield quality results for researchers and tribes in Indian Country. The team developed the list by comparing what had been effective in conducting research with tribes and engaging in an ongoing dialogue with local tribes about what they wanted to see.

The guiding research principles include the following 11 areas: (a) native centered, (b) respect, (c) self-reflection and cultural humility, (d) authentic relationships, (e) honoring community time frames, (f) building on strengths, (g) colearning and ownership, (h) continual dialogue, (i) transparency and accountability, (j) integrity, and (k) community relevance. These principles are strikingly different from those taught in research classes in psychology graduate programs. Except for a few references on participatory action research and community-based participatory research, all other considerations were written by Indigenous authors and tribal organizations about respect in research and who owns the data. In other words, the references were about research and data sovereignty. The principles did not come about as the result of examining liberation psychology or decolonial literature; they came through examining Indigenous strengths in the authors' communities (see M. A. García et al., 2017). Notably, they are compatible with other authors' descriptions (see Beltone et al., 2016; Comas-Díaz & Torres Rivera, 2020; Smith, 2012).

Following the principle of being native centered, the team decided to self-publish rather than submit to the editorial process from current psychological journals with colonial orientations that would have likely diluted what they had to say and how they said it. Additionally, respecting the Indigenous principle of generosity, the guiding principles are published in open access format (Straits et al., 2012). Using these principles as a guide, the Society of Indian Psychologists concurrently engaged in a two-year study of the APA Ethics Code. This process resulted in the society's commentary on the APA's Ethics Code (M. A. García & Tehee, 2014) and the articulation of the following ethical values for the practice of psychology:

1. All things are sacred. Sacredness is not religiosity but a recognition that everything has an important role to play in the universe. This idea of sacredness is respectful of reciprocal relationships, family, the community, environment, and of the past, present, and future.

2. Life and development are understood in terms of cycles as opposed to a linear process.

3. Everything is connected. All beings (including the Earth, the environment, and events in the past, present, and future) respond to each other's actions. Every living system is a whole in itself, as well as part of a larger system. This explanation is an essential concept of full circle understanding.

4. Events in life can best be understood as lessons. That this moment is part of the lesson of whom we were, are, and whom we are to become is acknowledged.

5. Respect and honoring are essential to true or long-lasting relationships. These need to be demonstrated in a way that recognizes the cultural context of the individual and the community.

6. Relevant healing places emphasis on the social, historical, and political contexts that have shaped Indigenous experiences, lives, and perceptions.

7. Relevant healing encourages balance and harmony within a person's life and in relationship to others; it encourages the growth of positive elements in a person's life and emphasizes the strengthening of resilience.

8. Individuality is valued by how it improves the community. Collaboration is more highly valued than autonomy. Competition should enhance collaboration.

9. Sustainability is essential for all of us to survive and thrive. This generation is not the most important for all time. It is important to question. How can we live in a way that allows others to live? How can we live in a way that reflects respect to all those whom we impact?

10. Mystery, awe, wonder, intuition, and miracles occur naturally in everyday life. The fact that Western culture has not yet figured out how to measure them is irrelevant.

11. The best way to understand one's place and identity is in the context of past, present, and future within one's community. Any action may have broad consequences. It is important to consider how to act deliberately and thoughtfully.

12. Compartmentalism misses the beauty of the whole. The whole is often much more complex and functional than the sum of each individual part. Working with the whole acknowledges the mystery of those things still unknown and that cannot be readily observed or measured (M. A. García & Tehee, 2014, pp. 13–14).

These twelve values stem from a way of relating to the world that differs sharply from a compartmentalized, Western, or European view of health. To illustrate this perspective, the commentary provides the following summary:

> Indigenous people have a holistic and inter-relational view of health. This view means that the Western-based concepts of body, emotions, mind, spirit, community, and land cannot be separated and that an individual cannot be separated from their relationships, including the generations before them and the generations to come. There are no distinctions between physical health, mental health, and spiritual health, which also means that, "my physical health, mental health, and wellbeing are related to yours" ("we are all related"). Indigenous people consider the land and environment to be living, breathing beings in their own right. In the Indigenous context, healing is transpersonal and as such, extends beyond the physical person and applies to their place or environment, housing, education, work, and even the society in which they are a part. (M. A. García & Tehee, 2014, p. 13)

A complex, holistic, and interrelational view of health has been integral to Indigenous people for thousands of years. Health interventions encourage character growth, resilience, and the development of a person's unique strengths to support the community (National Institutes of Health, 2019). This notion is related to the pre-Columbian Náhuatl concept of *In Ixtli, In Yóllotl* (Náhuatl), *Rostro Sabio, Corazón Firme* (Spanish), or Wise Face and Firm Heart, discussed in the following sections.

Pre-Columbian Mexicans Had Psychologists?

According to the Náhua, the ideal mature person possessed "a Wise Face and a Firm Heart" (León-Portilla, 1980b). The Wise Face, or Wise Countenance, refers to the person's outward behavior in public and private. The heart was where choices were made based on the culture's values. The mature person possessed a heart that was "firm like stone, a heart resilient as the trunk of a tree" (p. 193). In other words, someone with a firm heart displayed high morals and great integrity. The *tlamatinime* (plural, *tlamatini:* singular) were one of the categories of guides who taught people to achieve this.

The *tlamatinime* gave form to the countenance of men and women, helping to bring forth their personalities, educating them to confront adversities in life, showing love to others, and cultivating their hearts (León-Portilla, 1980b). They were the "masters of the word" who taught both in the *calmécac* (place of higher learning) and the *telpochcalli* (school for warriors and hunters; p. 199). They had exceptional writing skills and were in charge of vast libraries of books. They were described as "owners of noble language and careful expression," in other words, as knowledgeable and precise. They were poets and caretakers of sacred songs and taught literature, humanities, philosophy, and rhetoric (León-Portilla, 1980b).

León-Portilla (1980a) noted that although their translation refers to "he," *tlamatinime* (plural) were not always male. When this information was gathered in the 16th century, the scribes were already indoctrinated into Spanish ideas of gender through their education in the Franciscan college. The translators stated that they did not know whether the informants used "he" or a gender-neutral term, but only that the scribes wrote "he." In the following section, the description from the Náhuatl is italicized and followed by my comments.

The Ideal Image of the Náhuatl Sage (Tlamatini)

The wise man: a light, a torch, a stout torch that does not smoke. (Illumination for others, who does not obfuscate.)

A perforated mirror, a mirror pierced on both sides. (The *tlamatini* sees the mundane world as well as the spiritual.)

His are the black and red ink, his are the illustrated manuscripts, he studies the illustrated manuscripts. (A learned and educated person. The black ink was for facts like demographics, weather, socioeconomic data, or geography. The red ink was for philosophical and spiritual teachings and insights.)

He himself is writing and wisdom. He is the path, the true way for others. (Teaching by example.)

He directs people and things. He is a guide in human affairs.

The wise man is careful (like a physician) and preserves tradition.

His is the handed-down; he teaches it; he follows the path of truth. Teacher of the truth, he never ceases to admonish. (Admonish here means to warn, point out, guide, and do so in a good way.)

He makes wise the countenances of others; to them, he gives a face [personality]; he leads them to develop it.

He opens their ears. He enlightens them.

He is the teacher of guides. He shows them their path.

One depends on him.

He puts a mirror before others; he makes them prudent, cautious; he causes a face [personality] to appear in them. He attends to things; he regulates their path; he arranges and commands.
He applies his light to the world.
He knows what is above us [and] in the region of the dead.
He is a serious man. (The *tlamatini* shares what he has learned with the community. He not only focuses on consensual reality, but is also actively tuned into the worlds above and below us. He is not frivolous or flighty.)
Everyone is comforted by him, corrected, taught.
Thanks to him, people humanize their will and receive a strict education.
He comforts the heart; he comforts the people; he helps, gives remedies, heals everyone.
Translation: Miguel León-Portilla, from the *Codex Matritensis*, fol. 118 (Tolosa Manuscript). (cited in León-Portilla, 1980a, p. 200)

This is the Náhuatl description of a person who did what psychologists do. More than 500 years ago, the Náhua knew that someone needed to have the function of helping people to bring forth their face and their heart (their identity) and to balance the two (González, 2019). Naturally, the concept of a psychologist is a modern Western European and North American compartmentalized idea that has removed the psychologist's function from cultural, sociopolitical, and spiritual contexts. Psychology can learn a great deal by looking at wisdom traditions discarded by the colonizers.

The *tlamatini* educated individuals and communities. They helped people know who they were and how to be upright. They actively helped their community by teaching them the traditions and sacred songs. They realized the spiritual world is as important as the waking world in understanding human behavior. They had both those worlds integrated inside themselves and helped others balance in all areas; they walked their talk. Literature, history, myth, theater, music, and culture were all areas that they used to help people have a Wise Face and a Firm Heart. None of them existed by themselves in a silo.

Contemporary Caribbean and Latin American scholars such as Quijano (2007) of Peru, Maldonado-Torres (2011) of Puerto Rico, and Dussel (2013) of Argentina have described an ethic of liberation related to the worldview of the Original Peoples of the Abya Yala, which means "mature land" or "land that flowers" in the language of the Kuna people of Panamá and Colombia. This term was used to indicate the North and South American continent. Caribbean and Latin American activists have adopted the name as an act of self-naming. This liberation ethic—transmodernity—promotes liberation from Western modernity's racism, patriarchy, capitalism, and neocolonialism (Dussel, 2013; Maldonado-Torres, 2011). In contrast to some scholars of liberation psychology who maintain that it is necessary to help the colonized reclaim critical consciousness (Torres Rivera, 2020), Indigenous wisdom keepers maintain that we have been awake, aware, and critical all along. Although intergenerational waves of genocide and ethnic cleansings, forced relocations, stolen resources, slavery, internment camps, deliberate federal policies of broken treaties, refusal to pay debts and continual underresourcing, judicial amnesia, and the government-sanctioned stealing of children have all contributed to tremendous poverty and hardships, they do not mean that colonized, and marginalized people do not have strengths, wisdom, or critical consciousness. It is incumbent on decolonial psychologists not to fall into the trap of playing the "external savior" because this approach disrespects colonized people's dignity, intelligence, and humanity (Tuck & Yang, 2012).

Potential Buddhist Contributions to Decolonial Psychology

Three significant teachings of Buddhism are important resources for the decolonial psychologist: the Eightfold Path, the Practice of Meditation, and the Bodhisattva. According to Buddhist tradition, Siddhartha Gautama, who became known as the Buddha (Awakened One) centuries after his death, was born in the 6th to 5th centuries BCE in what is now known as northern India. He lived for about 80 years, spending nearly 45 of them teaching a method to release suffering and thus escape the cycle of death and rebirth. The central tenets of his teachings are the Four Noble Truths: life has suffering; we need to recognize what we are doing that causes us to suffer; cessation of suffering is possible; the way to stop suffering is to follow the Noble Eightfold Path.

The Eightfold Path consists of practicing the following skills. These descriptions are taken from *The Heart of the Buddha's Teaching* by Thich Nâht Hanh (1998), a Zen Buddhist monk and teacher.

Right View. Our views are based on our perceptions, and erroneous perceptions lead to suffering. "The quality of our views can always be improved" (Hanh, 1998, p. 54), similar to the tenets of cognitive behavior therapy to see what is in front of us as it is.

Right Thinking. "Thinking is the speech of our mind. Right Thinking makes our speech clear and beneficial. . . . Right Thinking is needed to take us down the path of Right Action" (p. 55). The practice of Right Thinking involves sorting through our natural impulses to think in judgmental or harmful ways, noticing when those harmful ways come up, learning to pause rather than react, and correcting those thoughts. "'Image teaching' uses words and ideas. 'Substance teaching' communicates by the way you live" (p. 52).

Right Mindfulness. Mindfulness has to do with how we pay attention as well as what we focus our attention on. As psychologists, we can agree that we are always giving our attention to something. Hanh stated "Our attention may be 'appropriate' . . ., as when we dwell fully in the present moment or inappropriate . . ., as when we are attentive to something that takes us away from being here and now" (p. 59). The goal of this skill is to be able to be in the present moment all day long.

Right Speech. This skill area includes mindful speech to speak truthfully (no "white lies" here) in a way that increases understanding, joy, and hope, and deep listening. "Deep listening is at the foundation of Right Speech. . . . When communication is cut off, we all suffer" (p. 79).

Right Action. This skill area "is the practice of touching love and preventing harm" (p. 86). Right Mindfulness is the basis for Right Action, which includes four major areas: (1) reverence for life, (2) generosity, (3) sexual responsibility, and (4) mindful eating, drinking, and consuming.

Right Diligence. This skill area, which teaches the steps and point of view needed to pursue the Eightfold Path, is also known as Right Effort. Interestingly, the practice of Right Diligence is based on joy and interest; if your practice does not bring you joy, you are not likely to continue to pursue it.

Right Concentration. The goal of this practice "is to cultivate a mind that is one-pointed" (p. 96). Hanh described two types of concentration: active, when "the mind dwells on whatever is happening in the present moment" (p. 96), and selective, when "we choose one object and hold onto it" (p. 97). The point of Right Concentration is for the practitioner to be completely present, leading to greater happiness and Right Action.

Right Livelihood. "To practice Right Livelihood . . ., you have to find a way to earn your living without transgressing your ideals of love and compassion" (p. 104).

The components of the Eightfold Path are often presented to students as points in a circle with arrows going from each of them to the others, illustrating that the practice of one influences all of the others (Hanh, 1998, p. 53). It is important that Buddhism has as many variations as Christianity does. It is also important that Buddhism is an ancient spiritual tradition that encourages study and writing. Much as been written from multiple points of view for each of the matters described. The point of this chapter is to indicate contributions to decolonial psychology that have been overlooked precisely because of a continued perceptive lens shaped by colonization that psychological science should eschew spirituality or spiritual concepts to be valid.

Meditation is the primary method used to learn the Eightfold Path skills. Meditation is the practice of learning to "still" the mind, which moves restlessly from one thing to another whenever we are awake. In the United States, much confusion surrounds what meditation is. It is not guided imagery, and it is not a body scan for relaxation and stress reduction. It is not something that beginners can do lying down. The purpose is not to go to sleep. The goal is to train the undisciplined mind, sometimes called the monkey mind, to be still.

The other purpose is to cultivate nonjudging and respectful awareness. As the practitioner becomes more skillful, this understanding quality leads to mindfulness or attention to the present moment. In the present moment, it is possible to listen deeply (without composing a response or multitasking) and to respond skillfully rather than impulsively or automatically. This skill is crucial for decolonial psychologists because it allows for greater communication and collaboration with others. Regular meditation reduces stress by encouraging the practitioner to distinguish actual from imagined threats and distinguish unsafe situations from those that are uncomfortable (Harris, 2014). It is possible to realize that most daily events do not merit a panic response, absent a war zone or another life-or-death situation. (For an excellent and humorous description of the process, challenges, and benefits of learning to meditate skillfully, see Harris, 2014.)

Some branches of Buddhism include the path of the Bodhisattva. This Sanskrit word refers to a person who has taken a vow to pursue awakening, or enlightenment, and to step out of the cycle of reincarnation. Reincarnation is the belief that the spirit begins a new life in a new body following death. Depending on the moral quality of the actions of the previous life, the new life may take animal, human, or spirit form (Nagaraj et al., 2015). Bodhisattvas have postponed leaving the reincarnation cycle until all beings are awakened. This person commits to living their life in a way that benefits others. This is in direct contrast to the emphasis on the individual that forms the basis for Western psychology. The Tibetan Buddhist Bodhisattva vow, based on a teaching from the sixth century, bears some striking similarities to the description of the *tlamatini*.

> *May I be a guard for those who need protection*
> *A guide for those on the path*
> *A boat, a raft, a bridge for those who wish to cross the flood*
> *May I be a lamp in the darkness*
> *A resting place for the weary*
> *A healing medicine for all who are sick*
> *A vase of plenty, a tree of miracles*
> *And for the boundless multitudes of living beings*
> *May I bring sustenance and awakening*
> *Enduring like the earth and sky*
> *Until all beings are freed from sorrow*
> *And all are awakened.* (Kornfield, 2008, p. 355)

The ability to do no harm is necessary but not sufficient to define competence for decolonial psychologists (right action). Consistent work on and vigilance about our colonization is essential (right view, right mindfulness, right concentration). This process is not easy, it is not quick, and it is not comfortable (right diligence). It is impossible to do this internal work in a vacuum; it must be done in groups, with others who can be considered teachers (right speech, right view), and with great compassion for our reality as imperfect humans. The judges of our decolonial competence are the communities with whom we work instead of our academic peers and supervisors (right livelihood, right view).

Heal the Discipline

The teachings from the three wisdom traditions described come from spiritual paths. However, immersing oneself in a path to learn from it is not necessary. Traditional cultures worldwide include a relationship to that which cannot be seen and a relationship to the Earth and land. Each area presented is committed to healthy relationships with others, including the Earth, to improve their lives. They strongly encourage the practitioner to work on themselves to be a better helper to others.

The psychologist or social scientist is not a neutral actor. We enter this work with all the biases from our cultural backgrounds and education. We need to actively push ourselves to learn outside of the areas usually associated with psychology. Decolonizing our lens requires a great deal of work. It is far more than attending seminars or reading inspiring books. In the excellent sixth edition of *Ethics in Psychotherapy and Counseling*, Pope et al. (2021) pointed out that "Ethical awareness is a continuous and active process that involves constant questioning and personal responsibility" (p. 7). A few pages later, they reminded us, "We and our clients do not live in a vacuum. We live and develop in socio-cultural contexts" (Pope et al., 2021, p. 11). Taking this a step further, the report of the Warrior's Path Task Force (a Division 45 Task Force aimed to help shape psychology to become a decolonized, postcolonized, and decolonial discipline) maintains that Western psychology has historically ignored its sociocultural context as well as the context of the people with whom we work and study. For decolonial psychologists to be ethical, we need to actively work to radically change the field of psychology (Aiello et al., 2021; see also M. A. García et al., 2017).

Decolonial psychology continues to be too siloed and works in areas defined by Western psychology as "psychology" rather than looking at how colonization has affected the health of marginalized populations more broadly (Aiello et al., 2021). As a counterexample, Kinari Webb, a physician who has worked with local Indigenous people on successfully reclaiming endangered forests in Borneo and Madagascar, maintained that the communities know the local problems that contribute to poverty and deforestation, and they know what the solutions are. She insisted that the most important thing social scientists can do is radical listening (2021), similar to the deep listening described by Right Speech. Social justice issues are often linked with intersectional environmental problems resulting from centuries of colonialism. The local population does not need critical consciousness, and social scientists need to use radical listening to understand the existing consciousness. The social scientist can then help raise the money to bring in critical health care, infrastructure, alternative job training, or education while working with the local population to take over and manage that effort (Webb, 2021).

In another example, *Here and Now*, an NPR podcast, recently published an interview with Girardin Jean-Louis, a leading sleep researcher and psychologist at the University of Miami. "Anybody really sleeping six [hours] or less are at risk," he said. "In terms of Blacks and Brown folks of Latinx background, about 45% of them are sleeping six or less, which means therefore that the risk for cardiometabolic condition as well as early mortality are substantially higher" (Young & Muhammad, 2021, para. 4). A longer description of this research with communities of color is in *Science* (Pérez Ortega, 2021). In a study published in *Sleep Health*, Cheng et al. (2020) found that the experience of racial discrimination accounted for almost 58% of the relationship between race and the severity of insomnia symptoms in racial minority groups.

The factors contributing to the critical lack of sleep in Black and Brown Latinx people are directly related to hundreds of years of colonization. In direct response, Tricia Hersey (2022) teaches that rest is critical to liberation because it allows space for healing and invention. She notes that working Black people to exhaustion has been an essential element of capitalism (cited in S. E. Garcia, 2020). Fortunately for all of us, Hersey is skilled at teaching online as The Nap Bishop (Instagram @thenapministry). Hersey teaches individuals to recognize historical and systems-level patterns of oppression so that by changing their behavior, individuals disrupt systems. Decolonial psychologists have been conditioned not to look at something as fundamental as sleep as essential to liberation, even though treating people as disposable is a well-documented aspect of colonialism.

Decolonial writings often do not use the wisdom of the multicultural literature except as add-ons: liberation in the Black community, liberation in the

Latinx community, liberation in the Indigenous community, liberation and feminism, or liberation and "special" populations, which reinforces colonial separation and keeps us from learning from the wisdom of others. Multiculturalism and decoloniality are inherently interdisciplinary. Let us do work that eliminates antiquated disciplinary boundaries in our methodologies and practices. Let us commit to integrating multicultural and decolonial knowledge (e.g., see the description of Indigenous feminism in APA, Division 35, Section 6, 2021). Queer, trans, diversely abled, undocumented, and religiously marginalized populations and the Global South need to be in the conceptualization of what it means to be a decolonial psychologist as a matter of course and not as add-ons.

Healing the field of psychology includes two major actions. The first is acknowledging how communities and individuals have been pathologized for reacting to tremendous pressures placed on them by colonial forces, including migration and removal from traditional lands. The second is recognizing how our orientation and biases have been and continue to be complicit. It is crucial to recognize when efforts are performative or virtue signaling. It is just as important to hold ourselves and our colleagues accountable in ways that demonstrate the understanding that none of us has a perfect moral ground to stand upon. The process of accountability is messy and complex. Responsibility takes attention, intention, and practice (brown, 2020). As M. A. García and Tehee (2014) wrote,

> The abuse of power, whether intentional or unintentional, plays a major role in the harm experienced by Indigenous people as well as other marginalized and stigmatized people. It is essential that psychologists be alert to and aware of their position within different power structures as individuals and as a profession, and how that relates to the power and status of Indigenous individuals and communities or peoples with whom they work. While the APA Ethics Code encourages psychologists to be aware of their own biases, values, and sociocultural framework, in actual practice, this kind of awareness is rare. (p. 15)

Wise Face, Firm Heart: Committed, Sustained Action

Imagining a healthy decolonial society is more than pointing out what is not working in our current ones. Moreover, as pointed out earlier, it is not just looking at new technologies. We need to be able to welcome the old and the new, a practice which strengthened and protected our peoples since ancient times. To do that, we need to learn the histories of colonized and marginalized people. For BIPOC psychologists, this means understanding the histories of multiple groups in addition to one's own. This shows that we have respect for one another and recognize that we are all connected, and it gets away from the toxic competition for "who has the worst trauma" to justify a fight over scarce resources. Remembering that we are all sacred allows us to walk together to discover a balance and harmony that respects all beings and the Earth.

We have to commit to broadening our individual frameworks. We must work together outside the frameworks for psychology we were given in graduate school. This means looking to community participants, disciplines outside psychology, psychological research outside the Northern Hemisphere, the use of art and music, and alternative ways of communicating via social media. Any work that contributes to a forward movement in our discipline is meaningful. For example, the artist and former teacher Martin Lee has teamed with his brother, the psychologist Rich Lee, to draw a daily comic on Instagram that can be seen at @theotheronesbylee. The comic, illustrated in the style of the classic strip *Peanuts*, deals with the experience of macroaggressions and microaggressions on various marginalized populations. Through their use of social media to educate the public, the brothers illustrate the essential nature of media literacy for decolonization.

To claim the mantle of decolonial psychology with integrity is to commit oneself to cultivate a Wise Face and a Firm Heart for the good of all people. Being a decolonial psychologist is not an intellectual exercise or point of view. It does not mean working in isolation and keeping quiet despite continued settler colonial attitudes and policies. Dismantling Eurocentrism within psychology means taking a courageous look at "the norms that we have also inherited through colonial processes that deflect the hard questions of how we harm each other" (Aiello et al., 2021, p. 31). The decolonial psychologist commits to exploring these issues within themselves. "We must examine, interrogate, and struggle with our own internalizations of colonial values and processes" (p. 31). Decolonizing oneself is not an activity that can be done in isolation or by reading many books. It needs to be done by building learning communities devoted to establishing deep trust and safety among members, diligently excavating how we embody colonial attitudes and privilege, and confronting those behaviors constructively.

Dunford (2017) suggested that we use the following perspective to guide our efforts: "decolonial approaches reject abstract global designs in favour of inter-cultural dialogue amongst multiple people(s), including peoples who deem collective and non-human entities to be of fundamental moral importance. In addition, decolonial global ethics rejects universality in favour of 'pluriversality'" (p. 380).

To do that, we need to learn to disagree in ways that lead to a greater understanding of the intersectionality of colonized groups so that we can work together actively toward the invention of the new. Decolonial psychology must commit to interrogating and struggling with White supremacy and capitalism on an ongoing basis to educate other sectors of our society on why and how to do it. To this end, we should actively embrace the practice of Difficult Dialogues (for an excellent resource, see https://wwwdifficultdialoguesproject. org/). Difficult Dialogues encourage examination of the paradoxical, holding more than one point of view at a time on an issue and cultivating the third point of view. This is especially critical in our currently divided society, where ideas considered unpopular or unskillful are quickly and publicly condemned in social and mainstream media. Decolonial psychologists need to be able to hold complexity to create spaces for healthy disagreements and resolutions and invent ways to go forward. This is the modern embodiment of the *Tlamatini*, The Noble Eightfold Path, and the idea that everything is sacred.

It is more important to reenvision and cocreate care systems for our communities that respect their dignity than to focus on the discomfort of those currently holding power and privilege as embodied in Right Action and Right Livelihood (Hanh, 1998). It is vital to engage with transformative justice: "the work of addressing harm at its root, outside the mechanisms of the state, so that we can grow into right relationship with each other" (brown, 2020, p. 5).

No ideal society can be pointed to as a model of healthy decolonial practices. It is a mistake to idealize societies of the past because we do not have enough information to know their harmful sides. Moreover, it is a mistake to assume that past societies did not have harmful practices, just as idealizing traditional cultures is dangerous. As long as there has been recorded history, there have been stories of one group attacking and taking advantage of another (or many others). We are responsible for educating ourselves using integrity in dealing with others and looking at traditions that European-based colonial powers have dismissed for the fertilizing wisdom that can not only nurture that responsibility to actually do no harm, but also perhaps even be helpful.

Even though working to change systems of oppression caused by centuries of colonization can seem to be the purview of extroverts comfortable in the public eye, it is important to recognize the diverse roles, responsibilities, talents, and potential impact we all have. We can only build a healthy decolonial world together using all our talents; this is how to become good ancestors to the coming generations.

All My Relations.

RESOURCES

Kimmerer, R. W. (2013). *Braiding sweetgrass: Indigenous wisdom, scientific knowledge, and the teachings of plants.* Milkweed Editions.

Kimmerer, R. W. (2014, January 14). *Questions for a resilient future* [Video]. YouTube. https://www.youtube.com/watch?v=y4nUobJEEWQ

Penniman, L. (2018). *Farming while Black: Soul Fire Farm's practical guide to liberation on the land.* Chelsea Green Publishing.

Sacred Land Film Project. (2001). *In the light of reverence* [Film]. https://sacredland.org/in-the-light-of-reverence/

Simon, T. (Host). (2021, November 2). Embracing pleasure, fractal responsibility, and the power of our imagination [Audio podcast episode]. In *Sounds true.* Sounds True. https://resources.soundstrue.com/podcast/embracing-pleasure-fractal-responsibility-and-the-power-of-our-imagination/

Smith, L. T. (2020, February 5). *Decolonizing methodologies, 20 years on* [Video]. YouTube. https://www.youtube.com/watch?v=YSX_4FnqXwQ

Webb, K. (2016, February 19). *Saving lives by saving trees* [Video]. YouTube. https://www.youtube.com/watch?v=tJkeZ_4wuYg

REFERENCES

Adames, H., & Chavez-Dueñas, N. (2021, August 12–14). A unified framework of decolonial psychology: Implications for psychotherapy. In L. Comas-Díaz (Chair), *Decolonial psychotherapy: Healing in context* [Symposium]. American Psychological Association Annual Convention [Virtual], United States.

Aiello, M., Bismar, D., Casanova, S., Casas, J. M., Chang, D., Chin, J. L., Comas-Díaz, L., Salvo Crane, L., Demir, Z., García, M. A., Hita, L., Leverett, P., Mendez, K., Morse, G. S., shodiya-zeumault, s., O'Leary Sloan, M., Weil, M. C., & Blume, A. W. (2021). Protecting and defending our people: Nakni tushka anowa (The Warrior's Path) final report. APA Division 45 Warrior's Path Presidential Task Force (2020). *Journal of Indigenous Research, 9*(2021), Article 8. https://digitalcommons.usu.edu/kicjir/vol9/iss2021

American Psychological Association. (2017). *Ethical principles of psychologists and code of conduct* (2002, amended effective June 1, 2010, and January 1, 2017). https://www.apa.org/ethics/code/

American Psychological Association. (2021). Apology to People of Color for APA's Role in promoting, perpetuating, and failing to challenge racism, racial discrimination, and human hierarchy in U.S. Resolution adopted by the APA Council of Representatives on October 29, 2021. https://www.apa.org/about/policy/racism-apology

APA Division 35, Section 6. (2021). Skywoman, Spider Woman, Corn Maiden, White Buffalo Calf Woman, Tonantzín: A description of Indigenous feminism. American Psychological Association. https://www.apadivisions.org/division-35/sections/section-six/indigenous-feminism

Association of Black Psychologists. (2021, November 24). The APA apology: Unacceptable, official statement. https://abpsi.org/abpsis-official-statement-to-the-apa-apology/

Belone, L., Tosa, J., Shendo, K., Toya, A., Straits, K., Tafoya, G., Rae, R., Noyes, E., Bird, D., & Wallerstein, N. (2016). Community-based participatory research for cocreating interventions with Native communities: A partnership between the University of New Mexico and the Pueblo of Jemez. In N. Zane, G. Bernal, & F. T. L. Leong (Eds.), *Evidence-based psychological practice with ethnic minorities: Culturally informed research and clinical strategies* (pp. 199–220). American Psychological Association. https://doi.org/10.1037/14940-010

brown, a. m. (2020). *We will not cancel us: And other dreams of transformational justice.* A. K. Press.

Campbell, L. (2021a, February 26–28). Status of Ethics Task Force slides. APA Council of Representatives Meeting. https://www.apa.org/ethics/task-force

Campbell, L. (2021b, February 26–28). Updates on ethics code revisions from ECTF chair. APA Council of Representatives Meeting. https://www.apa.org/ethics/task-force

Cheng, P., Cuellar, R., Johnson, D. A., Kalmbach, D. A., Joseph, C. L. M., Cuamatzi Castelan, A., Sagong, C., Casement, M. D., & Drake, C. L. (2020). Racial discrimination as a mediator of racial disparities in insomnia disorder. *Sleep Health, 6*(5), 543–549. https://doi.org/10.1016/j.sleh.2020.07.007

Comas-Díaz, L., & Torres Rivera, E. (Eds.). (2020). *Liberation psychology: Theory, method, practice, and social justice.* American Psychological Association. https://doi.org/10.1037/0000198-000

de Sahagún, B. (Writer and Editor), Dibble, C. E. (Translator), & Anderson, A. J. O. (Translator). (1969). *Florentine codex: General history of the things of New Spain: Book 6: Rhetoric and moral philosophy.* The University of Utah Press.

de Sahagún, B. (Writer and Editor), Dibble, C. E. (Translator), & Anderson, A. J. O. (Translator). (1981). *Florentine codex: General history of the things of New Spain: Book 10: The people.* The University of Utah Press.

de Sahagún, B. (Writer and Editor), Dibble, C. E. (Translator), & Anderson, A. J. O. (Translator). (1982). *Florentine codex: General history of the things of New Spain: Book 1: Introduction and indices.* The University of Utah Press.

Dunford, R. (2017). Toward a decolonial global ethics. *Journal of Global Ethics, 13*(3), 380–397. https://doi.org/10.1080/17449626.2017.1373140

Dussel, E. (2013). *Ethics of liberation: In the age of globalization and exclusion.* Duke University Press.

García, M. A., Loft, S. L., Palmer, M. A., & Morse, G. (2020). Competent discernment. In G. Morse & V. Lomay (Eds.), *Understanding Indigenous perspectives: Visions, dreams, and hallucinations* (pp. 51–64). Cognella.

García, M. A., Morse, G. S., Trimble, J. E., Casillas, D. M., Boyd, B., & King, J. (2017). A Partnership with the people: Skillful navigation of culture and ethics. In S. L. Stewart, R. Moodley, & A. Hyatt (Eds.), *Indigenous cultures and mental health counseling: Four directions for integration with counseling psychology.* Routledge/Taylor & Francis.

García, M. A., & Tehee, M. (Eds.). (2014). *Society of Indian Psychologists commentary on the American Psychological Association's (APA)* Ethical Principles of Psychologists and Code of Conduct. https://www.nativepsychs.org/product-page/sip-ethics-commentary

Garcia, S. E. (2020, June 18). Rest as reparations. *The New York Times.* https://www. nytimes.com/2020/06/18/style/self-care/healing-trauma-racism-wellness.html

González, J. (2019). Rostro y Corazón: o la busqueda del verdadero yo: Filosofía Náhuatl. *Difusión Norte,* February 20. https://clasico.difusionnorte.com/filosofia-Náhuatl/

Hanh, T. N. (1998). *The heart of the Buddha's teaching.* Parallax Press.

Hanh, T. N. (2004). *Taming the tiger within: Meditations on transforming difficult emotions.* Riverhead.

Harris, D. B. (2014). *10% Happier: How I tamed the voice in my head, reduced stress without losing my edge, and found self-help that actually works—A true story.* HarperCollins.

Henrich, J., Heine, S. J., & Norenzayan, A. (2010). The weirdest people in the world? *Behavioral and Brain Sciences, 33*(2–3), 61–83. https://doi.org/10.1017/S0140525X0999152X

Hersey, T. (2022). *Rest is resistance: A manifesto.* Litte, Brown Spark.

Johnson, C. R. (2014). *Taming the ox: Buddhist stories and reflections on politics, race, culture and spiritual practice.* Shambhala Publications.

Kabat-Zinn, J. (2013). *Full catastrophe living: Using the wisdom of your body and mind to face stress, pain and illness* (Rev. Ed.). Bantam Books.

King, R. (2018). *Mindful of race: Transforming racism from the inside out.* Sounds True.

Kornfield, J. (2008). *The Wise Heart: A guide to the universal teachings of Buddhist psychology.* Bantam Books.

Léon-Portilla, M. (Ed.). (1980a). *Native MesoAmerican spirituality.* Paulist Press.

Léon-Portilla, M. (1980b). *Toltecayotl: Aspectos de la cultura Náhuatl* [Toltecáyotl: Aspects of Nahuatl culture]. Fondo de Cultura Económica.

Maldonado-Torres, N. (2011). Enrique Dussel's liberation thought in decolonial turn. *Transmodernity: Journal of Peripheral Cultural Production of the Luso-Hispanic World, 1*(1), 1–30. https://escholarship.org/uc/item/5hg8t7cj

Manuel, Z. E. (2015). *The way of tenderness: Awakening through race, sexuality and gender.* Wisdom Publications.

Nagaraj, A. K. M., Nanjegowda, R. B., & Purushothama, S. M. (2015). The mystery of reincarnation. Retracted from the *Indian Journal of Psychiatry, 57*(4), 439. https://doi.org/10.4103/0019-5545.105519

National Institutes of Health (NIH). (2019). *2019 traditional medicine summit report: Maintaining and protecting culture through healing.* https://dpcpsi.nih.gov/sites/default/files/NIH-THRO-2019-Traditional-Medicine-Summit-Report.pdf

Owens, R. (2020). *Love and rage: The path of liberation through anger.* North Atlantic Books.

Pérez Ortega, R. (2021, October 28). Divided we sleep: Poor sleep disproportionately undermines the health of Communities of Color. Researchers want to figure out why—and find solutions. *Science.* https://www.science.org/content/article/poor-sleep-takes-heavy-toll-communities-color-can-scientists-help

Pope, K. S., Vasquez, M. J. T., Chavez-Dueñas, N. Y., & Adames, H. Y. (2021). *Ethics in psychotherapy and counseling: A practical guide* (6th ed.). John Wiley & Sons.

Quijano, A. (2007). Coloniality and modernity/rationality. *Cultural Studies, 21*(2–3), 168–178.

Smith, L. T. (2012). *Decolonizing methodologies: Research and Indigenous peoples* (2nd ed.). Zed Books.

Straits, K. J. E., Bird, D. M., Tsinajinnie, E., Espinoza, J., Goodkind, J., Spencer, O., Tafoya, N., Willging, C., & the Guiding Principles Workgroup. (2012). *Guiding principles for engaging in research with Native American communities,* Version 1. UNM Center for Rural and Community Behavioral Health & Albuquerque Area Southwest Tribal Epidemiology Center.

Torres Rivera, E. (2020). Concepts of liberation psychology. In L. Comas-Díaz & E. Torres Rivera (Eds.), *Liberation Psychology: Theory, method, practice, and social justice* (pp. 41–52). American Psychological Association. https://doi.org/10.1037/0000198-003

Tuck, E., & Yang, K. W. (2012). Decolonization is not a metaphor. *Decolonization: Indigeneity, Education & Society, 1*(1), 1–40.

Webb, K. (2021). *Guardians of the trees: A journey of hope through healing the planet.* Flatiron Books.

Williams, A. K., Owens, R., & Syedullah, J. (2016). *Radical dharma: Talking race, love and liberation.* North Atlantic Books.

Young, R. (Host), & Muhammad, J. (Producer). (2021, November 8). Black and Brown communities aren't getting enough sleep compared to White people, report reveals [Audio podcast episode]. In *Here & Now*. WBUR. https://www.wbur.org/hereandnow/2021/11/08/black-brown-communities-sleep

PART **IV** PSYCHOTHERAPIES

12 DECOLONIAL PSYCHOTHERAPY

Joining the Circle, Healing the Wound

LILLIAN COMAS-DÍAZ AND FREDERICK M. JACOBSEN

Decolonial psychotherapy is a healing approach that addresses colonialism's effects on individuals, groups, and communities' psychological, physical, and spiritual health. Within this perspective, Del Castillo et al. (2012) defined decolonial therapy as "a healing process, a space where wounded spirits and souls from disenfranchised racial groups recover from historical trauma, racism, and other collective social ills caused by long-term negative effects of colonization. It is a spiritual cleansing process, an acceptance of self" (p. 8).

Decolonial psychotherapy is grounded in the understanding that European American mainstream psychotherapy's individualist approach is limited in addressing the needs of those affected by colonization. Therefore, decolonial psychotherapists use a pluriversal healing approach to syncretize the epistemologies of the Global South with those of the Global North (Escobar, 2018; Mignolo & Walsh, 2018). Decolonial therapists embrace the Two Eye Seeing perspective to facilitate such syncretistic healing, learning to see from one eye with the perspective of Indigenous knowledge and from the other

https://doi.org/10.1037/0000376-013
Decolonial Psychology: Toward Anticolonial Theories, Research, Training, and Practice,
L. Comas-Díaz, H. Y. Adames, and N. Y. Chavez-Dueñas (Editors)

with Western knowledge (Bartlett et al., 2012; Jeffery et al., 2021). Indeed, Native American psychologist Eduardo Duran (2019) interpreted the Two Eye Seeing perspective as an alchemical amalgamation of Western knowledge and Indigenous wisdom. Thus decolonial therapy expands the Western concept of curing by including Indigenous knowledge, folk healing, cultural practices, and spiritual healing.

Interestingly, talk therapy originated in the Global South (Adames & Chavez-Dueñas, 2017), a fact seldom recognized in mainstream psychotherapy. Although European American therapy and Native American healing have certain similarities, some aspects of mainstream therapy—such as emphasis on individualism, lack of sociopolitical and historical contexts, and silence regarding systemic oppression—are colonizing (Comas-Díaz, 2007; Linklater, 2014; Trejo Mendez, 2021). In contrast, decolonial therapists go beyond mainstream therapeutic approaches to include psychosocial interventions, community approaches, cultural healing practices, liberatory arts such as artivism or art for social justice purposes (Sandoval & Latorre, 2008), and spiritual healing (Comas-Díaz, 2006; Fine 2018). In this fashion, they aim to dismantle the colonization, racism, and oppression embedded in the mainstream mental health system. Decolonial psychotherapy is unique because it addresses coloniality—the ongoing effects of a history of colonization (Quijano, 2000), colonial mentality, historical and intergenerational trauma, racial trauma, and intersecting forms of oppression. Unfortunately, coloniality results in Black, Indigenous, and People of Color (BIPOC)'s adherence to Eurocentric individualist values as healthy, normative, and desirable while identifying sociocentric values as unhealthy, abnormal, and undesirable. Similarly, colonial mentality is an internalized oppression that BIPOC adopt as negative and inferior views of themselves resulting from a history of colonization (David & Okazaki, 2006; see Chapter 1 in this volume). Indeed, coloniality hurts the body, mind, and spirit (Maldonado-Torres, 2007). Because coloniality fragments and dehumanizes BIPOC, Indigenous and cultural emancipatory practices are paths to decolonization. These practices include ancestral spirituality and folk healing methods such as *curanderismo* (traditional Latin American holistic healing), *espiritismo* (Latinx syncretistic spiritualism and healing), *Santería* (Latin American syncretism of Yoruba religion and healing into some Catholic elements), and Hawaiian healing (*Ho'oponopono*; Comas-Díaz, 2012), among others. Interestingly, *curanderismo* (Trejo Mendez, 2021) and *espiritismo* (Olmos & Paravisini-Gebert, 2003) have been proclaimed decolonial and liberatory methods. Indeed, decolonial psychotherapists incorporate Global South concepts into their work.

DECOLONIAL PSYCHOTHERAPY'S GUIDING CONCEPTS

To promote decolonization, therapists endorse the Global South's concepts of *ancestrality*, spirituality, *vincularidad*, and *desenvolvimiento*. Ancestrality refers to the process of connecting with our ancestral memory, knowledge, wisdom, and healing. Because colonization and oppression disrupt our bond with ancestrality, connecting with ancestors helps us remember and preserve our ancestral wisdom. Moreover, relating to ancestors helps decolonize our minds (Esa, 2021) because it promotes empowerment and liberation (Norat, 2005). Thus, when we bond with ancestral guidance, intuition, and corporeal wisdom, we experience a sense of being grounded, supported, and self-confident (Trejo Mendez, 2020). To illustrate, research highlights how thinking about our ancestors—known as the ancestor effect—enhances our intellectual performance (Fischer et al., 2011). As ancestrality increases our connection with our progenitors, it also deepens our connection with our authentic selves. In other words, when we connect with our ancestors, we unearth our historical memory, become empowered, nurture self-determination (Neeganagwedgin, 2020), and work toward liberation (Martín-Baró, 1994).

Spirituality is another decolonial psychotherapy guiding concept. Most Indigenous and African groups consider spirituality the first component of every physical and emotional healing (Mehl-Medrona, 2003; Monteiro & Wall, 2011), illustrating the intimate relationship between healing and spirituality (Portman & Garrett, 2006). Interestingly, Carl Jung (1989) identified spirituality as a requirement for human transformation. Likewise, Ignacio Martín-Baró (1994), a priest and psychologist, recommended that psychologists assist clients in identifying with a higher power. Similarly, Eduardo Duran (2019), a Native American psychologist, advised therapists to shift from psychologizing to spiritualizing. As a pathway to meaning-making, spirituality alleviates trauma because it helps sufferers connect with positive emotions such as compassion, gratitude, love, and hope. For instance, a qualitative study found hope to be an emerging clinical model for trauma victims (Wood, 2015). Based on this research, hope is a healing factor that helps connect with the sacred (Martín-Baró, 1994). Following this notion, a BIPOC and Global South radical hope orientation can instill positive changes at the individual and societal levels (Mosley et al., 2019). Besides promoting healing, spirituality can encourage liberation and a commitment to social justice (Rodriguez, 1999). Unlike religion, spirituality denotes an intimate connection with the sacred, wherein all living entities are considered sacred (Marks, 2006). For instance, as Indigenous healer Ratu Civo explained, "we feel love for others because they are part of the sacred web of the universe; it's an unconditional love that does not demand that we agree with that person's lifestyle or even like that person" (Katz, 2017, p. 259). This message also relates to the notion of *vincularidad*.

As a decolonial psychotherapy concept, *vincularidad* is a Latin American construct that transcends the meaning of interconnectedness. Rooted in Indigenous cosmovision, *vincularidad* relates to the indivisible nature of all beings, emphasizing the close bond we share with others, nature, and the spirit world (Mignolo & Walsh, 2018). In this fashion, *vincularidad* connotes an awareness of the integral relationship between all organisms, the environment, and the cosmos (Mignolo & Walsh, 2018). Known as kin-centric ecology, this Indigenous cosmovision holds that existence is viable only when people view life surrounding them as kin (Salmon, 2000). Likewise, *vincularidad* illustrates the relational interdependence of all beings in their search for balance and harmony in life (Mignolo & Walsh, 2018), helping restore equilibrium between body, mind, emotions, spirit, and environment. Anchored in a pluriversal practice, *vincularidad* exemplifies the Native American concept of *All Our Relations*. Even more saliently, *vincularidad* fosters mutual healing and development.

Desenvolvimiento, another decolonial therapeutic concept, is a Spanish-Portuguese concept meaning spiritual development within healing and liberation. Nurturing a lifelong spiritual developmental process, *desenvolvimiento* denotes a psychospiritual transformation rooted in enlightenment, evolution, and transcendence. Decolonial therapists nurture clients' bonding with ancestral spirituality (Diaz, 2022) and practice *desenvolvimiento* to connect with the inner healer to assist in this process. As an Indigenous psychiatrist and psychologist, Lewis Mehl-Madrona (2003) asserted that "the foundation for healing among Indigenous cultures is recognizing that you are the healer" (p. 63). So, within an Indigenous healing paradigm, *desenvolvimiento* enables the deepening of spirituality and, therefore, the development of spiritual faculties, such as *la facultad.* According to Anzaldua (1987), *la facultad* is a spiritual intuition and particular sensitivity that oppressed individuals develop to perceive and understand systems, especially power dynamics. Along these lines, while discussing colonial wounds and healing, decoloniality scholar Walter Mignolo (2019) indicated that a person who has *la facultad* is exquisitely alive. Consistent with this notion, *desenvolvimiento* fosters *buen vivir*— the Aymara concept of living a life in full and with a psychospiritual purpose (Acosta, 2016). In this way, *desenvolvimiento* nurtures critical consciousness, encourages empowerment, and promotes what Anazaldua (2002) called spiritual activism—activism with a spiritual vision.

The described decolonial therapy concepts interconnect cyclically. In other words, decolonial healing can be initiated through any of these principles. Because Indigenous Medicine Wheel approaches are typically described as decolonization methods (Linklater, 2014), we conceive decolonial healing principles as a Medicine Wheel. To illustrate, we use Garrett and Garrett's (1994) model. Within this representation, clients and sufferers engage in a healing path at any of the four directions of the Medicine Wheel. The East represents family, community, and nation; the South denotes our abilities and interests; the West signifies our sources of strength and limitations; and the North represents what we offer and receive. When we apply this framework to decolonial psychotherapy concepts, ancestrality may represent East (ancestors or family); spirituality may be associated with West (strengths and limitations); *vincularidad* may correspond with South (what you do well, what you have); and *desenvolvimiento* may be associated with the North (what we offer and receive; see Figure 12.1).

FIGURE 12.1. Decolonial Psychotherapy Medicine Wheel

NORTH: Desenvolvimiento

Psychospiritual development
Connection with the inner healer
Psychospiritual faculties
Buen vivir

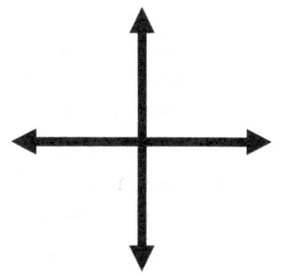

WEST: Spirituality

Positive emotions
Spiritual healing
Sacredness
Spiritual activism

EAST: Ancestrality

Ancestor effect
Ancestral memory
Ancestral healing
Ancestral wisdom

SOUTH: Vincularidad

Relatedness
Interdependence
All Our Relations
Kincentric Ecology

In an example of pluriversal healing, decolonial therapists address historical trauma, racial trauma, and systemic oppression, all aimed at healing the Wound. We identify the Wound as the cumulative intersecting traumas affecting BIPOC. The following section introduces the Wound as a compendium of intergenerational oppression and intergenerational resistance.

NAMING THE WOUND

A history of colonization exposes people to sociopolitical trauma (Ward, 2013). Most BIPOC experience systemic oppression from birth to death (Gee & Verissimo, 2016). Systemic oppression includes the cumulative effects of historical trauma, racial trauma, race-related stress, gendered racism, racial microaggressions, heterosexism, homophobia, transphobia, xenophobia, and other forms of oppression trauma. Racial trauma refers to the events of danger, real or perceived experiences of racial discrimination, threats of injury, damage, and humiliating, shaming events (Carter, 2007; Comas-Díaz et al., 2019). Racial trauma also entails vicarious racial trauma (Comas-Díaz et al., 2019). A related syndrome, ethnoracial trauma, refers to the individual and collective emotional distress and fear resulting from experiencing and or witnessing discrimination, intimidation, threats of harm, violence, and intimidation directed at ethnoracial groups (Chavez-Dueñas et al., 2019). Even more salient, ethnoracial trauma highlights the role of intersectionality, such as the effects of ethnocentrism, xenophobia, racism, nativism, sexism, and heterosexism, among other oppressions in the development of ethnoracial trauma (Chavez-Dueñas et al., 2019).

BIPOC may also experience a legacy of oppression before birth. A product of a history of colonization and oppression, colonization trauma is transmitted intergenerationally. It is a unique phenomenon because, as an intergeneration syndrome, it is exacerbated by contemporary oppression. Indeed, trauma resulting from a history of colonization gives birth to the Wound. As indicated, the Wound is a complex, continuous, collective, cumulative, and compounding interaction of the effects of colonization, coloniality, oppression, and racism. The colonizers used racism to designate Indigenous, Blacks, and other People of Color as nonhuman to justify their abuse and exploitation of the colonized and the environment (Quiñones-Rosado, 2020). Racism remains well and alive today.

Born of intergenerational subjugation and nurtured by contemporary oppression, colonial trauma relates to the phenomenon whereby the descendants of a person and or a group who experienced horrific events manifest adverse psychological, behavioral, physiological, and spiritual reactions to events such as their ancestors' traumatic experiences (Reed, 2021b). For example, the prolonged collective historical trauma inflicted on Native Americans affects their wellness and intensifies their lifespan, leading to increased stress syndromes (Sotero, 2006). The Wound offers a framework to understand what Mitchell et al. (2019) articulated as the relationship between health disparities and the traumagenic effects of colonization. Specifically, the disparities in health and well-being, in addition to socioeconomic and political disparities among First Peoples (Hawaiians, Native Americans, and Maori), are consequences of soul wounds (Peters, 2001). Definitively, colonial trauma generates soul wounds—the intergenerational transmission of oppression (Duran, 2019). Furthermore, soul wounds extend to individuals and groups with historical oppression, such as enslavement. Resmaa Menakem (2017) defined soul wounds among African Americans as the intergenerational transmission of trauma: "Through families in which one member abuses or mistreats another member. Through abusive systems, and structures and/or cultural norms. Through our genes. Recent work in human genetics suggests that trauma is passed on in our DNA" (p. 10).

Colonial or historical trauma and soul wounds are manifested via blood memory. Even though the term generally refers to a genetic connection to ancestors, Thomas Reed (2021b) described blood memory as the intergenerational transmission of traumatic memories, especially among Native Americans and other groups with a history of colonization, leading to colonial trauma. A documentary, *Blood Memory: A Story of Removal and Return* (see the Resources at the end of this chapter), presents a Native American woman's experience of blood memory. Colonial trauma is a collection of the historical effects of colonization, such as war, enslavement, genocide, displacement, abuse, ethnic cleansing, broken treaties, and oppression, among many other historical traumatic events. Colonial trauma is not limited to people with a history of colonization. For instance, Kenneth Clark (1989), the first Black president of the American Psychological Association (APA), identified the condition of African Americans in the United States as one of colonization. In this vein, the concept of colonization can be extended to oppressed people. Therefore, the intergenerational effects of colonial, ancestral, and historical trauma include soul wounds, suppressed and distorted memories, blood memory, and the embodiment of trauma. Additionally, colonial trauma can metamorphose into intergenerational syndromes such as colonial mentality, postcolonial stress disorder (PCSD), and posttraumatic slave syndrome (PTSS). PCSD refers to the effects of coloniality and the subsequent internalization of mainstream culture as superior (Comas-Díaz, 2000). In addition to exhibiting colonial mentality, individuals suffering from PCSD identify with the oppressor and, thus, oppress marginalized individuals and groups. Coined by African American psychiatrist Joy DeGruy (2005), the construct of PTSS refers to an intergenerational trauma that originated in the history of slavery among African Americans. However, the concept of PTSS has been criticized for its negative attributions, such as associating African American poverty with criminality (Kendi, 2016).

In summary, we identify the Wound as the cumulative colonial, historical, and contemporary racial oppression that BIPOC experience. Because trauma can be transmitted via DNA (Menakem, 2017), the Wound can be transmitted intergenerationally. Epigenetics studies can help elucidate the concepts of transgenerational trauma, soul wounds, and blood memory, which we discuss in the next section.

EPIGENETICS

In what many consider to be one of the most groundbreaking developments of the last half century, ongoing work in the burgeoning field of epigenetics is fundamentally changing the scientific and lay public's understanding of biology and its relationship with our environment. The science of epigenetics is strictly defined as the study of relatively stable phenotypic changes that do not involve alterations in DNA (genotypic) sequences but instead can affect gene activity and expression. Recently, however, particularly in the social sciences and the popular press, the epigenetics concept (and theoretical reach) is often extended to describe any potentially heritable phenotypic change.

Thousands of articles have been published explicating long-term heritable epigenetic effects on aspects of human health and disease. One of this chapter's authors (Frederick Jacobsen) recently conducted numerous PubMed literature searches exploring the overlap of epigenetics with various subject areas. This returned nearly 23,000 results for epigenetics and human health: 1,864 articles were found under "epigenetics and cultural differences," 958 under "epigenetics and human illness," but substantially fewer to have investigated interactions directly relating to themes often considered under the umbrella of coloniality, for example, "epigenetics and poverty" (86 references) or "epigenetics and racism" (35 references).

Developmental psychology has described the epigenetic interplay between heredity and the environment (Erikson, 1968; Gottlieb, 1991). The physical and emotional traumas suffered over recorded human history as a result of uncontrolled exposure to massive sociocultural events (wars, genocides, famines, and so on) are considered likely to cause epigenetic modifications that could function as a biological mechanism for transgenerational trauma (Yehuda & Lehrner, 2018). The recent development of the field of social epigenetics expands sociocultural consideration to both transgenerational and intergenerational epigenetic marks (small chemical tags that instruct genes to switch on or off) to better understand racial and social inequities (Mulligan,

2021). Bierer et al. (2020) reported that transgenerational epigenetic transmission of traumatic stress can affect stress-regulation pathways, and numerous social epigenetics studies are exploring direct correlations of epigenetic variations occurring secondary to adverse social experiences or inequities and resulting in population health inequalities (Martin et al., 2022).

Some difficulties in drawing broad, potentially social policy-altering conclusions from epigenetic studies stem from the sometimes complex interpretations of the trauma data itself. Although a sizable number of behaviorally focused studies have found results that suggest adverse effects of social inequalities, most have been inadequately structured or insufficiently powered to directly address the downstream epigenetic effects of poverty or racism per se, not to mention potentially multifactorial downstream effects of colonization. Moreover, although many social epigenetic studies have found that offspring of extremely traumatized or stressed parents are at higher risk for mental and physical illnesses, studies have also found that genetically identical subjects raised in similar environments can show remarkably different outcomes after social stress, from disease and illness vulnerability to resilience (Nestler, 2016).

Given that parents and offspring often share a living environment and similar constant long-term environmental stressors (such as poverty or racism), it may be difficult to distinguish between parental biology versus parental behavior as mediators of offspring effects (Bowers & Yehuda, 2016). Moreover, most research on transgenerational trauma has focused on maternal transmission, where differences have been noted between stress exposures occurring before conception, at the time of conception, during pregnancy, or in the early postnatal period, whereas the contribution by the paternal transmission of stress or posttraumatic stress disorder (PTSD) has been substantially less researched but may add (several) interacting levels of complication (Bowers & Yehuda, 2016).

Evolution tends to favor fitness adaptations to the environment, even—or perhaps especially—in the face of traumatic occurrences. Thus, some societally based trauma-induced epigenetic alterations will likely result in beneficial compensatory (and protective) factors such as resilience and posttraumatic growth (Youssef, 2022). While psychological traumas may uniquely induce in some individuals both short and long-term biological changes and PTSD or other anxiety or mood disorders, other individuals may show no disease or disability, or, as described in this and other chapters, may experience alternate culturally based fitness reactions such as forms of intergenerational resilience and resistance. However, given the accumulating evidence that colonizing factors such as racism or racial discrimination and socioeconomic disparities can have adverse effects on both general health (Okeke et al., 2022) and on specific aspects of brain health (Fani et al., 2022) from a public health perspective such as colonizing factors are now increasingly understood to carry adverse downstream (generational) epigenetic effects.

INTERGENERATIONAL RESILIENCE AND RESISTANCE

Fortunately, despite their colonial trauma, many BIPOC inherit cultural resilience and, more important, resistance. Even though cultural resilience refers to a composite of strengths, values, and practices that promote coping mechanisms and adaptive reactions to traumatic oppression (Elsass, 1992), it is important to decolonize the concept of resilience among BIPOC. A concrete example is that the mainstream concept of resilience may support addressing oppression without necessarily engaging in systemic transformation. In contrast, resistance entails opposition to oppression aimed at systemic change. In other words, many oppressed groups have historically resisted oppression, reviving and using methods their ancestors used to survive and oppose oppression (Chavez-Dueñas et al., 2019; Martín-Baró, 1994). Because intergenerational trauma is embodied (Rosenthal, 2022), so is intergenerational resistance. Notably, intergenerational resistance includes survivance, cultural wealth, activism, enhanced wisdom, and spiritual development. *Survivance* refers to the effect of healing stories that Native Americans share in honoring cultural strengths and counteracting a sense of victimhood (Hartman et al., 2019; Vizenor, 2008). Cultural wealth relates to a collection of knowledge, skills, behaviors, and abilities that communities of color use to resist racism and other forms of oppression (Yosso, 2006).

BIPOC also engage in social justice activism against colonial, ethnic, and racial trauma. As a resistance strategy, many People of Color enhance their wisdom by developing open-mindedness, humility, and empathy (Dorfman et al., 2021). Equally important, numerous BIPOC develop and intensify their connection with spirituality. Through this process, various BIPOC engage in spiritual activism—social justice actions with a spiritual vision that requires self-reflection, compassion, and a thirst for social change (Anzaldua, 2002). Significantly, BIPOC frequently evidence intergenerational flowering. We define flowering as a process much like the lotus flower's blooming in a precarious environment, such as "The Lotus flower blooms most beautifully from the deepest and thickest mud" (Leading Lotus, 2018, para. 7). In our experience, flowering nurtures spiritual and psychic abilities such as *la facultad*, prophecy, energy healing, and empathic connectedness.

In sum, many BIPOC bond with ancestral resistance, such as survivance, cultural wealth, enhanced wisdom, spiritual development, and *flowering*. Of particular importance, decolonial therapists aim to address clients' intergenerational trauma while supporting sufferers' intergenerational resistance. Table 12.1 shows colonial trauma's origins, intergenerational wounds, and resistance.

TABLE 12.1. Colonial Trauma: Origins, Wounds, Syndromes, and Resistance

Origins	Intergenerational wounds	Intergenerational resistance
Colonization	Soul wounds	Survivance
War	Historical trauma	Cultural wealth
Genocide	Blood memory	Antiracism and antioppression
Enslavement	Suppressed and distorted memories	Social justice activism
Broken treaties		Enhanced wisdom
Ethnic cleansing	Somatic memory (embodiment of trauma)	Spiritual development
Displacement		Flowering
Forced assimilation	Increased stress symptoms	
	Colonial mentality	
	Postcolonization stress disorder	
	Posttraumatic slave syndrome	
	Racial trauma	
	Ethnoracial trauma	

Despite BIPOC's intergenerational resistance, the Wound continues to affect them negatively. Consequently, decolonial psychotherapists address the Wound from a Two Eye perspective. The following section uses the Two Eye perspective to compare decolonial psychotherapy to a healing circle.

JOINING THE CIRCLE

Our ancestors knew that healing comes in cycles and circles. One generation carries the pain so that the next can live and heal. One cannot live without the other, each is each other's hope, meaning, and strength. (Benton, 2016, as cited in Clark, 2021, p. 91)

Decolonial psychotherapists strive to decolonize mental health care by integrating cultural and communal approaches into pluriversal healing practices. To achieve this goal, they embrace the Indigenous meaning of the circle. A sacred element, the circle symbolizes healing the mind, body, spirit, and environment. The circle process incorporates ceremony and storytelling, inviting people to sit in a circle where one by one share their stories without being interrupted. Participants commit to creating a space infused with safety, respect, sacredness, acceptance, and transformation. Such a sharing process is like *testimonio*, a liberation psychology healing where the sufferers share their stories of trauma and sociopolitical oppression (Aron, 1992). As a result, participants feel accompanied. Another liberation psychology concept, *acompañamiento* (accompaniment), refers to standing alongside oppressed clients who need witnessing, advocacy, and a safe space to summon *conocimiento* (ancestral knowledge; Watkins, 2015) and engage in social justice action. Thus healing is conceptualized as reconstituting the self, relationally and collectively (Fernandez, 2022). Equally significant, circle practices are infused with decoloniality because they have a spiritual core that serves as a social justice vehicle (Reed, 2021a).

Healing circles are popular among the public (Baldwin, 1998) and thus are growing among BIPOC individuals. To illustrate, healing circles for African American women focus on intersectional forms of oppression (Richardson, 2018) and on womanism—a Black woman feminism (Bryant-Davis & Comas-Díaz, 2016). Moreover, many healing circles specialize in the recovery of trauma (Healing Justice, 2018); several healing circles are race focused (Initiatives for Change, 2019). Healing circles are now increasingly recognized as a communal approach to healing trauma and a conduit for restorative justice.

Research findings attest to the efficacy of healing circles. To illustrate, a primary care medical team incorporated a talking circle as a treatment modality and studied the effects of the intervention. The research findings indicated significant statistical improvement in reported symptoms and quality of life among Native American patients (Mehl-Madrona & Mainguy, 2014). Healing circles are also attracting interest among health practitioners. For instance, Meg Jordan (2014) discussed an application of a healing circle within an integrative medicine model. The circle included a client and several health practitioners of diverse specialties. Following circle procedures, the practitioners engaged in active listening and communicated empathetically and nonjudgmentally. Significant findings of this 8-year ethnographic study resulted in a client-centered focus, participatory process, minimization of clinician's control, egalitarian relationships, and enhanced multidisciplinary knowledge (Jordan, 2014).

Because many mainstream therapies tend to be ahistorical, individualistic, and decontextualized, decolonial therapists join a symbolic (or real) circle to practice holistic social justice healing. In addition to mainstream psychotherapeutic practices, decolonial therapists use psychospiritual approaches such as guided image, visualization, meditation, and connection with inner guidance, among other modalities. As healing is facilitated when we bond with ancestral and spiritual guidance (Trejo Mendez, 2020), decolonial therapists mentally invite clients' ancestors and invoke clients' spiritual guides into the therapy (Comas-Díaz, 2022). Based on *vincularidad*, ancestors and spiritual guides of both client and therapist can be spiritually invited to join the healing circle. Such invitations are accomplished by setting an intention (Baldwin, 1998). Even individual therapy can function as a healing circle (Duran, 2019) when client and therapist include *All Our Relations*. As decolonial therapists join the circle, they engage in healing informed by racial trauma.

HEALING THE WOUND: A RACIAL TRAUMA-INFORMED THERAPY

We consider racial trauma to be an archetypical aspect of the Wound. This assertion is based on the colonial and postcolonial practice of equating dark skin color with inferiority, thus differentiating the White colonizer from the Red, Black, Brown, and Yellow colonized (Grosfoguel & Georas, 2010; Quijano, 2000). Moreover, racism is alive today, and as such, it has been declared a mental health crisis (Mendez et al., 2021). Consequently, healing racial trauma requires acknowledging the effects of a history of colonization and oppression and the subsequent effects of colonial mentality and coloniality that perpetuate the colonial-racial trauma. As a result, we need a decolonial therapy informed by racial trauma to heal the Wound. Unfortunately, aspects of mainstream trauma therapy are colonizing because the mainstream definitions of trauma, traumatic stress, and trauma therapy are rooted in Western Eurocentric models (Hernandez-Wolfe, 2011). This is an example of coloniality of knowledge—also known as epistemic violence—the belief that Eurocentric knowledge is superior to Indigenous or ancestral wisdom (Quijano, 2000). Moreover, mainstream therapy is often silent about sociopolitical causes, thus, ignoring the role of broader systemic violence (Linklater, 2014). The concept of racial trauma is often subsumed under PTSD because many effects of racial trauma, such as anxiety, depression, suicidal ideation, poor concentration, self-medication, hypervigilance to threat, substance abuse, anger, despair, and physiological reactions are also PTSD symptoms (Comas-Díaz, 2007; Comas-Díaz et al., 2019). However, despite these similarities, racial trauma significantly differs from PTSD. To illustrate, although posttraumatic often implies that the traumatic event is a single occurrence, due to systemic racism, BIPOC often suffer from longitudinal continuing racial wounding inflicted by racial trauma, racial violence, racial microaggressions, vicarious racism, and reexposure to race-based stress (Comas-Díaz et al., 2019). Therefore, when the mainstream mental health system excludes racial trauma and race-related stress as separate diagnostic entities from PTSD, it colonizes, oppresses, and retraumatizes BIPOC. Additionally, mainstream trauma therapy lacks the crucial sociopolitical and cultural relevance for most BIPOC (Bryant-Davis & Ocampo, 2006; Comas-Díaz, 2016; Comas-Díaz et al., 2019). Consequently, most mainstream therapists rarely address colonial and historical trauma and tend to misdiagnose racial trauma as PTSD.

To address colonial trauma, racial trauma, race-related stress, and sociopolitical oppression, in addition to helping clients restore their dignity, decolonial practitioners infuse antiracism and antioppression into therapy. Decolonial healing is a racial trauma-informed therapy, the goals of which are to empower, decolonize, heal, and liberate. Linklater (2014) stated that Indigenous approaches to healing trauma are culture specific. To illustrate, when U.S. Army psychiatrists during the Korean War observed that Puerto Rican soldiers engaged in a fighting fit (*mal de pelea*), they coined the term Puerto Rican syndrome to diagnose the soldiers' behavior, which included hyperkinesis, aggressiveness to self and others, hyperventilation, partial loss of consciousness, psychotic behaviors, forgetfulness, among other symptoms (Fernandez-Marina, 1961; Mehlman, 1961). The American Psychiatric Association (2000) initially classified the Puerto Rican syndrome as a culture-bound syndrome; in contrast, Latin American psychologist Patricia Gherovici (2003), who worked with continental Puerto Rican clients, identified such psychiatric classification as racism. Alternatively, she suggested using *espiritismo*, a cultural folk healing, to assist those suffering from Puerto Rican Syndrome (Gherovici, 2003). Noteworthy, given that Puerto Rico remains the oldest colony in the Americas (Trias-Monje, 1999), Gherovici's perspective is consistent with earlier proponents of Puerto Rican independence who practiced *espiritismo* as a decolonial method (Olmos & Paravisini-Gerbert, 2003).

Fortunately, several therapists of color have developed racial trauma–informed approaches consistent with decolonial therapy. For example, Bryant-Davis and Ocampo (2006) advanced a race-informed trauma therapy that entails creating a safe environment for clients to share traumatic racial incidents, examine internalized racism, enhance self-care, and demand equality. Likewise, Comas-Díaz (2007, 2016) developed an ethnopolitical healing approach to racial trauma using (a) *testimonio* for assessment, (b) holistic ethnic healing and self-healing for desensitization, (c) eye movement desensitization reprogramming for reprocessing, (d) critical consciousness to challenge coloniality and multiple forms of oppression, (e) solidarity with other oppressed individuals, and (f) advocacy for social justice and equity. Moreover, it is essential for decolonial therapists to include an antiracism component to inoculate and resist racial trauma (Mosley et al., 2020). Table 12.2 illustrates such decolonial therapy's components.

TABLE 12.2. Decolonial Therapy: A Racial Trauma-Informed Healing

Assessment	Decoloniality	Self-healing	Social justice action
Safety and trust	Ancestral spirituality	*Testimonio*	*Acompañamiento*
Desensitization	Mind-body approaches	Ethnic healing	Artivism
Reprocessing	*Concientización*	Agency	Collective self-care
Advocacy	Antioppression	Racial equity	Global solidarity

Decolonial therapists recognize the centrality of the decolonial therapeutic relationship as a crucial variable in healing. In the following section, we discuss the decolonial therapeutic relationship and the relevance of mutuality, therapist self-care, and the therapist's decolonization.

DECOLONIAL THERAPEUTIC RELATIONSHIP

We disclose our decolonial positionalities as we introduce the parameters of a decolonial therapeutic relationship to our clients. Following the principles of ancestrality and *vincularidad*, this practice is a central aspect of decolonial psychotherapy in that it addresses and demystifies the power differential inherent in mainstream therapeutic relationships.

Within this context, I, Lillian Comas-Díaz, am a mixed-race, cisgender, heterosexual, Puerto Rican woman with Taíno, African, and Iberian ancestry. Growing up in the oldest colonized nation in the Americas inspired my thirst for decolonization. I, Frederick Jacobsen, am a White, cisgender, American man with Danish, German, Cherokee, and British ancestry who experienced transformative transculturation while living in Brazil.

Following Kluckhorn and Murray, the decolonial therapeutic relationship is in certain respects like all therapeutic alliances, like some other therapeutic relationships, and like no other therapeutic relationship. Like mainstream therapists, decolonial therapists are guided by the American Psychological Association's Ethics Code. Decolonial therapists additionally observe the Society of Indian Psychologists' comments on the APA Ethics Code (Garcia & Tehee, 2014; see Chapter 11 in this volume). Like other therapists who endorse liberation, humanist, and social justice approaches, decolonial therapists accompany their clients in a mutually agreed (shared) therapeutic endeavor, support reclaiming historical memory, foster critical consciousness, nurture spirituality, cultivate creativity, and foment social justice action.

Despite commonalities with other therapists, decolonial therapists embrace *vincularity* by relating to sufferers as kin to facilitate healing. To achieve this objective, they adopt a healer identity within a liberation spirituality. Anzaldua's (2002) concept of spiritual activism—activism with a spiritual vision that requires self-reflection, compassion, and a thirst for social change—is a guiding format for spiritual liberation activism. Decolonial therapists may also incorporate Indigenous and Global South cultural healing practices into therapy to enhance the therapeutic relationship. Striving to foster a healing space where oppressed, traumatized, and marginalized clients feel safe and trust the therapeutic process. Following the concept of ethics and positionality in qualitative research with marginalized individuals (Shaw et al., 2020), decolonial therapists recognize and honor clients' needs to feel respected and heard, aspiring to act as a "container" that holds a safe place while witnessing *testimonios* and promoting liberation (Comas-Díaz, 2020). To help achieve these goals, decolonial therapists engage in radical listening (Winchell et al., 2016), as illustrated by the description of traditional counseling by Mary Lee, a Cree Elder, as "listening with respect and without judgment" (cited in Katz, 2017, pp. 280–281). Such radical listening means that therapists listen to clients' verbal, nonverbal, and energetic-intuitive communication (Comas-Díaz, 2022). In a healing journey, decolonial therapists encourage clients' creativity—including artivism—as decolonial, social, and cultural-political activism (Barson, 2019).

When decolonial therapists endorse a healer identity, they recognize the central role of mutuality within healing relationships. In other words, decolonial therapists engage in participatory healing relationships. As an example, African American psychologist Maureen Walker (2004) advised therapists to be cotravelers in the healing journey and to *"show up* with an authentic presence and open themselves to the possibility of healing and change" (p. 36). Following this orientation, decolonial therapists aim to develop a deep communion with their clients while addressing colonial trauma, soul wounds, and racial trauma, allowing a mirroring process that fosters permeability (Comas-Díaz, 2016) and honors *vincularidad*. Consequently, exhibiting radical empathy, decolonial therapists use their *facultad,* among other spiritual-psychic abilities, to intuitively feel their client's pain, creating a shared field of sensation (Koss-Chioino, 2007). Such radical empathy helps therapists "embody" the client's distress to help sufferers connect with their inner healer (Comas-Díaz, 2022).

Because healing is mutual, decolonial therapists commit to lifelong decolonization and *desenvolvimiento*. As noted, *desenvolvimiento* goes beyond the mainstream development concept to include flourishing within a communal or collectivist context. As decolonial therapists challenge coloniality and multiple intersecting forms of oppression, they radically transform themselves to connect with their inner healer. In this way, they aim to listen with an open heart, feel with an embodied spirit, connect with ancestral wisdom, bond with ancestral spirituality, and become a healing vessel. To become a healing vessel, psychiatrist Judith Orloff (1996) advised connecting with positive emotions by invoking the Peace Prayer (aka Saint Francis Prayer): "make me a channel of thy peace, that where there is hatred, I may bring love; that where there is error, I may bring truth; that where there is despair, I may bring hope" (Prayer of Saint Francis, n.d., paragraph 1). Ultimately, decolonial therapists aim to integrate their therapeutic role into their public persona, extending the healing principle to every aspect of their lives. Indeed, decolonial therapists aim to embody a healer-warrior-liberator identity. Articulated by the American Psychological Association Society for the Psychological Study of Culture, Ethnicity, and Race (Division 45) Task Force on The Warrior's Path (Protecting and Defending our People; Aiello et al., 2021), a warrior identity means that we defend the peace, liberty, health, and well-being of all marginalized people. In this way, decolonial therapists accompany their clients in a healing, emancipatory, and liberation journey. However, decolonial practitioners are frequently subject to compassion fatigue—a by-product of working with racially traumatized clients. Consequently, when BIPOC therapists engage in decolonial self-care, they aspire to heal their clients' Wound and their own. Hence, unlike the mainstream concept of self-care, decolonial self-care is collective, communal (see Chapter 16 in this volume), and spiritual.

As decolonial therapists acknowledge the existence of mutuality in healing, they understand that taking care of themselves enhances their ability to care for their clients, often embracing ancestral and spiritual guidance to join a healing circle. Indeed, connecting with ancestors heals. To illustrate, during a constellation family therapy (Cohen, 2006) session, I (Lillian) learned about my ancestral family intergenerational trauma, how to address it, and thus became a trauma therapist (Comas-Díaz, 2022). Constellation therapy is grounded in the belief that we inherit our ancestors' trauma because of epigenetics. According to this approach, to heal, we need to connect with our ancestral family energy through what is called *morphic resonance* within a psychodrama format (Cohen, 2006). Advanced by biologist Rupert Sheldrake, the concept of morphic resonance refers to a kind of collective memory inherited in nature through the interconnection between organisms (Sheldrake, n.d.). Along these lines, constructing an ancestral genogram helps identify intergenerational traumas (Wolynn, 2016). Moreover, Indigenous wisdom teaches that when we heal our ancestral trauma, we heal seven generations before us as well as seven generations after us (Comas, 2018).

A remarkable quality of decolonial therapists is that they assist clients in connecting with the inner healer, warrior, or liberator. Thus decolonial therapists promote psychospiritual inner approaches, such as contemplation, meditation, guided imagery, breathwork, hypnosis, and dream work, among other self-generative practices. Such psychospiritual function requires removing what has been appropriated from BIPOC's ancestral healing and wisdom while conscientiously acknowledging the sources (see Chapter 16 in this volume). Additional examples include Latinx *baños* and *limpias* (spiritual cleansings), *yerbas* (healing plants; Esa, 2021), *dichos* (proverbs), *consejos* (advice), as well as Native American sweat lodges, drumming, smudging, journeying, following the red path (harmony with nature; see Rybak & Decker-Fitts, 2009). Similarly, rooted in *desenvolvimiento*, decolonial therapists nurture clients' psychospiritual abilities such as *la facultad*. Based in *vincularidad*, decolonial therapy becomes a mirror reflecting the Latinx Indigenous belief: *You Are My Other Me* (Comas-Díaz, 2020).

If you experience compassion fatigue when working with BIPOC individuals, we recommend consulting a decolonial-liberation therapist. Likewise, you can also compose your *testimonio*, create your ancestral genogram, engage in artivism, and practice spiritual activism. Nonetheless, if you want to become a decolonial therapist, we urge you to embark on your own decolonization.

To achieve this goal, we suggest you engage in several decolonial stages, namely, reclaim, battle, transform, and evolve. (For a similar process, see Angelique Nixon's *Elements of Decolonial Healing Justice*.) When you journey a decolonial path, you first reclaim your ancestrality, recover your historical memory, and aim to connect with ancestral guidance, spirituality, and wisdom. Then you battle by becoming a decolonial warrior, fighting oppression, and following the Warrior's Path (Aiello et al., 2021), in other words, committing to defend and protect the oppressed. Paradoxically, as a decolonial warrior, you aim to become an instrument of peace. In the next stage, you transform by bonding with your inner healer, liberator, or warrior. Finally, you honor your *desenvolvimiento* when you choose decolonization in an evolving life-long personal, professional, and public journey.

CONCLUSION

Decolonial therapists assist oppressed people in healing their Wounds. This approach addresses colonial historical wounds, intergenerational, racial, ethnoracial trauma, and contemporary oppression trauma and race-related stress. Using pluriversal perspectives, decolonial therapists integrate Indigenous and Global South healing practices into mainstream psychotherapy. In this way, decolonial therapists join the circle—to heal the Wound—a compendium of multiple intersecting colonial, racial, and ethnic oppressions. In conclusion, decolonial therapists assist clients in composing *testimonios*, connecting with ancestrality, celebrating *vincularidad*, practicing and enhancing spirituality, nurturing *desenvolvimiento*, engaging in social justice action, and exercising spiritual activism. Finally, the psychospiritual effects of connecting with positive emotions—such as hope, gratitude, compassion, and love—nurture and sustain decolonial therapists' commitment to work toward creating a socially just and equitable world.

RESOURCES

Foor, D., with Bright, B. (2017, October 15). *Ancestral healing: Insights on animism and shamanism* [Video]. YouTube. https://www.youtube.com/watch?v=Mf-xpEdclbA

Nicholas, D. (Director). (2020, November 17). *Blood memory: A story of removal and return* [Film]. America ReFramed. https://www.bloodmemorydoc.com

Nixon, A. (2020, November 18). *The elements of decolonial healing justice* [Video]. TEDxPortofSpain. https://www.youtube.com/watch?v=7J_BDOJjk5c&t=350s

REFERENCES

Acosta, A. (2016). Rethinking the world from the perspective of *buen vivir*. https://www.degrowth.info/en/dim/degrowth-in-movements/buen-vivir/

Adames, H. Y., & Chavez-Dueñas, N. Y. (2017). *Cultural foundations and interventions in Latino/a mental health: History, theory, and within groups differences*. Routledge/Taylor & Francis Group.

Aiello, M., Bismar, D., Casanova, S., Casas, J. M., Chang, D., Chin, J. L., Comas-Diaz, L., Salvo Crane, L., Demir, Z., Garcia, M. A., Hita, L., Leverett, P., Mendez, K., Morse, G. S., shodiya-zeumault, s., O'Leary Sloan, M., Weil, M. C., & Blume, A. W. (2021). Protecting and defending our people: Nakni tushka anowa (The Warrior's Path) final report. APA Division 45 Warrior's Path Presidential Task Force 2020. *Journal of Indigenous Research, 9*(8). https://doi.org/10.26077/2en0-6610

American Psychiatric Association. (2000). *Diagnostic and statistical manual of mental disorders* (4th ed.).

Anzaldua, G. (1987). *Borderlands/La Frontera: The new Mestiza*. Spinster/Aunt Lute.

Anzaldua, G. (2002). Now let us shift . . . the path of conocimiento . . . inner work, public acts. In G. E. Anzaldua & A. L. Keating (Eds.), *This bridge we call home: Radical visions for transformation* (pp. 540–570). Routledge.

Aron, A. (1992). *Testimonio*, a bridge between psychotherapy and sociotherapy. *Women & Therapy, 13*(3), 173–189. https://doi.org/10.1300/J015V13N03_01

Baldwin, C. (1998). *Calling the circle: The first and future culture*. Bantam Books.

Barson, B. (2019, September 5). *Artivism and decolonization: A brief theory, history and practice of cultural production as political activism*. https://nmbx.newmusicusa.org/artivism-and-decolonization-a-brief-theory-history-and-practice-of-cultural-production-as-political-activism/

Bartlett, C., Marshall, M., & Marshall, A. (2012). Two-Eyed Seeing and other lessons learned within a co-learning journey of bringing together Indigenous and mainstream knowledges and ways of knowing. *Journal of Environmental Studies and Sciences*, *2*(4), 331–340. https://doi.org/10.1007/s13412-012-0086-8

Benton, G. B. (2016). *Then she sang a willow's song: Reclaiming life and power with the Ancestors*. CreateSpace Independent Publishing Platform.

Bierer, L. M., Bader, H. N., Daskalakis, N. P., Lehrner, A., Provençal, N., Wiechmann, T., Klengel, T., Makotkine, I., Binder, E. B., & Yehuda, R. (2020). Intergenerational effects of maternal Holocaust Exposure on *FKBP5* methylation. *The American Journal of Psychiatry*, *177*(8), 744–753. https://doi.org/10.1176/appi.ajp.2019.19060618

Bowers, M. E., & Yehuda, R. (2016). Intergenerational transmission of stress in humans. *Neuropsychopharmacology*, *41*(1), 232–244. https://doi.org/10.1038/npp.2015.247

Bryant-Davis, T., & Comas-Díaz, L. (Eds.). (2016). *Womanist and mujerista psychologies: Voices of fire, Acts of courage*. American Psychological Association. https://doi.org/10.1037/14937-000

Bryant-Davis, T., & Ocampo, C. (2006). A therapeutic approach to the treatment of racist incident-based trauma. *Journal of Emotional Abuse*, *6*(4), 1–22. https://doi.org/10.1300/J135v06n04_01

Carter, R. T. (2007). Racism and psychological and emotional injury: Recognizing and assessing race-based traumatic stress. *The Counseling Psychologist*, *35*(1), 13–105. https://doi.org/10.1177/0011000006292033

Chavez-Dueñas, N. Y., Adames, H. Y., Perez-Chavez, J. G., & Salas, S. P. (2019). Healing ethno-racial trauma in Latinx immigrant communities: Cultivating hope, resistance, and action. *American Psychologist*, *74*(1), 49–62. https://doi.org/10.1037/amp0000289

Clark, K. B. (1989). *Dark ghetto: Dilemmas in social power* (2nd ed). Wesleyan University Press.

Clark, S. E. (2021). *Hope . . . is the thing*. Welbeck Publishing.

Cohen, D. B. (2006). Family constellations: An innovative systemic phenomenological group process from Germany. *The Family Journal*, *14*(3), 226–233. https://doi.org/10.1177/1066480706287279

Comas, L. (2018, July 24). Healing my ancestors, healing myself. *SageWoman Blogs*. https://witchesandpagans.com/sagewoman-blogs/an-invitation/healing-my-ancestors-healing-myself.html

Comas-Díaz, L. (2000). An ethnopolitical approach to working with People of Color. *American Psychologist*, *55*(11), 1319–1325. https://doi.org/10.1037/0003-066X.55.11.1319

Comas-Díaz, L. (2006). Latino healing: The integration of ethnic psychology into psychotherapy. *Psychotherapy: Theory, Research, Practice & Training*, *43*(4), 436–453.

Comas-Díaz, L. (2007). Ethnopolitical psychology: Healing and transformation. In E. Aldarondo (Ed.), *Promoting social justice in mental health practice* (pp. 91–118). Lawrence Erlbaum.

Comas-Díaz, L. (2012). *Multicultural care: A clinician's guide to cultural competence.* American Psychological Association. https://doi.org/10.1037/13491-000

Comas-Díaz, L. (2016). Racial trauma recovery: A race-informed therapeutic approach to racial wounds. In A. N. Alvarez, C. T. H. Liang, & H. A. Neville (Eds.), *The cost of racism for people of color: Contextualizing experiences of discrimination* (pp. 249–272). American Psychological Association. https://doi.org/10.1037/14852-012

Comas-Díaz, L. (2020). Journey to psychology: A *mujerista testimonio. Women & Therapy, 43*(1–2), 157–169. https://doi.org/10.1080/02703149.2019.1684676

Comas-Díaz, L. (2022). Decolonization: A personal manifesto. *Women & Therapy, 45*(4), 304–319. https://doi.org/10.1080/02703149.2022.2125617

Comas-Díaz, L., Hall, G. N., & Neville, H. A. (2019, January). Racial trauma theory, research, and healing: Introduction to the special issue. *American Psychologist, 74*(1), 1–5. https://doi.org/10.1037/amp0000442

David, E. J. R., & Okazaki, S. (2006). Colonial mentality: A review and recommendation for Filipino American psychology. *Cultural Diversity and Ethnic Minority Psychology, 12*(1), 1–16. https://doi.org/10.1037/1099-9809.12.1.1

DeGruy, J. (2005). *Post traumatic slave syndrome: America's legacy of enduring injury and healing.* Uptone Press.

Del Castillo, R., Wycoff, A., & Cantu, S. (2012, March 17). *Curanderismo* as decolonization therapy: The acceptance of *mestizaje* as a *remedio.* NACCS Annual Conference Proceedings, Chicago, IL, United States. https://scholarworks.sjsu.edu/naccs/2012/Proceedings/7

Diaz, J. (2022). *The altar within: Radical devotional guide to liberate the divine self.* Row House Publisher.

Dorfman, A., Moscovitch, D. A., & Grossman, I. (2021). Pathways for adversity to wisdom. In F. J. Infurna & E. Jayawickreme (Eds.), *Redesigning research on post traumatic growth: Challenges, pitfalls and new directions* (pp. 259–279). Oxford University Press.

Duran, E. (2019). *Healing the soul wound: Trauma informed counseling for Indigenous communities* (2nd ed.). Teachers College Press.

Elsass, P. (1992). *Strategies for survival: The psychology of cultural resilience in ethnic minorities.* New York University Press.

Erikson, E. H. (1968). *Identity: Youth and crisis.* W. W. Norton.

Esa, E. (2021, October 12). Beginner's guide to spiritual practice to start connecting with your ancestors. *HipLatina.* https://hiplatina.com/connecting-ancestors-guide/

Escobar, E. (2018). *Designs for the pluriverse: Radical interdependency, autonomy and the making of worlds.* Duke University Press.

Fani, N., Harnett, N. G., Bradley, B., Mekawi, Y., Powers, A., Stevens, J. S., Ressler, K. J., & Carter, S. (2022). Racial discrimination and White matter microstructure in trauma-exposed Black women. *Biological Psychiatry, 91*(3), 254–261. https://doi.org/10.1016/j.biopsych.2021.08.011

Fernandez, J. S. (2022). A *mujerista* psychology perspective on *testimonio* to cultivate decolonial healing. *Women & Therapy, 45*(2–3), 131–156. https://doi.org/10.1080/02703149.2022.2095101

Fernandez-Marina, R. (1961). The Puerto Rican syndrome: Its dynamics and cultural determinants. *Psychiatry, 24*(1), 79–82. https://doi.org/10.1080/00332747.1961.11023256

Fine, M. (2018). *Just research in contentious times: Widening the methodological imagination.* Teachers College Press.

Fischer, P., Sauer, A., Vogrincic, C., & Weisweiler, S. (2011). The ancestor effect: Thinking about our generic origin enhances intellectual performance. *European Journal of Social Psychology, 41*(1), 11–16. https://doi.org/10.1002/ejsp.778

Freire, P. (1992). *Pedagogy of hope: Relieving pedagogy of the oppressed.* Continuum.

Gantt, L., & Tripp, T. (2016). The image comes first: Treating preverbal trauma with art therapy. In J. L. King (Ed.), *Art therapy, trauma and neuroscience: Theoretic and practical perspectives* (pp. 67–99). Routledge.

Garcia, M. A., & Tehee, M. (2014). *Society of Indian Psychologists commentary of the American Psychological Association's (APA) Ethical Principles of Psychologists and Code of Conduct.* Society of Indian Psychologists.

Garrett, J. T., & Garrett, M. W. (1994). The path of good medicine: Understanding and counseling Native American Indians. *Journal of Multicultural Counseling and Development, 22,* 139–144.

Garrett, M. T., Garrett, J. T., & Brotherton, D. (2001). Inner circle/outer circle: A group technique based on Native American healing circles. *The Journal for Specialists in Group Work, 26*(1), 17–30.

Gee, G. C., & Ontniano Verissimo, A. D. (2016). Racism and behaviroal outcomes over the life course. In A. N. Alvarez, C. T. H. Liang, & H. A. Neville (Eds.), *The cost of racism for people of color: Contextualizing experiences of discrimination* (pp. 133–152). American Psychological Association. https://doi.org/10.1037/14852-007

Gherovici, P. (2003). *The Puerto Rican syndrome.* Other Press.

Gottlieb, G. (1991). Epigenetic systems view of human development. *Developmental Psychology, 27*(1), 33–34. https://doi.org/10.1037/0012-1649.27.1.33

Grosfoguel, R. (2007). The epistemic decolonial turn: Beyond political-economic paradigms. *Cultural Studies, 21*(2–3), 211–223.

Grosfoguel, R., & Georas, C. S. (2010). Coloniality of power and racial dynamics: Notes toward a reinterpretation of Latino Caribbeans in New York City. *Identities, 7*(1), 85–125. https://doi-org.ezproxy.bucknell.edu/10.1080/1070289X.2000.9962660

Hartman, W. E., Wendt, D. C., Burrage, R. L., Pomerville, A., & Gone, J. (2019). American Indian historical trauma: Anticolonial prescriptions for healing, resilience, and survivance. *American Psychologist, 74*(1), 6–19. https://doi.org/10.1037/amp0000326

Healing Justice. (2018, November 16). *The origin of our healing circles.* https://healingjusticeproject.org/news/2019/2/26/healing-circles

Hernandez-Wolfe, P. (2011). Decolonization and mental health: A Mestiza journey in the borderlands. *Women & Therapy, 34*(3), 293–306.

Initiatives for Change. (2019). *Racial healing circle training.* https://us.iofc.org/news/2019/3/racial-healing-circle-training-for-iofc-alumni

Jeffery, T., Kurtz, D. L., & Jones, C. A. (2021). Two-Eyed Seeing: Current approaches and discussion of medical applications. *BC Medical Journal, 63*(8), 321–325.

Jordan, M. (2014). Healing circles: An ethnographic study of interactions among health and healing practitioners from multiple disciplines. *Global Advances in Health and Medicine, 3*(4), 9–13.

Jung, C. G. (1989). *Memories, dreams, reflections* (Rev. ed.). Vintage Books.

Katz, R. (2017). *Indigenous healing psychology: Honoring the wisdom of the First Peoples.* Healing Arts Press.

Kendi, I. X. (2016, June 21). Post-traumatic slave syndrome is a racist idea. *Black Perspectives.* https://www.aaihs.org/post-traumatic-slave-syndrome-is-a-racist-idea/

Kluckhohn, C., & Murray, H. A. (1953). *Personality in nature, society and culture* (2nd ed.). Knopf.

Koss-Chioino, J. (2007). Spiritual transformation, ritual, healing, and altruism. *Journal of Religion & Science, 41*(4), 877–892.

Leading Lotus. (2018). *Leading from the mud and beyond: About the Lotus.* https://www.leadinglotus.com/article/leading-from-the-mud-and-beyond

Linklater, R. (2014). *Decolonizing trauma work: Indigenous stories and strategies.* Fernwood Publishing.

Maldonado-Torres, N. (2007). On the coloniality of being: Contributions to the development of a concept. *Cultural Studies, 2*(2–3), 240–270. https://doi.org/10.1080/09502380601162548

Marks, L. (2006). Global health crises: Can indigenous healing practices offer a valuable resource? *International Journal of Disability, Development and Education, 53*(4), 471–478.

Martin, C. L., Ghastine, L., Lodge, E. K., Dhingra, K., & Ward-Caviness, C. K. (2022). Understanding health inequalities through the lens of social epigenetics. *Annual Review of Public Health, 43*(1), 235–254.

Martín-Baró, I. (1994). *Writings for a liberation psychology: Ignacio Martín-Baró* (A. Aron & S. Corne, Eds. and Trans.). Harvard University Press.

Mehl-Madrona, L. (2003). *Coyote healing: Miracles in Native medicine.* Bear & Company.

Mehl-Madrona, L., & Mainguy, B. (2014). Introducing healing circles and talking circles into primary care. *The Permanente Journal, 18*(2), 4–9.

Mehlman, R. D. (1961). The Puerto Rican syndrome. *The American Journal of Psychiatry, 118*(4), 328–332.

Menakem, R. (2017). *My grandmother's hands: Racialized trauma and the pathways to mending our hearts and bodies.* General Recover Press.

Mendez, D. D., Scott, J., Adodoadji, L., Toval, C., MacNeil, M., & Sindhu, M. (2021). Racism as a public health crisis: Assessment and review of municipal declarations and resolutions across the United States. *Frontiers in Public Health, 9*, 686807. https://www.ncbi.nlm.nih.gov/pmc/articles/PMC8385329/

Mignolo, W. D. (2019). *Colonial wounds, decolonial healing* [Video]. Vimeo. https://vimeo.com/337899001

Mignolo, W. D., & Walsh, C. E. (2018). *On decoloniality: Concepts, analytics, praxis.* Duke University Press.

Misra, G., & Gergen, K. J. (1993). In the place of culture in psychological science. *International Journal of Psychology, 38*(2), 225–253.

Mitchell, T., Arseneau, C., & Thomas, D. (2019). Colonial trauma: Complex, continuous, collective, cumulative, and compounding effects on the health of Indigenous people in Canada and beyond. *International Journal of Indigenous Health, 14*(2), 74–94.

Monteiro, N. M., & Wall, D. J. (2011, September 15). African dance as healing modality throughout the diaspora: The use of ritual and movement to work through trauma. *Journal of Pan African Studies, 4*(6), 234–252. https://link.gale.com/apps/doc/A306357808/LitRC

Mosley, D. V., Hargons, C. N., Meiller, C., Angyal, B., Wheeler, P., Davis, C., & Stevens-Watkins, D. (2020). Critical consciousness of anti-Black racism: A practical model to prevent and resist racial trauma. *Journal of Counseling Psychology, 68*(1), 1–16. https://doi.org/10.1037/cou0000430

Mosley, D. V., Neville, H. A., Chavez-Dueñas, N. Y., Adames, H. Y., Lewis, J. A., & French, B. H. (2019). Radical hope in revolting times: Proposing a cultural relevant psychological framework. *Social Personal Psychology Compass, 14*(1), e12512. https://doi.org/10.1111/spc3.12512

Mulligan, C. J. (2021). Systemic racism can get under our skin and into our genes. *American Journal of Physical Anthropology, 175*(2), 399–405. https://doi.org/10.1002/ajpa.24290

Neeganagwedgin, E. (2020). Indigenous systems of knowledge and transformative learning practices turning the gaze upside down. *Diaspora, Indigenous, and Minority Education, 14*(1), 1–13. https://doi.org/10.1080/15595692.2019.1652815

Nestler, E. J. (2016). Transgenerational epigenetic contributions to stress responses: Fact or fiction? *PLOS Biology, 14*(3), e1002426. https://doi.org/10.1371/journal.pbio.1002426

Norat, G. (2005). Latina grandmothers. Spiritual bridges to ancestral lands. *Journal of the Association for Research on Mothering, 7*(2) 98–111.

Okeke, O., Elbasheir, A., Carter, S. E., Powers, A., Mekawi, Y., Gillespie, C. F., Schwartz, A. C., Bradley, B., & Fani, N. (2022). Indirect effects of racial discrimination on health outcomes through prefrontal cortical white matter integrity. *Biological Psychiatry: Cognitive Neuroscience and Neuroimaging, 8*(7), 741–749. https://doi.org/10.1016/j.bpsc.2022.05.004

Olmos, M. F., & Paravisini-Gebert, L. (2003). *Creole religions of the Caribbean: An introduction from Voodu and Santería to Obeah and Espiritismo*. New York University Press.

Orloff, J. (1996). *Second sight: An intuitive psychiatrist tells her extraordinary story and shows you how to tap your own inner wisdom*. Warner Books.

Peters, W. M. K. (2011). *The Indigenous soul wound: Exploring culture, memetics, complexity, and emergence* (Publication no. 3474460) [Doctoral dissertation, Institute of Transpersonal Psychology]. ProQuest Dissertations. https://www.proquest.com/docview/898334092

Portman, T. A. A., & Garrett, M. T. (2006, December). Native American healing traditions. *International Journal of Disability, Development, and Education, 53*(4), 453–469.

Prayer of Saint Francis. (n.d.). https://www.ewtn.com/catholicism/devotions/prayer-of-st-francis-837

Quijano, A. (2000). Coloniality of power, Eurocentrism and Latin America. *Nepantla: Views from South, 1*(3), 533–580.

Quiñones-Rosado, R. (2020). Liberation psychology and racism. In L. Comas-Díaz & E. Torres Rivera (Eds.), *Liberation psychology: Theory, method, practice, and social justice* (pp. 54–68). American Psychological Association. https://doi.org/10.1037/0000198-004

Reed, T. (2021a). A critical review of the Native American tradition of circle practices. In R. Throne (Ed.), *Indigenous research of land, self, and spirit* (pp. 132–152). IGI Global. https://doi.org/10.4018/978-1-7998-3729-9.ch009

Reed, T. (2021b). Intergenerational trauma and other unique challenges as barriers to Native American educational success. In R. Throne (Ed.), *Indigenous research of land, self, and spirit* (pp. 180–199). IGI Global. https://doi.org/10.4018/978-1-7998-3729-9.ch009

Richardson, J. L. (2018). Healing circles as Black feminist pedagogical interventions. In O. Perlow, D. Wheeler, S. Bethea, & B. Scott (Eds.), *Black women's liberatory pedagogies: Resistance, transformation, and healing within and beyond the academy* (pp. 281–294). Palgrave Macmillan.

Rodriguez, J. (1999). Towards an understanding of spirituality in U.S. Latina leadership. *Frontiers: A Journal of Women's Studies, 20*(1), 137–146.

Rosenthal, M. (2022). Intergenerational trauma: An embodied experience. *International Body Psychotherapy Journal, 20*(2), 80–86.

Rybak, C., & Decker-Fitts, A. (2009). Understanding Native American healing practices. *Counselling Psychology Quarterly, 22*(3), 333–342. https://doi.org/10.1080/09515070903270900

Salmon, E. (2000, October). Kincentric ecology: Indigenous perceptions of the human–nature relationship. *Ecological Applications, 10*(5), 1327–1332. https://doi.org/10.2307/2641288

Sandoval, C., & Latorre, G. (2008). Chicana/o artivism: Judy Baca's digital work with youth of color. In A. Everett (Ed.), *Learning, race, and ethnicity: Youth and digital media* (pp. 81–108). MIT Press.

Shaw, R. M., Howe, J., & Beazer, J. (2020). Ethics and positionality in qualitative research with vulnerable and marginal groups. *Qualitative Research, 20*(3), 277–293.

Sheldrake, R. (n.d.). *Morphic resonance and morphic fields—An introduction.* https://www.sheldrake.org/research/morphic-resonance/introduction

Sotero, M. M. (2006). A conceptual model of historical trauma: Implications for public health: Practice and research. *Journal of Health Disparities, 1*(1), 93–108.

Trejo Mendez, P. (2020). *Volver a la cuerpa: Endometriosis y salud autogestiva* [Back to the body: Endometriosis and self-managed health]. La Catártica ediciones. https://lacatartica.files.wordpress.com/2020/09/volver-a-la-cuerpa-libro.pdf

Trejo Mendez, P. (2021, December 16). Decolonizing healing: Weaving the *curandera* path. *Globalizations, 20*(2), 316–331. https://doi.org/10.1080/14747731.2021.2009306

Trias Monje, J. (1999). *Puerto Rico: The trials of the oldest colony in the world.* Yale University.

Tubbs, S. (2020). *The Black girls healing circle workbook: A guide to healing through sisterhood & connection: Vol. 1. Foundations.* Independently published.

Vizenor, G. (2008). Aesthetics of survivance: Literary theory and practice. In G. Vizenor (Ed.), *Survivance: Narratives of Native presence* (pp. 1–24). University of Nebraska Press.

Walker, M. (2004). Walking a piece of the way: Race, power, and therapeutic movement. In M. Walker & W. B. Rosen (Eds.), *How connections heal: Stories from relational-cultural therapy* (pp. 35–52). Guilford Press.

Ward, A. (2013). Understanding postcolonial traumas. *Journal of Theoretical and Philosophical Psychology, 33*(3), 170–184. https://doi.org/10.1037/a0033576

Watkins, D. (2020). Critical consciousness of anti-Black racism: A practical model to prevent and resist racial trauma. *Journal of Counseling Psychology, 68*(1), 1–16. https://doi.org/10.1037/cou0000430

Watkins, M. (2015). Psychosocial accompaniment. *Journal of Social and Political Psychology, 3*(1), 324–341. https://doi.org/10.5964/jspp.v3i1.103

Winchell, M., Kress, T. M., & Tobin, K. (2016). Teaching/learning radical listening: Joe's legacy among three generations of practitioners. In M. F. Agnello & W. M. Reynolds (Eds.), *Practicing critical pedagogy: The influences of Joe Kincheloe* (pp. 99–112). Springer.

Wolynn, M. (2016). *It didn't start with you: How inherited family trauma shapes who we are and how to end the cycle.* Penguin Books.

Wood, L. (2015). Hoping, empowering, strengthening: Theories used in intimate partner violence advocacy. *Affilia: Journal of Women & Social Work, 30*(3), 286–301. https://doi.org/10.1177/0886109914563157

Yehuda, R., & Lehrner, A. (2018). Trauma across generations and paths to adaptation and resilience. *Psychological Trauma, 10*(1), 22–29. https://doi.org/10.1037/tra0000302

Yosso, T. J. (2006). Whose culture has capital: A critical race theory discussion of community cultural wealth. *Ethnicity and Education, 8*(1), 69–91.

Youssef, N. A. (2022). Potential societal and cultural implications of transgenerational epigenetic methylation of trauma and PTSD: Pathology or resilience? *Yale Journal of Biology and Medicine, 95*(1), 171–174.

13 DECOLONIZING PSYCHOANALYSIS

Anti-Blackness, Coloniality, and a New Premise for Psychoanalytic Treatment

DANIEL JOSE GAZTAMBIDE, FABIÁN E. FELICIANO-GRANIELA, JOSÉ LUIGGI-HERNÁNDEZ, AND EDLYANE VERONICA MEDINA ESCOBAR

Race is no more mythical and fictional than gender–both are powerful fictions.
                                                        –Lugones, 2007, p. 12

Psychoanalysis seems a strange bedfellow for a text on decolonial psychology. It has been scrutinized as the example par excellence of colonial psychology, mired in racist, sexist, queerphobic, and classist practices (Aron & Starr, 2013; Gaztambide, 2019; Tummala-Narra, 2016). Although research has established a growing evidence base for psychodynamic treatment processes (therapeutic alliance, addressing ruptures, and the like) and psychodynamic therapies (CBT, humanistic), much of this research relies on predominantly White samples (Leuzinger-Bohleber et al., 2020). Parallel to this research turn is a decolonial turn, unearthing the progressive history of psychoanalysis (Danto, 2005) and its contributions to postcolonial theory (Beshara, 2021), anticapitalist studies (Pavón-Cuéllar, 2018), and liberation psychology (Gaztambide, 2019). Scholars and clinicians in the United States have also called for a community psycho-analysis (González & Peltz, 2021), catching up to developments already taking place in psychoanalysis of the Global South (see Noboa Ortega, 2019).

https://doi.org/10.1037/0000376-014
Decolonial Psychology: Toward Anticolonial Theories, Research, Training, and Practice,
L. Comas-Díaz, H. Y. Adames, and N. Y. Chavez-Dueñas (Editors)

In this chapter, we contextualize the colonial complicity and decolonial potential of psychoanalysis in Sigmund Freud's anxieties as a Jewish man in an anti-Semitic, colonial world whose racist fantasies (falsely) equated Jewishness, Blackness, and queerness and how he participated in them in pursuit of cis-heteronormative Whiteness and social mobility (Brickman, 2017; Tate, 1996). We paint a nuanced yet no less fraught view of psychoanalysis that underscores how anxieties around race, class, sexuality, and the body led Freud to articulate important insights on the psyche and society while leaving behind an unfinished decolonial project that we need to continue in his stead. We will accomplish this by rereading Freud through the lens of Martiniquan Black psychiatrist Frantz Fanon, whom Edward Said referred to as Freud's "most disputatious heir" (Beshara, 2021). It is not disputed that Fanon "transcended" psychoanalysis (Maldonado-Torres et al., 2021), but we claim him as an ancestor who evolved psychoanalytic practice—seeing patients five to six times a week, using the couch, and drawing from techniques similar to contemporary relational approaches, alongside his experiments in community intervention (Gaztambide, 2021; Manuellan, 2017; see also Turner & Neville, 2020).

We find in Fanon's work a unique opportunity for a decolonial reimagining of psychoanalytic treatment both in the clinic and the community. We argue that reading Freud through Fanon yields a framework that resists easy bifurcations between traditional and decolonial psychoanalysis. Instead of such a split—mirroring our field's broader division between general and culturally competent therapy—we integrate existing theory *within* a decolonial framework. As a project that includes but extends beyond the consulting room, we offer illustrations of this approach in both clinical and community settings and outline implications for future work. In relation to this chapter, we begin by positioning ourselves as a team of Puerto Rican scholars, clinicians, and activists.

POSITIONALITY STATEMENT

Daniel Jose Gaztambide: I was born in San Juan, Puerto Rico, to a White Cuban mother and a Brown Puerto Rican father. In childhood, my father's skin was suspect beside my White body—"Is he the father or a kidnapper?" On morning drives to school, my mother and I, inside the car, were White. The indigent outside were Black and Brown, with skin and socioeconomic structure inscribing a language of inequality without words. My mother introduced me to psychoanalysis in this context; my father taught me about his past as a decolonial socialist. Psychoanalysis became a tool to decode the language of the colony, naming the ghosts haunting my community.

José Luiggi-Hernández: I am a mixed-race, light-skinned, queer Puerto Rican from a working-class family. It was my grandmother who highlighted my Black features and encouraged me to enhance my Whiteness despite my skin color. It was not until university that I learned about the history of colonialism and racism in Puerto Rico and the United States, my White privilege, and the difficulties of living as a queer person in a predominantly conservative society. Freudo-Marxism was my introduction and liberation from how neoliberalism privatizes suffering as an individual instead of collective experience. Yet, it failed to account for other idioms of suffering, such as coloniality, racism, sexism, and queerphobia, among others. Through Fanon's (1952/2008) work, I found a psychoanalytic practice informed by a decolonial ethics.

Edlyane Veronica Medina Escobar: I was born in Moca, a rural town on the west side of Puerto Rico, to a Brown, low-income family on my father's side and a lighter-skin, low-income family on my mother's. My father is Brown like myself; my mother has lighter skin, straight hair, and green eyes. Her eyes were a constant reminder of what I *could* have looked like, "if you had your mother's eyes . . . you would have been even *more* beautiful . . . but that's okay; your children might inherit them." Family members developed nick-names for me out of endearment and the anxiety that my skin evoked in them. My grandmother and mother endearingly called me *Prieta* (Black), and my lighter-skin sister *Blanqi sal* (white as salt). Nameless aside from my skin color, I struggled to find the meaning of this condition. As an adult who migrated to the country colonizing my homeland, I return to the identi-fication of *prieta* as a way to both honor my non-White ancestral heritage and, at the same time, name the fact that I am the realization of a larger Whitening project in the larger Americas. Educated from frameworks such as liberation psychology, feminist and queer studies, Intersectionality, and a socialist perspective, I approach my calling as a clinical psychologist with a commitment to decolonize practice, research, and scholarship. My clini-cal, academic, and personal efforts aim to tackle and dismantle the familiar silencing in families, institutions, communities, and therapy rooms.

Fabián E. Feliciano-Graniela: I was born in Ponce and brought up in a family from Peñuelas that consisted of Black Puerto Ricans that worked with sugar cane and textiles on my dad's side and White(ned) Puerto Ricans that worked in chemical and pharmacological industries on my mother's. Growing up queer with this history from which I bloomed in the Puerto Rico metropolitan area is not without profound contradictions. It is here that I encountered feminist psychoanalytic critique while collaborating in lesbian, gay, bisexual, trans-gender, queer, intersex, asexual plus (LGBTQIA+), feminist and pro–student activism. The first person to shape my learning was my mentor Carlos García, whose teachings on leftist Lacanian thinkers from the geopolitical South are immortalized in my notebooks. I can still hear him say, "If we are to change society's structures, we must be willing to face the unconscious components that safekeep and reproduce these structures." This phrase informs my work and the kind of world I build alongside the people I love dearly. Currently, I am one of the few in my family to pursue graduate studies in clinical psychology at the University of Puerto Rico. Here, I am part of Siempre Vivas Metro— a transdisciplinary effort by students and faculty to eradicate gender and sexual violence, where I facilitate workshops to explore new forms of masculinity.

We wrote this chapter as Puerto Rican scholars and clinicians who grew up in the shadow of the world's oldest colony. Although beyond the scope of this chapter, it is essential to underscore how capitalism, colorism, and patriarchy collide in our experience growing up on the island and in our approach to psychoanalysis. Through collaborative writing, we articulated a desire to move beyond the contradictions that prevent honest dialogue about psychoanalytic practice's challenges and promises. Further, we explored our indebtedness to multicultural psychology (see Sue et al., 2019) alongside the limitations we experience within that framework—in particular, a sometimes rigid bifurcation between Western and non-Western approaches to psychology. We turn here to provide further context for our work.

PSYCHOANALYSIS IN BROADER HISTORICAL CONTEXT

First, we recognize that although Freud formulated psychoanalysis as a product of the European Enlightenment, he was not the originator of psychoanalytic ideas per se. Indeed, recent Indigenous scholarship has shown that notions of the individual, interiority, or the psyche are not uniquely or originally European (see Mann, 2001; Sioui, 1992; Steckley, 2014). On the contrary, these ideas are present across the Global South, evidence showing that European notions of the individual psyche reflect a distorted theft of Indigenous political and spiritual philosophies. Further, Indigenous notions of individual freedom, gender equality, and democracy were frequently distorted by European political theorists into abstracted forms of individualism (see Graeber & Wengrow, 2021, for a review). For example, the Wendat and Iroquois peoples of North America spoke of the soul's "other desires," hidden from the conscious mind. Reports by missionaries and direct accounts by First Nations peoples show that these desires are

> known by means of dreams, which is its language. Accordingly, when these desires are accomplished, it is satisfied; but, on the contrary, if it be not granted what it desires, it becomes angry, and not only does not give its body the good

and the happiness that it wished to procure for it, but often it also revolts against the body, causing various diseases, and even death. (cited in Graeber & Wengrow, 2021, p. 453)

Some Indigenous peoples believed these "concealed desires" are expressed through an indirect, symbolic language, often by consulting spiritual guides who interpreted these wishes in dreams and shed light on the relationship between unconscious desire and the body. Other examples include ancient Egypt and wider Africa, where ideas such as *sekhem* (libido), dream interpretation, and a dynamic unconscious influenced diverse mystical and intellectual traditions, including psychoanalysis (Bynum, 1999). Freud's use of the word *seele* (soul) to refer to the mind also reflects this genealogy, sharing root words with the Greek word for soul, associated with the goddess Psyche, and the Egyptian *khe* for soul and the female pronoun *su*—"su-khe" (Bynum, 1999, p. 160). Hence we see psychoanalysis having deeper roots that came before and go beyond Freud, compatible with diverse cultural contexts (see also Comas-Díaz, 2021).

We also want to name the broader historical and contemporary context in which we practice. Following Robinson (2021), we refer to our current global system as racial capitalism, a "colonial materiality" (Beshara, 2021, p. 2), which began with Europe's extraction of wealth and labor from Indigenous and African peoples and instituted racial hierarchy to justify oppression and division. This violence also disrupted the diverse gender and sexual expressions of Global South peoples, replacing them with rigid gender norms positioning colonized men as dominators of colonized women and erasing queer subjectivities (Adames & Chavez-Dueñas, 2021; Lugones, 2007; Oyěwùmí, 1997). In our theorizing, we give primacy to racism not to minimize other oppressions but because racial discourse and, in particular, anti-Blackness structures other hierarchies around class, gender, and sexuality (Fanon, 1952/2008; Turner & Neville, 2020). It structures the desire for social mobility by positioning Blackness as an ontological bottom one should fear falling into, and Whiteness as the heights one aspires to (see Gaztambide, 2022; Helms, 2020)—as we will see in the case of Freud himself.

An important caveat is in order before proceeding. Rather than presenting decolonial psychoanalysis as an alternative to traditional psychoanalysis, purified of oppressive tendencies, we argue that all psychotherapy—psychodynamic or not—must engage in an ongoing decolonial process. We also resist making too neat a distinction between Western and non-Western intellectual traditions because this erases the fact that many categories seen as European—the individual, the unconscious, and so on—have decidedly non-European origins (Bynum, 1999; Graeber & Wengrow, 2021). Further, we follow the founder of liberation psychology, Ignacio Martín-Baró (1994), in rejecting this tension as a false dilemma—a theory's demographic origins do not determine how colonial or decolonial they are. Instead, what is essential is whether the theory helps shed light on our world and serves a decolonial function. With this in mind, we turn to the history of psychoanalysis itself.

PROTO-DECOLONIAL PSYCHOANALYSIS: AN ABBREVIATED HISTORY

Historical research has recovered how Freud and the early analysts—the majority being Jews with socialist-left politics (Danto, 2005)—engaged in dialogues around psyche, race, and class that would later inform postcolonial and liberation psychology (Gaztambide, 2019). Sandor Ferenczi, a forerunner of relational psychoanalysis, wrote to Freud about the political implications of psychoanalysis, "we investigate the *real* conditions in the various levels of society . . . just as they are mirrored in the individual" (cited in Gaztambide, 2019, p. 34). They recognized the unconscious as a repository of repressed feelings and a collective dynamic associated with oppressed groups—particularly Jewish, Black, and queer people (Aron & Starr, 2013).

The 19th-century European world in which psychoanalysis was born linked anxieties around the White-male body with racist fantasies positioning the Jewish body as queered "mulattos" or "White negroes" existing between masculinity and femininity, heterosexuality and queerness, Whiteness, and Blackness (Aron & Starr, 2013; Brickman, 2017). Analysts such as Otto Fenichel (1940) wrote about how anti-Blackness—the association of Black people with degraded, "nonhuman" status—underlined anti-Semitic discourses that racialized Jews as Black due to the "foreignness" of their culture and texture of their hair. But Fenichel (1940) also recognized that anti-Blackness scapegoated Black people in unique ways (p. 28) that Fanon (1952/2008) would later echo and emphasize. Fenichel pointed out how anti-Blackness structured anti-Semitism, with racism fulfilling a psychopolitical function—to foment racial division while facilitating an identification with the capitalist elite, a formulation shared by other psychoanalytic writers of the time (Hirschfeld, 1938; Reich, 1933/1970).

Although the progressive tradition of the early psychoanalytic movement was destroyed during World War II (Danto, 2005), other practitioners outside American psychoanalysis drew attention to the sociopolitical context of psychic suffering. In the United States, Karen Horney described how capitalism foments status anxiety and competition to rise to the top. Harry Stack

Sullivan studied the impact of segregation on Black youth and worked alongside Black novelist Ralph Ellison, who joined Richard Wright and Fredric Wertham in developing a psychoanalytic understanding of how racism exerts a psychic and material cost on both oppressor and oppressed (see Ahad, 2010). In the Francophone world, Mannoni (1950/1990) wrote the first psycho-analytic study of colonialism but was resoundingly critiqued by Fanon (1952/2008) for its "psychologising" focus on the colonized's passive "depen-dency." To understand Fanon's critique, we review his engagement with Freudian revisionist Jacques Lacan.

Lacan (1955/2002) argued that postwar psychoanalysis assimilated to White American capitalism, transforming it into a colonial duality between the analyst "who knows" and the patient "who does not" (p. 109). He called for a "return to Freud," centering the role of language, desire, and *jouissance*. Briefly (see Fink, 1999, for a review), the self is constituted through lan-guage, meaning that when we speak, we do so not as isolated individuals but are "spoken through" by our sociocultural world. We desire not only the other's love but also what the Big Other—culture and society—tells us to desire. *Jouissance* refers to how desire provides a balm for our pain even as it results in pain. For example, one may take a drug to reduce anxiety, then consume more even if it results in side effects. *Jouissance* is thus a "pleasure in pain," a relief derived from our attempts to avoid pain even when these attempts also lead to suffering.

Although originally a clinical concept applied to a wide range of human behaviors, *jouissance* provides a framework for understanding our attachment to oppressive structures, "[working] unconsciously against social betterment. . . . It also acts as the source of our enjoyment" (McGowan, 2013, p. 2). Whiteness, hegemonic masculinity, and class mobility are "master discourses" structuring the desire of oppressed peoples who, despite the brutality of the oppressor, identify with them as a way of achieving "human" status. Fanon's (1952/2008) critique of Mannoni involved the recognition that the colonized are not pas-sive objects that become dependent on the colony, but instead active sub-jects whose desire itself becomes colonized by socioeconomic structures. He argued the materiality of the colony is "epidermalized" (p. 4) on the Black body, "fixed" by the White gaze as an ontological "bottom," providing *jouis-sance* for those seeking to "move up" within the colony. This review suggests that racism provides exploited non-Black male and female, heterosexual, and queer workers a *jouissance* compensating their suffering under patriarchal capitalism with the enjoyment of Whiteness and anti-Blackness. If the early analysts and Fanon developed such a theory of race and *jouissance*, what about Freud? What "pleasure in pain" did race offer him?

FREUD'S ANTI-BLACKNESS AS COLONIZED ENJOYMENT

In his paper "The Unconscious," Freud's (1915) racial ontology is evident. Outlining the topography of the psyche—unconscious as repressed "bottom," conscious as what "passes into" awareness—he distinguished the preconscious as an "in-between" space of thoughts and feelings that "break into" consciousness but are "incapable of becoming conscious. . . . Their origin is what decides their fate":

> We may compare them with individuals of mixed race who, taken all round, resemble white men, but who betray their coloured descent by some striking feature or other, and on that account are excluded from society and enjoy none of the privileges of white people. (p. 191)

This psychic hierarchy positioning Blackness at the bottom and mixed-race people, as Jews were framed in Freud's time (Gilman, 1993), in the middle is key to understanding his thinking on race. In his more lucid theorizing on race and class, Freud (1927) maintained that inequality "was imposed on a resisting majority by a minority which understood how to obtain possession of the means to power and coercion," evolving to effect "a certain distribution of wealth [and] maintaining that distribution" (p. 6). Although the ruling elite benefit from a surplus of wealth and enjoyment, the exploited "develop an intense hostility towards a culture whose existence they make possible by their work, but in whose wealth they have too small a share" (p. 12). Like others in the psychoanalytic movement, Freud saw how anti-Semitism and anti-Blackness offer a shared *jouissance* that nurtures an "identification of the suppressed classes with the class who rules and exploits them . . . the suppressed classes can be emotionally attached to their masters; in spite of their hostility to them they may see in them their ideals" (p. 13). The exploited can enjoy racism as a salve for their pain, "since the right to despise the people outside [their culture] compensates them for the wrongs they suffer within their own unit" (p. 13).

Freud (1927) thus posited a triangulation between the elite capitalist class, the White working class, and racial Others, including the Jew and the African, with anti-Blackness facilitating Whiteness as a desire for upward mobility. This flows naturally into his critique of religion—the reward of "going up" to Heaven as compensation for suffering on Earth mirrors the reward of moving up the racial-economic hierarchy and becoming like the ruling class. Freud called for the oppressed to renounce the *jouissance* of "the other world" and focus their "liberated energies" on transforming this one, "achieving a state of things in which life will become tolerable for everyone and civilization no longer oppressive to anyone" (p. 50). Citing Heine, he advocated, "We leave Heaven to the angels and the sparrows" (p. 63).

But did Freud renounce the *jouissance* of the other world promised by Whiteness? African American philosopher Claudia Tate (1996) showed how he unconsciously equated the analyst–patient relationship with the White master–Black slave relationship (cf. Brickman, 2017), not unlike his equating the unconscious, preconscious, and conscious with Blackness, mixed-race Jewishness, and Whiteness. In this equation, Freud both evoked and erased his anxieties as a Jewish body in an anti-Semitic world, seeking to symbolically "ascend" into White masculinity, an ontological form of social mobility facilitated by anti-Blackness itself, helping him "master" his anxieties around his queered, "mixed-race" body as a Jew in turn-of-century Vienna.

FREUD THROUGH FANON'S EYES

Freud saw how racism maintains inequality and psychic suffering yet turned away from fully articulating its implications for psychoanalysis as a clinical practice. Here, Fanon's (1952/2008) analysis of colonialism presents a unique opportunity to put Freud on Fanon's couch. Like the early analysts, Fanon recognized how the wealthy exploited racism to facilitate a White identity among the working class, preventing the latter from "sinking any lower" than the "Black" (p. 64). Fanon (1952/2008) embraced solidarity with Jews as "brother[s] in misery," remembering a mentor's words, "Whenever you hear anyone abuse the Jews, pay attention, because he is talking about you . . . an anti-Semite is inevitably anti-Negro" (p. 92). But, like Fenichel, he also noted a critical difference between Black people, Jews, and other People of Color such as Arabs. "The Arab is told," Fanon wrote, "'if you are poor, it is because the Jew has . . . taken everything from you.' The Jew is told: 'You are not of the same class as the Arab *because you are really white*' . . . *the Negro is told nothing because no one has anything to tell him*" (p. 77, emphasis added). This difference had profound implications.

Fanon (1952/2008) cited Sartre's remark that Jews are "poisoned by the stereotype that others have of them . . . from the inside" (p. 87). Echoing Freud's anxieties as a Jew positioned between Whiteness and Blackness, Fanon stated that "apart from some rather debatable characteristics, [Jews] can sometimes go unnoticed [as White]." "Simple enough," he wrote, "*one has only not to be a [n-word]*" (p. 87, emphasis added). Fanon was cognizant of how Jews—and non-Black People of Color—suffer violence and persecution but argues that anti-Blackness positions him differently, "I am overdetermined from without. I am the slave not of the 'idea' that others have of me but of my own appearance" (p. 87). Even though racism "places [the Negro] beside the Jew," Jewish people and non-Black People of Color can "get out" of this emplacement by performing anti-Black racism (p. 133).

As if circling back to Freud's unconscious, Fanon (1952/2008) writes that under racial capitalism, "the lowest values is represented by the Negro . . . the unconscious representing the base and inferior traits is colored black" (p. 146). Speaking of the Jewish physician Michel Salomon in words that could be applied to Freud, Fanon writes, "He is a Jew, he has a 'millennial experience of anti-Semitism,' and yet he is a racist" (p. 156) enjoying the eucharist of anti-Blackness transubstantiating his Jewish body into a "White" one, an unconscious ritual that both Black and non-Black colonized people can also partake in (p. 147). Being oppressed does not inoculate one from desiring the *jouissance* that comes from pursuing Whiteness, masculinity, and wealth, even if that means "climbing" over other oppressed people—including one's own.

THEORETICAL IMPLICATIONS OF DECOLONIZING PSYCHOANALYSIS

Decolonizing Freud leads us to broaden "our understanding of what psychoanalysis is, has actually been, and what it can become" (González & Peltz, 2021, p. 411), with powerful implications for psychoanalytic practice relevant to other decolonial psychotherapies, blurring the arbitrary line between inner and outer, clinical and political, general and culturally competent psychotherapy. We outline those implications as follows.

Racial capitalism subordinates both privileged and underprivileged groups, fostering an "allegiance" to the system that disrupts "bonds of practical solidarity" (Lugones, 2007, p. 189). The system, borrowing from Lugones (2007), has a light and dark side. The light side constructs hegemonic race, gender, or sexual relations, elevating the middle-upper class White man and subordinating middle-upper class White women. Whiteness presents an unreachable ideal that promises wholeness, even as it is fleeting and incomplete (see Helms, 2016). One can achieve the American Dream through hard work yet be saddled with debt and fear of being one medical bill away from precarity. One might also aspire to the role of the male breadwinner, stoic, capable and invulnerable, yet unable to provide for one's family. These failures lead to desperate attempts to reclaim *jouissance*—including symbolic and literal violence toward women, LGBTQ people, and People of Color. The dark side of racial capitalism results from this violence—destruction of the Global South's notions of gender and sexuality, upending of ancestral traditions, genocide, slavery, exploitation, and forced labor (Lugones, 2007).

Alongside these two sides is "an ambiguous in-between zone" for those who fall short of the sex-gender binary and Whiteness, "racialized . . . but not as white" (p. 208).

We derive two conclusions from reading the colonial materiality of racial capitalism through Freud and Fanon. First, the oppressed—whether Black, Indigenous, and other People of Color, women, queer, and working-class people—are no less vulnerable to being seduced by the *jouissance* of relative privilege, with anti-Blackness a foundational source of enjoyment. Cis-heterosexual men of color, for example, may attempt to repair hegemonic masculinity, a symptom of symbolic and literal wounding by White supremacy, through the oppression of cis-heterosexual and queer Women of Color—especially those with darker skin (see Chavez-Dueñas et al., 2014; Comas-Díaz, 2021). Second, the suffering of the privileged is different though related to that of women and non-White, poor, and queer people. Although patriarchy privileges men, and antiwoman queerphobia provides a *jouissance* that ratifies one's "being a man," men suffer because of the cis-heterosexist structure of racial capitalism.

Put bluntly, there would be no "fear of falling to the bottom," of losing one's masculinity, whiteness, wealth, and the like—if there were no bottom. This fear maintains elite power, weaponizing our suffering against one another while offering an unreachable *jouissance*—"you too can be like us." The ethics of psychoanalysis, whether clinical or communal, are "to call each other to reject this [racial capitalist] system as we perform a transformation of communal relations" (Lugones, 2007, p. 189), following Freud, to value one another and leave Whiteness, toxic masculinity, and wealth "to the angels and the sparrows." This theoretical position, we argue, has a bearing on clinical and communal work.

A DECOLONIZING PSYCHOANALYTIC APPROACH TO CLINICAL AND COMMUNITY WORK

This understanding of suffering articulates how the suffering of colonizer and of colonized groups are different and distinct though indelibly related. It also recontextualizes analytic principles such as attunement, defensive functioning, containment, analytic listening, mentalization, multiplicity, transference or countertransference, and so on, in collective and systemic contexts (González & Peltz, 2021). One is not intervening on a "patient" but a relational system embedded within a political-economic structure. In what follows, we elucidate a brief theoretical and research-informed sketch of decolonial psychoanalysis in clinical and communal work.

Research on attachment and cultural humility supports the effectiveness of a "not-knowing" stance that allows therapists "to keep their minds open and allow a space for their patients to reflect on their own" (Talia et al., 2020, p. 14) and to be "other-oriented (or open to the other) in relation to aspects of cultural identity that are most important to the client," (Davis et al., 2018, p. 91). This stance strengthens the patient–therapist bond while helping them survive, process, and repair ruptures when power and status become salient (Davis et al., 2018), decolonizing the subjectivity of both patient and therapist. To accomplish this, we advocate paying close attention to both verbal and body language in the clinical encounter, integrating Lacanian (Pavón-Cuéllar & González Equihua, 2013) and relational (Wachtel, 2011) psychoanalytic perspectives on language. This clinical approach calls on us to complement our clinical listening for the language of attachment and relationship with listening for the language of power, status, and hierarchy in words and action (Gaztambide, 2022).

Decolonizing psychoanalysis must also be integrative in considering the unconscious as an embodied phenomenon. As noted, colonialism produced racial, gender, and sexual divisions that distorted the cultures of Global South peoples (Oyěwùmí, 1997), reflected in the dualism establishing the primacy of mind over body. Pavón-Cuéllar (2018) showed how this dichotomy establishes intellectual labor as superior to physical labor, in turn licensing those who consider themselves "superior" to force those who are "inferior" to engage in physical, motoric "body" labor. Mainstream psychoanalysis' historical preference for words over action similarly emplaces certain forms of clinical work as superior, marginalizing Global South people as not "psychologically minded" (Aron & Starr, 2013; Gaztambide, 2019). Conversely, other analytic thinkers, such as Reich (1933/1970) and Fenichel (see Gaztambide, 2019), located the unconscious in the body as a material reality, with symptoms as our body's attempt to communicate what we must change in our lives. This idea transcends psychoanalysis itself to ancestral and Indigenous knowledge (see Gaztambide, 2019). Trauma, for example, becomes archived in the body through postures and motoric gestures that seek to protect people from retraumatization.

One contemporary approach for listening to the body is the use of *rituales de reflexividad* (rituals of reflexivity; Moreno & Lozano, 2014), in which participants in a group are invited to breathe and connect with their bodies while reflecting on the elite discourses we have internalized, normalized in a way that limits our imaginative capacities. During such rituals, mindfulness and bodily exercises are employed to deepen reflection. Noboa Ortega (2019) illustrated a similar clinical-political dynamism through the work of the Legal Psychological Clinic in Puerto Rico after Hurricane Maria. Community group discussions "create a common space where people can talk to each other about their suffering . . . [build] proximity and trust, and enhance one's social support network." Alongside community discussions around policy change, individual therapy helps "elaborate through words the pain and sadness they are dealing with" (p. 282). Such examples of community psychoanalysis illustrate a form of "political mentalization" (Gaztambide, 2019), the process of reflecting dynamically on self and others in relational and sociopolitical contexts. We now provide three case examples—two clinical and one community focused—that illustrate the principles just elucidated.

CLINICAL ILLUSTRATIONS

In these cases, we strive to show how (a) psychoanalytically informed therapists and activists attend to issues of power and identity, (b) how the suffering of marginalized and privileged groups are distinct though related, and (c) how reflecting on this dynamism promotes therapeutic and communal change.

Case One

Noora (pseudonym) was a young adult Black Muslim woman I (José Luiggi-Hernández) saw in psychotherapy for generalized anxiety, depressed mood, and a sense of helplessness. She presented as shy, made little eye contact, and spoke with a soft voice that made it difficult for me to hear her. At the time, she could not identify the cause of her anxiety but recognized that it affected her relationships. Through free association, she became aware of her fear she would upset others if she expressed her opinions, choosing to be silent or "[telling] people what they want[ed] to hear." She felt it futile to express her needs, not trusting that her voice could be heard or her knowledge seen as having value. Through further exploration, Noora linked her anxiety, fear, and passivity to an early life experience in which her voice was negated. She witnessed an emergency at home and tried to alert her father. At the time, he was in deep conversation with a guest and, when Noora interrupted, aggressively told her not to disrupt them. Her plea to listen was cut down by her father yelling that women and children do not interrupt men while they speak. Throughout her life, Noora felt silenced by male peers, supervisors, and romantic partners; her voice trampled, her intellect belittled or rejected.

Noting the possibility of both a relational and a status-based transference, I focused on building a relationship with Noora in which she could speak her mind while I reflected her words and mirrored her body language without assuming their meaning. The relationship with me—as someone who presents as White and male—could provide a corrective experience in which she could exert her voice while someone positioned as "higher" on a gender or race hierarchy bore witness without intruding on her agency in a way that demanded she "tell [me] what [I] want to hear." In subsequent sessions, Noora expressed grievances about her father and other men in her life, often raising her voice, which was followed by increased assertiveness at work and her romantic relationship at the time. Although her symptoms improved, Noora still felt a degree of impotence with a work supervisor and her partner. Noora was ignored, spoken over, or silenced despite her attempts at voicing her opinions with these men. She felt stuck both in therapy and the position a racist and sexist society emplaced her in as a Black woman.

Traditional formulations could interpret Noora's helplessness as the result of intrapsychic or relational dynamics, but this would only partially explain her symptoms and risk of "unlink[ing] the psychic from the social" (Layton, 2020). I needed to help Noora link her experience to the sociopolitical structures in which she lived, conditions enacted through her speech. Noora asked in one of our sessions, "Why are men like this? Why is my dad like this? I feel like if they don't change, things won't change." I reflected this statement back to her, accentuating particular words and adding language she used in previous sessions, "If *men* don't change if your *father*—an *orthodox Muslim man*—doesn't change, things won't change." Noora let out a deep sigh, becoming reflective in the silence that ensued. Rather than silencing Noora's experience, the intervention oriented her back to her own knowledge as valid and valuable, which she used to fill the silence that emerged. She talked about her father's experience as a Black Muslim man in the United States, and how patriarchy provided him with relative power within a structure that disempowers Black men. She explored how his power, and that of other men in her life, subjugated her and other Black women.

Mentalizing about her father within their political context helped Noora empathize with him while understanding his role in upholding Black patriarchy, and thus complicity in her distress. She appreciated his complex position as someone who, in navigating and surviving White supremacy, also upheld beliefs that erased her subjectivity. This led Noora to communicate her feelings to her father, leading to a more gratifying relationship. She also began a new relationship with a man who could really hear her. At work, she began talking about her experience with her male supervisor with women coworkers who revealed they shared her experience while noting his pointed hostility toward her. They reported this to human resources and organized around ways of making their voices heard at work. Notably, Noora began a series of art projects highlighting women's struggles and other issues she was invested in. In this sense, she "[chose] action with respect [to] the social structures" (Fanon, 1952/2008, p. 80).

Case Two

"Mr. R" (pseudonym) is a middle adult cisgender heterosexual White male who was in treatment with me (Edlyane Veronica Medina Escobar) after moving from another state where he lost a high-paying job in a tech startup. At the time of our work together, he was unemployed and having difficulty finding work in his field. He often started sessions presenting himself as cordial, asking "how are *you*?" and embodying contradictory affect by smiling and looking wide-eyed as if he were on high alert. During our sessions, Mr. R would become distressed about his professional instability, having lost work opportunities central to his identity and self-worth. He often mentioned his terror about finding work but struggled to elaborate on his feelings and thoughts. When I attempted to probe deeper, he irritated me, stating he would instead "move on" than dwell on his experience. Although he was initially open to exploring his anxiety around finding work, by midtreatment, he became deeply uncomfortable whenever it came up. He was increasingly dissatisfied with our work and made it known by resisting exploration as a way to "take back" some of the power he had lost in social status. A White, cis, heterosexual middle-class male, he was seen by a person who presents as non-White and femme.

I could feel Mr. R's need to control the treatment. He would demand that I give him tools to cope with his "anxiety," but when exploring his symptoms, he asked to change topics, often stating that "there is no use" dwelling on his struggles, remarking that he "is better than this." I felt a deep empathy for his financial struggles, as someone who has been of low socioeconomic status all my life but felt pushed away whenever I tried to know more about his experience. He was signaling we had nothing in common and were not on the same "level." As a budding clinician, I felt his discomfort with having me as a therapist and felt nervous addressing his reactions to me. He seemed to enjoy feeling powerful in the room, shifting from helplessness to tyranny. I became his object of aggression as a young woman of color, a degraded being he—a White man—could not imagine being a source of healing and relief. As we neared termination, I stressed the importance of exploring the end of our work together. Appalled, he stressed, "I don't want to talk about that *with you*; I think I'm done." He grabbed his bookbag and motioned to get up from his chair but did not, stuck between valuing me as someone who offered care and relationship and as someone devalued as "beneath" him.

Looking back on this case, I realize I experienced firsthand the most common form of racial enactment—the silencing of race (Leary, 2000). This was my first experience of racial silencing in the therapeutic sense. I was rendered silent in naming myself as more than my racial stimulus value and kept silent about my client's Whiteness in the room. In silencing me, he reproduced a privileged enjoyment that simultaneously silenced his own needs, fears, and yearnings that did not fit within White, capitalist masculinity. I still reflect on why I did not broach the silencing of race in this therapy, being left with more questions than answers: What is the role of White rage in the therapeutic room? Do therapists of color have to scaffold White rage, or can we denounce White power in the room? What are therapists and patients enacting in pursuing "human status" (Fanon, 1952/2008)? Although I felt racialized in this context, I am mindful that I inhabit an ambiguous space with my Brown skin and can use my stimulus value as a clinical tool to explore a client's fantasies about these hierarchies. A Black femme clinician might have been the target of degradation to the extent that I might never experience. This example conveys the ever-present *jouissance* of pursuing power and place present in both clients and therapists, highlighting the importance of challenging the silence around Whiteness, hegemonic masculinity, and class mobility, including—and especially—with White clients.

Case Three

In the Puerto Rico metropolitan area, a group of parents sought guidance from my (Fabián E. Feliciano-Graniela's) team in working through their guilt and ambivalence after responding negatively to their queer children "coming out."[1] Although they wanted to repair their parent–child relationships, they felt conflicted due to their conservative values. We joined with the parents using an intervention drawn from reflexivity rituals (Moreno & Lozano, 2014) and body-based exercises to assist in processing their experiences and seeing them in a new light. Our interventions consisted of four meetings. We explored their conceptions of sexuality and gender to generate dialogue and critical reflection; used body-based exercises to help them process and liberate tensions built up due to guilt, fear, and shame; and created opportunities for self-forgiveness and acceptance. We carried out these interventions in hybrid modalities, one team member meeting the mothers in person and another team member and I assisting asynchronously due to social distancing during the pandemic and some participants' being unable to leave their home. We worked around these and other daily obstacles to manage our work, professional development, and maternal duties when the earthquakes

---

[1] This team was a collaboration within the Diplomado Internacional Latinoamericano de Psicología Corporal, Teoría de la Praxis y Psicopolítica de la Liberación, led by a collaboration between Mónica Cintrón (Puerto Rico) and Érico Roberto Schleu (Brazil).

and the poor government management were wreaking havoc throughout the south of the archipelago of Puerto Rico.

During the first encounter, we introduced a guided visualization exercise[2] to help the parents imagine what it would be like to live a day in the shoes of those who are othered because of their sexual orientation. The exercise involved narrating an alternate world in which the cis-heterosexual majority was now the ostracized minority needing to hide "in the closet." Following the guided visualization, we explored the somatic experience of the feelings evoked by imagining themselves in their children's shoes. The parents reported feeling sad and uncomfortable for having to hide who they really were during the visualization process, which helped them understand how terrible and uncomfortable it was for their children to be othered.

The second encounter consisted of reflexivity rituals to deepen exploration of the group's conceptions of gender and sexuality, and promote critical consciousness about the distortions and hierarchical scripts we have internalized, problematizing them in structural context. In doing so, we opened space for organizing and action. Through the rituals, the parents reflected on the fact their children belong to an oppressed group, attending to the somatic impact of this insight on their bodies, which helped them become aware of how avoidance of conflicted emotions manifested in muscular tension, irregular breathing, and feelings of fatigue. The third meeting focused on helping the parents stay present with their bodily experience of repressed guilt, shame, and fear. We used movement to "shake off" and dissipate this stress, allowing for a newfound recognition of how these feelings had been "archived" in the body—the *jouissance* of a privileged cis-heterosexual position drawn into conflict with their attachment to their children.

By the end of the third encounter, the parents had developed a communal identity and were conscious of the commonalities and struggles that united them. They were able to transform their feelings of guilt and shame into self-compassion and forgiveness, anchored in the awareness that their LGBTQ+ prejudices and fears were not innate but the product of patriarchy and conservative religion. As a result, the parents were able to heal the rupture that occurred when their children came out, valuing familial bonds over the *jouissance* offered by the cis-heterosexism that stood in the way of their attachment to their loved ones.

During this process, I was torn by the imposition of having to earn a livelihood while dedicating my time to an act that I was not only passionate about

---

[2] The exercise was written by Miguel Vázquez Rivera, a psychologist who specializes in queer affirmative therapy and works closely with the LGBTQIA+ community in Puerto Rico.

but also implied a step toward decolonizing the archipelago of patriarchal norms imposed by colonial invasion. To be nonbinary and nonheterosexual in this colony is to walk on the margins of abjection, yet being a White Puerto Rican confers privileges that "soften the blow" of being queer. I reflected on how I longed for the safety of being in communion with queer folks growing up and how different my life would have been if I had received support earlier in life. In assisting these mothers with their conflict between their feelings of love and their colonized moralism, I assisted their healing process and healed as well. It felt awkward, at first, to be a fresh college graduate in psychology doing the kind of work that I deemed ethically and politically necessary to help build a society free from the shackles of patriarchal and colonial violence. The system does not allow us to imagine what work outside the clinic can look like, but we dared to dream and design that work together.

PRACTICE RECOMMENDATIONS

Based on our clinical experience, drawn from the previous three cases, we offer a series of practice recommendations. First, we advocate for a synthesis of what we call political mentalization (Gaztambide, 2019) and political action. Although psychoanalysis has historically focused on the individual patient and the psychic causes of their symptoms, psychoanalytic clinicians often fail to address how the sociopolitical issues influence the development of symptoms and their treatment. Addressing these issues does not imply rejecting interpersonal or intrapsychic dynamics that influence psychic suffering, but amplifies the complexity of lived experience and human suffering, aids in deepening contextual self-understanding, and fosters mentalization about how the sociopolitical influences the psychological experience of self and other. Moreover, it opens an avenue of exploring engagement in not only changing one's immediate context/environment but also the macro level determinants of suffering. Although psychoanalytic work has often focused on changing interpersonal and intrapsychic dynamics, a decolonial and Fanonian approach to psychoanalytic treatment must always move the patient toward changing the root of suffering—the social structure.

Second, we advocate for integrative psychoanalytic treatment, drawing from the skills, techniques, and interventions of other approaches to therapy to attend to the unique needs of the patient rather than limiting our work to psychoanalytic technique. At times, these tools address unique stressors that arise from the person's unique life world, including include body-oriented work as presented in the last case study.

CONCLUSION

In what follows, we offer practice recommendations for psychoanalytic training, theory, and future scholarship. First, psychoanalytically oriented training needs to teach its history frankly, acknowledging its liberationist potential and colonial complicity (Ahad, 2010; Brickman, 2017; Danto, 2005). Second, existing theories need to be recontextualized in a social and political context. Tummala-Narra (2016) and Comas-Díaz (2021), for example, drew on "traditional" relational theory reinterpreted through a robust cultural perspective alongside the work of scholars of color. Third, psychoanalysis needs to be integrative, with other therapeutic schools such as cognitive behavior therapy (Wachtel, 2011), somatic and body-based approaches (Moreno & Lozano, 2014), and psychoanalysis from the Global South (Pavón-Cuéllar, 2018).

More fundamentally, we argue for a new premise in psychoanalytic thinking. As elucidated earlier, we seem to have multiple Freuds and in turn multiple psychoanalyses—a "proto-decolonial and cultural" Freud who wrote about culture, race, religion, and capitalism, and a "colonial and clinical" Freud who wrote about child development and clinical treatment, but without addressing the sociocultural context. What if we instead understood Freud himself as torn and conflicted precisely by his relation to race in a capitalist world? What if we took on the task of integrating these two Freuds—and thus psychoanalysis? Reading Freud through Fanon would suggest that to the extent we attend to early attachment and the language of relationships, we must do so in the context of another language—the language of power, identity, and status.

In essence, the premise of psychoanalysis should not be an unconscious solely preoccupied with one's relations to others but an unconscious that exists in a matrix of political-economic relationships textured by race, class, gender, and sexuality within a racial capitalist world. Our fundamental premise is that human beings are as much concerned with where we stand on a given hierarchy and in the community as we are with relationships, attachment, and care. This would mean that if one takes the unconscious seriously, one should also attend to those ways, ever so subtle and implicit, in which our relatedness is always already taking place in, and infused by, a context of power. To be clear, to address this not only when some axis of difference between patient and therapist is perceived (e.g., patients of color, LGBTQ+, working-class, female), but as a matter of course with all patient–therapist configurations (Sue et al., 2019).

Outside of the consulting room, our perspective dovetails with race-class research showing how racism functions as a weapon of class warfare, empowering racist politicians and policies that harm all of us (Helms, 2016; McGhee,

2021). As a form of messaging and a political analysis, this work calls on us to reject racism, call out elites fomenting division, and come together to build a world for *all* of us, Black, White, and Brown (López, 2019). To clarify, we do not subscribe to an "all lives matter" discourse. On the contrary, we find the race-class approach echoes a core insight of the decolonial tradition in psychoanalysis—that the suffering of oppressed and privileged peoples are structurally different, though at the same time structurally related. If the primary purpose of racism within a racial capitalist world is to foment division and shore up the power of wealthy elites, then this work invites us to develop theories of suffering that can hold and deepen reflection on this tension. To paraphrase Paulo Freire (1972), the goal of such work should be to develop understandings of suffering that free ourselves and our oppressor as well (p. 28). Specifically, to develop tools that shatter the *jouissance* that maintains our attachment to this world and imagines a new world outside the colony.

We end both with and beyond Freud. For Freud, social justice "means that we deny ourselves many things so that others may have to do without them as well" (Gaztambide, 2019, p. 71). This opposes colonial desire—to visit violence upon the vulnerable in search of power and "moving up" in the system. Social justice, Freud tells us, involves our renunciation of the *jouissance* that harms all of us through "the influence of a common affectionate tie with a person outside the group" (Gaztambide, 2019, p. 71). By identifying with one another, we stand to enact a decolonial process inside and outside the session. We go beyond Freud's invitation to leave Heaven to "the angels and the sparrows" and end with the wisdom of the Indigenous Taino hero, Hatuey. When Hatuey was captured for rebelling against the Spaniards, he was asked if he would accept Jesus and "go to Heaven" before being burned at the stake. He asked if Spaniards went to Heaven. When told they did, Hatuey, without hesitation, replied he preferred to go to Hell. Beyond the clinic, Hell must be raised for Heaven to be torn down.

RESOURCES

Desplechin, A. (Director). (2013). *Jimmy P* [Film]. https://www.imdb.com/title/tt2210834/

Julien, I. (Director). (1995). *Frantz Fanon: Black skin, white masks* [Film trailer]. YouTube. https://www.youtube.com/watch?v=UOFLt_IhIfE

Winograd, B. (2020, July 22). *Black psychoanalysts speak* [Video]. YouTube. https://youtu.be/N8-Vli7tb44

REFERENCES

Adames, H. Y., & Chavez-Dueñas, N. Y. (2021). Reclaiming all of me: The racial queer identity framework. In K. L. Nadal & M. R. Scharrón-del Río (Eds.), *Queer psychology* (pp. 59–79). Springer. https://doi.org/10.1007/978-3-030-74146-4_4

Ahad, B. S. (2010). *Freud upside down: African American literature and psychoanalytic culture*. University of Illinois Press.

Aron, L., & Starr, K. (2013). *A psychotherapy for the people: Toward a progressive psychoanalysis*. Routledge. https://doi.org/10.4324/9780203098059

Beshara, R. K. (2021). *Freud and Said: Contrapuntal psychoanalysis as liberation praxis*. Palgrave Macmillan. https://doi.org/10.1007/978-3-030-56743-9

Brickman, C. (2017). *Race in psychoanalysis: Aboriginal populations in the mind*. Routledge. https://doi.org/10.4324/9781351718523

Bynum, E. B. (1999). *The African unconscious: Roots of ancient mysticism and modern psychology*. Teachers College Press.

Chavez-Dueñas, N. Y., Adames, H. Y., & Organista, K. C. (2014). Skin-color prejudice and within-group racial discrimination: Historical and current impact on Latino/a populations. *Hispanic Journal of Behavioral Sciences, 36*(1), 3–26. https://doi.org/10.1177/0739986313511306

Comas-Díaz, L. (2021). AfroLatinx females: Coloniality, gender, and transformation. *Studies in Gender and Sexuality, 22*(4), 322–332. https://doi.org/10.1080/15240657.2021.1996741

Danto, E. A. (2005). *Freud's free clinics*. Columbia University Press. https://doi.org/10.7312/dant13180

Davis, D. E., DeBlaere, C., Owen, J., Hook, J. N., Rivera, D. P., Choe, E., Van Tongeren, D. R., Worthington, E. L., Jr., & Placeres, V. (2018). The multicultural orientation framework: A narrative review. *Psychotherapy, 55*(1), 89–100. https://doi.org/10.1037/pst0000160

Fanon, F. (2008). *Black skin, White masks*. Pluto Press. (Original work published 1952)

Fenichel, O. (1940). Psychoanalysis of antisemitism. *The American Imago, 1*(2), 24–39. https://www.jstor.org/stable/26300856

Fink, B. (1999). *A clinical introduction to Lacanian psychoanalysis: Theory and technique*. Harvard University Press.

Freire, P. (1972). *Pedagogy of the oppressed*. Continuum.

Freud, S. (1915). The unconscious. In J. Strachey, A. Freud, A. Strachey (Eds.), & A. Tyson (Trans.), *On the history of the psycho-analytic movement: Articles about metapsychology and other works (1914–1916): Vol. XIV. The standard edition of the complete psychological works of Sigmund Freud* (pp. 141–216). Hogarth Press.

Freud, S. (1927). The future of an illusion. In J. Strachey (Ed.), *The standard edition of the complete psychological works of Sigmund Freud: Vol. XXI (1927–1931)* (pp. 1–56). Hogarth Press.

Gaztambide, D. (2019). *A people's history of psychoanalysis: From Freud to liberation psychology*. Lexington Books.

Gaztambide, D. J. (2021). Do Black lives matter in psychoanalysis? Frantz Fanon as our most disputatious ancestor. *Psychoanalytic Psychology, 38*(3), 177–184. https://doi.org/10.1037/pap0000365

Gaztambide, D. (2022). Love in a time of anti-Blackness: Social rank, attachment, and race in psychotherapy. *Attachment & Human Development, 24*(3), 353–365. https://doi.org/10.1080/14616734.2021.1976935

Gilman, S. L. (1993). Freud, race, and gender. Princeton University Press.

González, F. J., & Peltz, R. (2021). Community psychoanalysis: Collaborative practice as intervention. *Psychoanalytic Dialogues, 31*(4), 409–427. https://doi.org/10.1080/10481885.2021.1926788

Graeber, D., & Wengrow, D. (2021). *The dawn of everything.* Penguin.

Helms, J. (2016). An election to save White, heterosexual male privilege (WHMP). *Latino Psychology Today, 3*(2), 6–7.

Helms, J. E. (2020). *A race is a nice thing to have: A guide to being a White person or understanding the White persons in your life* (3rd ed.). Cognella.

Hirschfeld, M. (1938). *Racism.* Port Washington.

Lacan, J. (1955/2002). The Freudian thing, or the meaning of the return to Freud in psychoanalysis. *Ecrits: A Selection.* W. W. Norton.

Layton, L. (2020). Attacks on linking: The unconscious pull to dissociate individuals from their social context. In M. Leavy-Sperounis (Ed.), *Towards a social psycho analysis: Culture, character, and normative unconscious processes* (pp. 34–44). Routledge. https://doi.org/10.4324/9781003023098-4

Leary, K. (2000). Racial enactments in dynamic treatment. *Psychoanalytic Dialogues, 10*(4), 639–653. https://doi.org/10.1080/10481881009348573

Leuzinger-Bohleber, M., Solms, M., & Arnold, S. E. (Eds.). (2020). *Outcome research and the future of psychoanalysis: Clinicians and researchers in dialogue.* Routledge. https://doi.org/10.4324/9780429281112

López, I. H. (2019). *Merge left: Fusing race and class, winning elections, and saving America.* The New Press.

Lugones, M. (2007). Heterosexualism and the colonial/modern gender system. *Hypatia, 22*(1), 186–219. https://doi.org/10.1111/j.1527-2001.2007.tb01156.x

Maldonado-Torres, N., France, M. F. M., Suffla, S., Seedat, M., & Ratele, K. (2021). Fanon's decolonial transcendence of psychoanalysis. *Studies in Gender and Sexuality, 22*(4), 243–255. https://doi.org/10.1080/15240657.2021.1996727

Mann, B. A. (2001). *Native American speakers of the eastern woodlands: Selected speeches and critical analyses.* ABC-CLIO.

Mannoni, O. (1990). *Prospero and Caliban: The psychology of colonization* (P. Powesland, Trans.). University of Michigan Press. (Original work published 1950)

Manuellan, M. J. (2017). *Sous la dictée de Fanon.* L'Amourier.

Martín-Baró, I. (1994). *Writings for a liberation psychology.* Harvard University Press.

McGhee, H. (2021). *The sum of us: What racism costs everyone and how we can prosper together.* One World.

McGowan, T. (2013). *Enjoying what we don't have: The political project of psychoanalysis.* University of Nebraska Press. https://doi.org/10.2307/j.ctt1ddr7nv

Moreno, A., & Lozano, L. (2014). Modelo de investigación-intervención y acompañamiento psicosocial a través de la metodología de los rituales de reflexividad [Research-intervention model and psychosocial support through the methodology of reflexivity rituals]. *Revista Latinoamericana de Psicología Social Ignacio Martín-Baró, 3*(1), 157–174.

Noboa Ortega, P. (2019). Psychoanalysis as a political act after María. In Y. Bonilla & M. LeBrón (Eds.), *Aftershocks of disaster* (pp. 271–284). Haymarket Books.

Oyěwùmí, O. (1997). *The invention of women: Making an African sense of western gender discourses.* University of Minnesota Press.

Pavón-Cuéllar, D. (2018). Marxism, psychoanalysis, and the critique of psychological dualism: From dualist repression to the return of the repressed in hysteria and class consciousness. *Theory & Psychology, 28*(3), 319–339. https://doi.org/10.1177/0959354318766415

Pavón-Cuéllar, D., & González Equihua, E. E. (2013). Subversive psychoanalysis and its potential orientation toward a liberation psychology: From a Lacanian reading of Martín-Baró to a committed use of Jacques Lacan. *Theory & Psychology, 23*(5), 639–656. https://doi.org/10.1177/0959354313494274

Reich, W. (1933/1970). *The mass psychology of fascism*. Macmillan.

Robinson, C. J. (2021). Black Marxism, revised and updated third edition: The making of the Black radical tradition. UNC Press Books.

Sioui, G. (1992). *For an Amerindian autohistory: An essay on the foundations of a social ethic*. McGill-Queen's University Press.

Steckley, J. L. (2014). *The eighteenth-century Wyandot: A clan-based study*. Wilfrid Laurier University Press.

Sue, D. W., Sue, D., Neville, H. A., & Smith, L. (2019). *Counseling the culturally diverse: Theory and practice*. John Wiley & Sons.

Talia, A., Muzi, L., Lingiardi, V., & Taubner, S. (2020). How to be a secure base: Therapists' attachment representations and their link to attunement in psychotherapy. *Attachment & Human Development, 22*(2), 189–206. https://doi.org/10.1080/14616734.2018.1534247

Tate, C. (1996). Freud and his "Negro": Psychoanalysis as ally and enemy of African Americans. *Psychoanalysis, Culture & Society, 1*(1), 53–62.

Tummala-Narra, P. (2016). *Psychoanalytic theory and cultural competence in psychotherapy*. American Psychological Association. https://doi.org/10.1037/14800-000

Turner, L., & Neville, H. A. (Eds.). (2020). *Frantz Fanon's psychotherapeutic approaches to clinical work: Practicing internationally with marginalized communities*. Routledge. https://doi.org/10.4324/9780429465307

Wachtel, P. L. (2011). *Therapeutic communication: Knowing what to say when*. Guilford Press.

14 DECOLONIZING FEMINIST THERAPY

THEMA BRYANT, CAROLYN ZERBE ENNS, AND
YUYING TSONG

Feminist therapy was established to transform and decolonize psychotherapy by linking personal challenges with social and political forces and barriers. It became an important tool for individuals to understand how they had internalized and become hostage to patriarchal and other oppressive values, and to reframe symptoms as efforts to cope and survive rather than as signs of intrapsychic pathology (Brown, 2018; Kirsh, 1974). This chapter examines the evolution of feminist therapy, its limitations, the ways in which it has been challenged, and the alignment of intersectional feminist therapy with decolonial aims. Ongoing critical examination of the decolonization of feminist practice is needed. We describe gaps between ideals and actual practice and highlight the contributions of those who have offered decolonizing perspectives for feminist therapy practice. We also build on relevant American Psychological Association (APA) guidelines (2018, 2019) to propose tenets for ongoing transformation.

Author's note: The authors contributed equally; the order of names is alphabetical.

https://doi.org/10.1037/0000376-015

Decolonial Psychology: Toward Anticolonial Theories, Research, Training, and Practice,
L. Comas-Díaz, H. Y. Adames, and N. Y. Chavez-Dueñas (Editors)

INTRODUCTION AND HERSTORY

The founding premise of feminist therapy was that psychotherapy, especially therapy for women, needed to be transformed. Early feminist criticism of mainstream therapy focused on challenging the patriarchal nature of the psychotherapy relationship (Chesler, 1972), rejecting traditional diagnosis (Rawlings & Carter, 1977), and calling for widespread social change and advocacy rather than an emphasis on individual change alone. Thus, many of the early ideals of feminist therapy aligned with the values and goals of decolonization. For example, radical Black feminists and activists, such as the Combahee River Collective (1983), formed in 1973, committed themselves to address sexism, racism, heterosexism, and economic oppression within capitalism. However, it is also clear that feminist theory and practice are not monolithic (Enns, 2004) but are situated and informed by diverse life experiences, social locations, and philosophical foundations.

By the mid-1980s, feminists of color pointed out the ethnocentrism and racism within White feminism and practice and called for more inclusive feminisms (Anzaldúa, 1987; Collins, 1986). bell hooks (1989) also expressed concern that White women were likely to use civil rights movements to gain prominence and power for themselves, which would reinforce "historical servant-served relationships where White women have used power to dominate, exploit, and oppress" (p. 179). Critics noted that frameworks for feminist therapy were developed primarily "by and with White women" (Brown, 1990, p. 3), based primarily on the realities of White, middle-class women, viewed gender oppression as a framework for understanding all or most other oppressions, and were inattentive to the perspectives of Women of Color as well other social experiences such as economic hardship, homophobia, racism, and classism. Audre Lorde (1984) and Aída Hurtado (1989) elaborated on women's different experiences of oppression, stating that whereas White women were often "seduced by the oppressor under the pretense of sharing power" (Lorde, 1984, pp. 118–119) with men, Women of Color remained subjugated as objects of rejection.

These critiques led to the recognition that feminism and feminist therapy need to address the different realities of women with diverse social identities, oppressions, and privileges. Lillian Comas-Díaz (1994) proposed using the term *colonization* rather than oppression to reflect ways in which People of Color are required to accept dominant cultural norms to survive, norms that require "inevitable sacrifice" (p. 288) of one's culture of origin. Painful adaptations to colonial realities often result in self-denial, alienation, identity conflicts, racialized objectification, and a definition of womanhood shaped by dominant cultural values. Comas-Díaz also proposed using an integrative approach for working with Women of Color. She described "a therapeutic decolonizing and empowering perspective that is aware of ethnicity, race, and gender" (p. 287). As a way of centering the perspectives of Women of Color, womanist and *mujerista* psychologies (e.g., Bryant-Davis & Comas-Díaz, 2016) challenged dominant forms of feminism. They emphasized collective forms of liberation, mutual caring, community, and global solidarity among Women of Color. Feminist scholars of color propose using decolonization, critical consciousness, and intersectionality concepts to challenge monocultural feminist practice (Bryant-Davis, 2019). More recent is the call to attend to the complex realities of global existence such as immigration, border crossings, displacement, refugee status, hybrid and third-culture identities, colonial legacies, various diasporic communities, and diverse Indigenous identities in transnational feminist practice (Enns et al., 2021). Transnational feminism also must cultivate a critical consciousness of race, coloniality, and culture as women-centered practices (Noh, 2003) and be attentive to the gendered impact of colonialism, imperialism, global structural forces that reinforce economic exploitation and the dominance of northern world regions over southern regions (Enns et al., 2021; Macleod et al., 2020).

Thus this chapter presents critical consciousness–informed feminist therapy practices as a decolonizing force through critical reflection (reflexive examinations of internalized colonialism and White supremacy as feminist therapists), critical awareness (awareness and knowledge of the herstory and evolution of feminist therapy, colonial patterns, and White supremacy in White feminist therapy and feminism, and so on), and critical actions (strategies and activism to resist colonization and injustices).

Definitions

Critical consciousness refers to oppressed and marginalized people's critical reflection and analyses of their social conditions and the individual or collective critical action to produce social change (Diemer et al., 2017; Freire, 1970; Watts et al., 2011). It was originally developed as a pedagogical tool for the oppressed to think critically about social inequalities and to take actions to change the status quo (Freire, 1973); through critical reflections and actions, oppressed individuals develop agency despite existing structural constraints (Diemer et al., 2017). Further, in a "transitive" relationship between critical reflection and critical action greater reflection leads to greater action and vice versa (Freire, 1970, 1973). We use the phrase critical consciousness–informed feminist therapy practices to emphasize that the process is ongoing and evolving and involves lifelong critical learning, reflection, and action. It starts with equipping oneself with tools to understand the world and the inequitable social conditions through a critical lens, interrogating one's acceptance and normalization of oppressions, and shifting one's relationship with White supremacy and patriarchy to dismantle systems of oppression and promoting healing and liberation for all people.

Colonizing refers to the "visible and invisible attempts to socialize and resocialize those at the margins to fit into dominant cultural values and experiences" and decolonization involves "examining the concepts of power and access to opportunities while critically questioning and disrupting the systems and structures that maintain inequities" (Singh et al., 2020, p. 262). Because feminist therapists work with clients to critically reflect and analyze inequalities and oppressions and the resulting mental health consequences, we should reflect on the colonizing messages we may have internalized and perpetrated. Critical reflection and questioning are particularly important for healing internalized colonization. They can remove the blame and shame and shift toward understanding the systematic roots of oppressions and lead to healing, empowerment, and critical actions.

CRITICAL REFLECTIONS OF HISTORICAL AND CURRENT ISSUES AND PRACTICE CHALLENGES

A decolonizing feminist therapy is built on ongoing critical reflection, reflexivity, and humility about areas in which feminist practices have fallen short of ideals. In this section, we discuss overlapping and related challenges that are necessary to address as feminist therapists work toward correcting and transcending omissions, incomplete visions, and inadequate actions. Many of the problems we describe involve failures of reflexivity, lack of awareness or humility about positionality, or limited awareness of or will to challenge social and institutional power structures.

At a personal level, reflexivity and the examination of one's positionality require challenging one's unconscious, implicit (as well as explicit) biases as they relate to how one's relationships within power structures may influence one's work, reworking one's worldviews, building trust, and increasing effectiveness and transforming practice. Disciplinary reflexivity, a companion to personal reflexivity, emphasizes the critical examination of psychology's knowledge-producing structures and professional practices (Macleod et al., 2020). Decolonization necessitates a sociohistorical frame not only of nations, communities, and individuals but also of fields, and calls on feminists to work toward erasing the legacies of institutional and disciplinary racism, sexism, and other isms.

Disconnections Between Ideals and Reality

During the early years of feminist practice, feminist therapy collectives as well as rape and domestic violence crisis centers offered egalitarian services within structures that worked toward social and personal change. They countered hierarchical institutional foundations and the ethnocentric, misogynistic, racist, and heterosexist assumptions embedded in these institutions. However, sustaining the energy, commitment, and finances necessary to maintain egalitarian structures was challenging, and feminist services were gradually characterized by greater specialization, professionalization, and bureaucracy (Matthews, 1994). Feminist therapy practice was also influenced by external pressures such as diagnostic challenges, managed care, health insurance reimbursement mandates and limits, narrow definitions of appropriate research support for treatment, and concerns about risk management versus optimal treatment (Brown, 2018). As a result, ideals, especially those related to social change, have been challenging to maintain.

The transformational and social change ideals that feminist therapists espouse have often been displayed inconsistently, which raises questions about the feasibility of transforming and decolonizing feminist practice within professional disciplines such as psychology (Brown, 2018). One study concluded that feminist therapists typically worked "within existing gender arrangements and social institutions and did not overtly challenge systems of power operating in society" (Marecek & Kravetz, 1998, p. 26). Dana Becker (2005), author of the *Myth of Empowerment*, added that as feminist therapy evolved, empowerment goals were most typically tied to liberal feminist-humanist concepts such as building individual self-esteem, self-care, self-fulfillment, self-confidence, self-knowledge, and self-determination. This depoliticized form of empowerment may reinforce status quo practices by focusing solely, both within sessions and out-of-session assignments, on individual and personal change, thus ignoring the social systems in which individuals live. This type of emphasis on individual change alone diverts attention from critical consciousness, collective well-being goals, and challenges to social power structures. Further, when self-empowerment strategies are disconnected from social change implications, clients may also be more likely to look exclusively inside themselves for clues about the origins of their problems, blame themselves for external contributors to their distress, experience self-doubt and self-criticism, silence themselves, change themselves to fit into existing realities, or overfunction to neutralize resistance. These outcomes are inconsistent with the original transformation goals of feminist therapy, which called for both personal and political change. Decolonized feminist therapy emphasizes goals of individual liberation and addresses social-structural issues such as institutionalized barriers, systemic racism, and historical injustices.

White Feminism, Fragility, and Internalized White Supremacy

Crenshaw (1989) noted, "The failure of feminism to interrogate race means that the resistance strategies of feminism will often replicate and reinforce the subordination of People of Color, and the failure of antiracism to interrogate patriarchy means that antiracism will frequently reproduce the subordination of women." White feminism, a term that feminists of color such as bell hooks, Audre Lorde, and Kimberlé Crenshaw have used since the 1970s, is the feminist practice that centers the problems of predominantly White, middle to upper class, heterosexual, and cisgender women, and views gender inequality as the primary source of all other societal oppressions. White feminism is the feminism that internalizes White supremacy, whether unconsciously or intentionally, that centralizes and assumes the superiority of White people (defined or perceived) and the behaviors and practices based on this assumption (DiAngelo, 2018). The White feminism colonial patterns of marginalization of the Indigenous people and People of Color have occurred since the suffrage movement. In interactions with colleagues or clients of color, today, White feminism may present as tone policing (how much Women of Color speak, what can be said, how much emotion is acceptable, and so on), universalism (we are all the same, we are all diverse in our own ways), a White savior complex, and centering on personal experience (making issues of racism or intersectionality about the White woman and their feelings).

Closely related to the marginalization and subordination of Women of Color is the reproduction of colonial approaches through the exportation of Euro-U.S.-centric feminisms across global contexts. This practice reinforces dominant power structures and beliefs that Western feminisms are universally applicable rather than situated in and limited to local Western Minority World realities (Macleod et al., 2020). In contrast, transnational feminisms reject notions of a romanticized global sisterhood that offers a single feminist viewpoint; that defines Euro-American worldviews, values, and strategies for change as normative; and that overemphasizes and overvalues individual agency, achievement, and fulfillment.

Transnational feminisms highlight diverse realities among women regarding circumstances, cultural values, oppressions, access to power, and priorities. They support decolonizing efforts by rejecting narrow lenses and framing liberation in alternative ways, such as by exploring and valuing forms of agency and resistance associated with collective well-being and relational values (Kurtiş & Adams, 2015). For example, instead of defining empowerment as individuation and separation from family and cultural institutions, collective empowerment encourages persons to remain connected to their communities.

DEFENSIVENESS, ETHNOCENTRISM, AND DIFFICULTIES ACKNOWLEDGING PRIVILEGE

Challenging one's relative privilege is often invisible to those who benefit from it, and "often, one is more aware and reflective of one's oppressed statuses than one's privileged statuses" (APA, 2019, p. 14). It is often easier for relatively privileged women (especially White middle-class women) to see how they have been oppressed due to patriarchy than to acknowledge their own participation in power structures. When confronted with reality, defensiveness and lack of cultural humility is a frequent response. One chapter on this topic (Bowman et al., 2001) described how White women often deny their associations with power and privilege; and when challenged, "they cry; they whine; they shut down" (p. 793), repeatedly closing off difficult dialogue and implying that Women of Color need to take care of them. Due to their privilege, "White woman's reality is visible, and acknowledged because of her tears, while a Woman of Color's reality, like her struggle, is invisible, overlooked, and pathologized" (Accapadi, 2007, p. 210). Some of the mechanisms contributing to painful dialogues related to gendered racism and other intersectional "isms" include White women's tendencies to deny implicit racism, rationalize their actions, emphasize their good intentions, or claim friendship with People of Color (Accapadi, 2007). To ensure that decolonization continues, active exploration of one's privileged statuses, a listening attitude, and a clear commitment to new behaviors are necessary.

Appropriation and Assumptions of Sameness

When does the claim that one has experienced colonization represent appropriation? Colonization typically refers to the long-term effects of membership in a community that another country or dominant group has colonized, involuntary displacement and colonization because of slavery, or colonization of Indigenous peoples and eradication of their cultures by explorers or a settler community. The potential assertion that colonization is common to all women can be seen as a form of appropriation reminiscent of claims of common oppression of all women and a single vision of sisterhood. When relatively privileged feminists refer to their oppression (such as by patriarchy) as colonization, the distinctive barriers and historical legacies of colonization remain unrecognized, thus reinforcing power imbalances and equating all forms of oppression. Feminists with more privilege need to be especially cautious about inappropriately borrowing concepts that may result in erasing the reality of many women's multiple oppressions or the long-term power abuses of colonialism. In contrast, decolonization and the dismantling of colonialism are the responsibility of all. Self-examination and self-reflexivity, and the decolonization of one's mind is an important first step. However, it is also important to respect the insider knowledge of those who have experienced colonization and avoid "savior" mentalities that are sometimes associated with feminist activism of northern countries, and that do not show respect for the agency and leadership of women in various transnational contexts.

CRITICAL AWARENESS OF EXISTING DECOLONIZATION PRACTICES

A decolonizing feminist therapy is built on an extensive interdisciplinary literature about social justice and the seminal contributions of feminists of color. In this section, we discuss the importance of gaining decolonizing literacy and embedding our work in foundational tenets for decolonized feminist psychology. Foundational to decolonization is the inclusion and centering of marginalized voices whose continued erasure is a detriment to the field of psychology.

Develop Decolonization Literacy

To decolonize feminist therapy, feminists can start by increasing our literacy in decolonization, which is the ability to accurately interpret and assess oppressive and colonizing experiences and information, challenge and examine stereotyped narratives, and engage in socially just decision-making and behaviors. Feminist therapists can develop decolonization literacy by actively learning and integrating principles of concepts that center the experiences of the traditionally marginalized, such as intersectionality (Collins, 2015; Crenshaw, 1989), liberation psychology (Comas-Díaz & Torres Rivera, 2020), and critical race feminism (Wing, 2000). Feminists of color have long argued the importance of attending to power relationships and social inequalities beyond gender. Patricia Hill Collins noted that race, class, gender, sexuality, ethnicity, nation, ability, and age do not operate as unitary or mutually exclusive entities. Instead, intersectionality is a reciprocally constructing phenomenon (2015). Black feminism has been focused on dismantling multiple social inequalities since the 1960s and 1970s (bell hooks, Audre Lorde, Angela Davis). Chicana/Latina feminism (Gloria Anzaldúa, Aída Hurtado, Lillian Comas-Díaz) raised patriarchal nationalism and the interconnectedness of race, gender, class, sexuality, and issues of border crossing and political boundaries. Asian American feminist scholars such as Mari Matsuda, credited as one of the originating critical race theory scholars, described concepts such as multiple consciousness as an awareness of oppression they face simultaneously due to their race, ethnicity, gender, and immigration history. Other Asian American feminists, such as Yuri Kochiyama and Grace Lee Boggs, have built their work around solidarity with other marginalized communities in the United States and globally.

Tenets of Decolonized Feminist Psychology

Decolonizing feminist psychology requires psychologists to acknowledge the pervasiveness and harm of patriarchy and the historical and contemporary traumas of colonization, exploitation, and domination of marginalized nations and peoples both materially and ideologically (Escobar, 2007). Decolonizing our feminist practice, we propose, entails three elements. One is to intentionally and actively counter systemic oppression in our assessment, conceptualization, and intervention. Second is to attend to the wounds of historical and contemporary oppression, including internalized intersectional oppression. Third is to adopt feminist therapeutic frameworks and strategies that are not culturally or racially avoidant or merely cultural or racial modifications of the psychology of White women, but that indigenize psychology by attending to the contributions of multicultural feminist, womanist, *mujerista*, womanista psychologists who have developed interventions that reflect and center the experiences of intersectional or marginalized women and girls. These frameworks are actively antiracism and antioppression in all of their forms, which aim to a holistic liberation. The work of decolonizing feminist practice extends beyond intellectual curiosity. Instead, it is rooted in an urgent ethical mandate to raise awareness of clients' sociopolitical and psychohistorical lives (Cruz & Sonn, 2015) and empower and encourage the adoption of acts of resistance for clients and therapists.

Centering Multicultural Feminist, Womanist, and *Mujerista* Psychologies

As we decolonize feminist psychology, we shift the voices of historically neglected feminist psychologists from the margins to the center. We also center the wisdom that emerged from targeted, disenfranchised, and systemically disempowered communities. In their text on multicultural feminist practice with adolescent girls of color, Thema Bryant-Davis and Shavonne Moore-Lobban (2020) proposed that the multicultural feminist approach promotes egalitarian relationships, self-definition, culture as medicine, sociopolitical consciousness in the form of intersectional awareness, empowerment, community support or interpersonal connection, growth and thriving, holistic integration spirituality, notions of sisterhood that are often problematized in White feminist circles, integration of the expressive arts, and resistance, activism beyond consciousness-raising. These core commitments are a decolonizing of feminist psychology as they were cultivated, centering on adolescent girls of color. In contrast, much feminist psychology literature has neglected girls in general and girls of color in particular. Along these lines, many of the principles of feminist psychology have primarily been researched in the context of women's lives with much less research on the psychology of girlhood from a feminist, multicultural feminist, or intersectional feminist perspective (Bryant-Davis & Moore-Lobban, 2020). Two specific decolonizing feminist psychological orientations are womanist psychology and *mujerista* psychology, and they emerge from the wisdom and lived experiences of Black and Latinx women, respectively (Bryant-Davis & Comas-Díaz, 2016). Even though these two traditions developed independently, salient overlapping themes stretch Western feminist psychology and deconstruct and co-construct something new.

Adopting these frameworks, we decolonize feminist psychology by genuinely making it holistic, inclusive of spirituality (Banks & Lee, 2016). White feminists have often promoted the notion that to be feminist is to discard religiosity because, at its root, religiosity is patriarchal and therefore counter to women's wellness. Women of Color are more likely to endorse spirituality and religiosity than both White women and mental health professionals in general. Consequently, it is colonizing to decide what is best for Women of Color to surrender their faith and trust White women-led organizations to "save" them. Psychological studies have documented over the years the important role that spirituality, religion, and faith have played in Women of Color's meaning-making, awareness of their sacred identity, hope, community and social support, coping, healing, and growth. Decolonized feminist psychology acknowledges and celebrates women's diverse ways of nourishing and connecting with their spirits as a potential act of liberation rather than assuming faith equates to domination. In *mujerista* psychology, Latinx women's reconnection with Spirita, including their intuition, signifies their healing (Comas-Díaz, 2016). Additionally, decolonizing for Latinas and Black women has called for a decolonizing of feminist discourse on the intersection of spirituality and positive sexuality (Lara, 2008; Malone & Hargons, 2021). In womanist psychology, Black women are challenged to see themselves in sacred text and see themselves in the image and reflection of the Creator of the Universe (Banks & Lee, 2016).

Womanist and *mujerista* psychologies also promote self-definition, voice, agency, and empowerment (Bryant-Davis & Comas-Díaz, 2016). Although in theory these are key elements in feminist psychology, in practice, both in organizational life and therapeutic life, the historic assumption has been that Women of Color are to be rescued and made in the image of womanhood based on predominately White datasets and models. Women of Color, impoverished women, women with disabilities, immigrant women, and queer women were historically marginalized and disempowered in feminist psychology circles and literature. To decolonize feminist psychology, privileged women do not have the duty or capacity to speak for marginalized women. Still, instead, they should pass the mic so that diverse women can speak for themselves.

At their roots, *mujerista* and womanist psychologies are intersectional (Comas-Díaz & Bryant-Davis, 2016). Intersectionality is not an afterthought or an addendum; it is the ethical mandate of care that requires seeing and attending to the diverse identities that people hold. The intersectional awareness and analysis is not only for the client but also for the practitioner, not just for the research participant but for the researcher, and not just for the community being served but also for the consultant herself (Shin, 2015). Reflexivity is a call and mandate to consider the ways women who are psychologists experience oppression and the identities by which they also hold privilege. Decolonized feminist psychology springs from a conscious urgency of the present moment (Bryant-Davis & Adams, 2016). Recognizing the pervasiveness and severity of intersectional oppression, including racism, classism, ableism, religious intolerance, and heterosexism, puts a demand on feminist psychologists to not remain content with consciousness-raising but to engage in observable, measurable action to oppose oppression in its diverse manifestations in both the life of the client and the life of the psychologist (Castañeda-Sound et al., 2016; Joosub & Ebrahim, 2020). Decolonizing feminist psychology is to disrupt hierarchies of oppression and utilize cultural resources to resist the intergenerational and ongoing wounds of colonization and disempowerment (KANU, 2021).

CRITICAL ACTION: A DECOLONIZED APPROACH TO EXISTING GUIDELINES

The American Psychological Association adopted its *APA Guidelines for Psychological Practice With Girls and Women* in 2018 (APA, 2018) and *APA Guidelines on Race and Ethnicity in Psychology* in 2019 (APA, 2019). The introduction to a recent special issue on decolonizing psychology noted that "the psychological study of social issues may require refusal of the discipline of psychology" (Adams et al., 2022, p. 255). One may wonder whether the aspirational statements in these APA-approved guidelines provide enough of a framework for transcending colonial disciplinary forces in psychology and decolonizing feminist psychology. Our goal is to use these guidelines as a starting point. We hope to honor and reinforce the voices of activists within psychology who have worked tirelessly to transform psychology from within. We offer a radical approach in interpreting the following selected guidelines as an example to take critical action to decolonize feminist psychology in our current practice.

Theme-Priority 1: Recognize Strengths and Resilience

Guideline 1 from the *APA Guidelines for Psychological Practice With Girls and Women* calls for recognizing the strengths and resilience of women and girls (APA, 2018). To decolonize feminist psychology is to appreciate rather than pathologize cultural roles and values. For example, Chicano affirmative psychotherapy encourages Latinas not to feel that they need to reject cultural roles and values but instead that they have the freedom to expand their notions of these roles. Colonized feminist psychology will screen for and praise only attributes White feminists have deemed praiseworthy, such as independence. Decolonized feminist psychology recognizes the cultural resources and strengths as potential pathways to liberation rather than as a burden or hurdle to women's freedom.

Theme-Priority 2: Reflexivity and Critical Consciousness in Assessment, Diagnosis, and Case Conceptualization

Guideline 7 from the *APA Guidelines for Psychological Practice With Girls and Women* challenges psychologists to use diagnoses only if and when a diagnosis is necessary and encouraged to be aware of the history of bias in diagnosis or assessment (APA, 2018). To decolonize psychology is to broaden our critique of the enterprise of psychotherapy to problematize the assessment and diagnostic norms and the overall work of practitioners. The practice of psychology makes a profit from the pain of marginalized people, especially women. Additionally, those most afflicted by marginalization are least likely to have access to quality, affordable mental health care. Feminist psychologists who engage in practice but not in advocacy need to decolonize their psychology. Feminist psychologists who engage in research and teaching but not in the dismantling of systems of oppression in the larger society and in the field of psychology itself need to decolonize their psychology. Finally, feminist psychologists who fail to acknowledge and share the cultural congruence of talk and relationship as healing Indigenously participate in the appropriation of cultural healing spaces that predate the formalization of psychology; they need to decolonize their psychology.

Guideline 9 from the *APA Guidelines on Race and Ethnicity in Psychology* cautions psychologists to provide assessment, intervention, and consultation free from the adverse effects of racial and ethnocultural bias (APA, 2019). Decolonized feminist psychology requires reflexivity, self-awareness, and cultural humility (Lykes & Távara, 2020). This enables decolonized feminist psychologists to diversify and deepen their relationships on a personal and professional level to have a richer, more nuanced understanding of the diverse experiences within racial and ethnic groups. To resist racism and ethnocultural bias requires an acknowledgment of each person's susceptibility to these biases. One cannot guard against what one believes is outside the realm of possibility. To decolonize feminist practice, psychologists need to be aware that the colonized view of marginalized women and girls is pervasive and influential in shaping the minds of all people, including well-intended feminists. Psychologists who have explored the intersection of African-centered psychology, decolonizing psychology, and feminist psychology urge for ongoing recognition and analysis of how notions of women and men are mainly colonial and within feminist psychology can promote racist notions of, for example, Black men as violent. Additionally, to decolonize feminist African-centered psychology requires attending not only to violence against those who identify as women but also to violence against members of the queer community while noting the need to (a) collaborate across genders for the equity and rights of all genders, (b) cultivate healthier relationships, and (c) highlight cultural notions of gender as expansive (Ratele et al., 2018).

Guideline 10 from the *APA Guidelines on Race and Ethnicity in Psychology* urges psychologists to engage in reflective practice by exploring how their worldviews and positionalities may affect the quality and range of psychological services they provide (APA, 2019). To decolonize psychology, feminist psychology needs to take an additional step to note not only that the individual practitioner has worldviews and positionalities, but also that the field in which they have been trained and indoctrinated has embedded values based on a worldview that is often incongruent with the lived realities of marginalized people (Gorski & Goodman, 2015). The framing of presenting problems, the mental status examination, and even the common treatment goals have within them assumptions, ideals, and priorities that psychologists have often not critiqued beyond subscribing to the myth of objectivity and neutrality, which can often be a cover for Western, White, or colonial priorities.

Theme-Priority 3: Holistic Healing Practices

Guideline 9 from the *APA Guidelines for Psychological Practice With Girls and Women* (APA, 2018) and Guideline 11 from the *APA Guidelines on Race and Ethnicity in Psychology* (APA, 2019) both remind practitioners to value, identify, and integrate holistic practices. Decolonized feminist psychology acknowledges and appropriately integrates without appropriating community resources, Indigenous perspectives, and complementary or alternative forms of healing. Feminist psychologists who only deem ethical, professional practice as taking place in a closed room with two people in their chairs talking for fifty minutes need to decolonize their idea of psychology and psychological practice. Decolonized feminist psychology is flexible, creative, culturally grounded, and innovative. It may include sessions that are out in nature; sessions seated on the floor; sessions that include elders, faith leaders, cousins, and chosen family or fictive kin; sessions with prayer, dance, poetry, and sustained silence; as well as sessions of talking while baking, craft making, protest sign decorating, storytelling, and even baby nursing (Bryant-Davis & Rajan, 2019; Gray et al., 2019; Weatherall, 2020). Decolonized feminist psychology shows up in all of the diverse ways that women and girls show up while reclaiming and revising how we identify ourselves, including activist healers (Lara, 2008).

Along these lines, Guideline 11 for race and ethnicity challenges psychologists to understand and encourage Indigenous and ethnocultural sources of healing within professional practice. To decolonize feminist psychology is to understand that women's liberation is therapeutic, culture is medicine. To that end, decolonized feminist psychologists assess for, conceptualize given, provide psychoeducation about, and integrate cultural resources and richness throughout the healing process. They do not see themselves as messiahs or rescuers but as respectful collaborators with community members who come with their own cultural resources, protective factors, coping strategies, and healing pathways. This includes a radical view of women's beauty, wisdom, dignity, and humanity facing gendered racism, for example, decolonized feminist psychologists' descriptions of body-positive views of Caribbean women that emancipate thick, voluptuous bodies (Gentles-Peart, 2020).

Theme-Priority 4: Advance Social Change, Social Justice, and Systemic Transformation

Guideline 10 from the *APA Guidelines for Psychological Practice With Girls and Women* calls for a commitment to change hostile environments and institutional, systemic, and global discrimination (APA, 2018). To decolonize feminist psychology requires that psychologists extend their reach as they cocreate treatment plans to acknowledge and combat individual discrimination and harassment and systemic and structural oppression, both local and global (Norsworthy & Khuankaew, 2020). Although in practice much of this work begins with the individual narrative, authentic consciousness-raising extends beyond the individual's story to encompass how the story intersects with others. To adopt this approach, decolonized feminist psychologists need to read across disciplines and cultures. The reality is that reading psychological texts alone will not prepare feminist psychologists to understand the sociopolitical and psycho, cultural, and historical landscape of people's lives. To decolonize feminist psychology is to commit to lifelong, multidisciplinary learning.

Complementary to this guidance is the challenge issued in Guideline 12 from the *APA Guidelines on Race and Ethnicity in Psychology*, which calls for psychologists to promote health and well-being by challenging negative racial and ethnic biases that perpetuate oppression in practice settings, systems, and methods (APA, 2019). Decolonized feminist psychologists are vocal and active in dismantling oppressive practices in research, teaching, consultation, health care policy, and organizational systems (Lara, 2008). Decolonizing feminist psychologists go beyond behind the scenes encouragement of marginalized persons after mistreatment has occurred to direct action in naming the inequity and calling for and creating corrective, life-giving, equity-based systems in place of the old ones. Decolonizing feminist psychologists, whether in administration, counseling centers, the academy, research institutes, nonprofit organizations, or governmental agencies, actively combat structural, intersectional oppression and seek to replace them with empowering, equitable, accessible, affordable quality systems that are accountable to those they claim to serve (Norsworthy, 2017).

FUTURE DIRECTIONS

It is important to consider three critiques of decolonizing psychology. The first is the argument that decolonizing centers colonists by framing people as either colonized or decolonized. In this way, identity centers the act and actors of colonization. A counter approach is to center the action rather than the response. Such approaches include liberation psychology and multicultural feminist psychology (Comas-Díaz & Torres Rivera, 2020). To this critique, we highlight the power in naming the need for deconstruction, uprooting, and opposing oppression. Often if this is not named, the work of resistance is overlooked. A second critique is the implied idealization of life before colonization, which can overlook patriarchy, violence against women, and objectification of girls and women. This argument highlights the need for a continuous commitment to intersectionality. Just as many racial justice movements have ignored and/or perpetuated sexism, likewise, many feminist movements have ignored or perpetuated racism and other forms of oppression. As we decolonize psychology, we need to attend to all forms of oppression entangled at their roots and in practice. The third critique is that decolonization is not a mere metaphor. In particular, American Indians and South African scholars and activists have noted that to call for decolonization symbolically with no discussion of land and rights is an act of betrayal of the colonized. We agree that decolonizing anything, including psychology, should not be merely symbolic or poetic but should also include tangible changes that protect the lives and enhance the quality of life of those colonized historically and in contemporary times.

Future directions for decolonizing feminist psychology include establishing undergraduate, graduate, and continuing education courses that both integrate and center decolonized feminist psychology; decolonizing feminist psychology organizations in representation, strategic planning, belonging, and power-sharing; creating training materials such as films to demonstrate decolonized feminist practice; conducting exploratory qualitative research to understand the experience and outcomes of decolonized feminist psychological practice and programming; and setting a policy agenda that decolonized feminist psychologists can advocate for and conduct relevant research to understand the dynamics underlying the research priorities. This work should continue as we consider the harmful impact of neoliberal feminist interventions that have been disempowering and counter to the ideals of decolonized feminist psychology (Kurtiş et al., 2016) and consider the healing, liberating work that has been done when our feminist psychology is decolonized (Comas-Díaz & Bryant-Davis, 2016).

RESOURCES

Adichie, C. N. (2013, April 12). *We should all be feminists* [Video]. TEDxEuston. YouTube. https://www.youtube.com/watch?v=hg3umXU_qWc

Bryant, T. (Host). (2020, January 5). Womanist healing: Learning from Black Women's journeys (No. 27) [Audio podcast episode]. In *The Homecoming Podcast with Dr. Thema.* https://youtu.be/g4d9oODcC0o

Bryant, T. (2021, November 20). *Mind, body, spirit healing workshop for young adult women of color* [Video]. YouTube. https://www.youtube.com/watch?v=mw8tKp2hm30

Bryant, T. (2022). *Homecoming: Overcome fear and trauma to reclaim your whole authentic self.* Tarcher Perigee.

Bryant, T., Arrington, E., & Nadal, K. (2022). *The antiracism handbook: Practical tools to shift your mindset and uproot racism in your life and community.* New Harbinger Press.

Bryant-Davis, T. (2020, October). *Healing and liberation: Addressing the trauma of racism* [Video]. Loyola Marymount University Forum. YouTube. https://www.youtube.com/watch?v=zpaYV7V634s

Bryant-Davis, T. (2022, June 2). *Liberation psychology: Trauma informed integrated behavioral health* [Video]. YouTube. https://www.youtube.com/watch?v=-VChKvgan50

Bryant-Davis, T., Singh, A., & Comas-Díaz, L. (2021, June 21). *Liberation psychology: Ethical considerations for practice with marginalized communities* [Webinar]. YouTube. https://www.youtube.com/watch?v=vxhcOL3TEDg

Carson, Q. (2017, August 25). *Pedagogy of the decolonizing pedagogy of the decolonizing* [Video]. TEDxUAlberta. YouTube. https://www.youtube.com/watch?v=lN17Os8JAr8

Castañeda-Sound, C., & Comas-Díaz, L. (Eds.). (2022). Feminist liberation practice with Latinx women: Introduction to the special issue. *Women and Therapy, 45*(2–3), 123–130. https://doi.org/10.1080/02703149.2022.2094611

Crenshaw, K. (2016, December 7). *The urgency of intersectionality* [Video]. YouTube. https://youtu.be/akOe5-UsQ2o

Lombardi, R. (Host). (2022, February 9). Narrative therapies, womanism and community (No. 3) [Audio podcast episode]. In *Voices from the expressive therapies summit*. The Creative Psychotherapist. https://www.youtube.com/watch?v=CkWb5evBgAO

Mullan, J. (2020, October 8). *Decolonizing therapy SCO's CARE Talk* [Video]. YouTube. https://www.youtube.com/watch?v=-JgEv7MHSa4

Nappy Head Club. (2020, May 30). The four bodies: A holistic toolkit for coping with racial trauma [Blog]. *Medium*. https://medium.com/nappy-head-club/the-four-bodies-a-holistic-toolkit-for-coping-with-racial-trauma-8d15aa55ae06

Peak Resilience Counselling. (2012, November 14). *Feminist therapy with Black women* [Video]. YouTube. https://youtu.be/ndEbfN2hqgw

Peak Resilience Counselling. (2022, March 6). *Feminist therapy Part 2: The evolution of feminism* [Video]. YouTube. https://www.youtube.com/watch?v=ylvWem_uAMQ

Vergès, F. (2019, April 23). *Decolonizing feminism* (Decolonizing the Human Lecture Series) [Lecture]. YouTube. https://www.youtube.com/watch?v=wO_xGz7U6W8

Zerbe Enns, C., Comas-Díaz, L., & Bryant-Davis, T. (Eds.). (2021). Transnational feminist theory and practice. *Women & Therapy, 44*(1–2), 1–233. https://doi.org/10.1080/02703149.2020.1774997

REFERENCES

Accapadi, M. M. (2007). When White women cry: How White women's tears oppress women of color. *The College Student Affairs Journal, 26*(2), 208–215.

Adams, G., Ratele, K., Suffla, S., & Reddy, G. (2022). Psychology as a site for decolonial analysis. *Journal of Social Issues, 78*(2), 255–277. https://doi.org/10.1111/josi.12524

American Psychological Association. (2017). *Multicultural guidelines: An ecological approach to context, identity, and intersectionality*. https://www.apa.org/about/policy/multicultural-guidelines.pdf

American Psychological Association. (2018). *APA guidelines for psychological practice with girls and women.* https://www.apa.org/about/policy/psychological-practice-girls-women.pdf

American Psychological Association. (2019). *APA guidelines on race and ethnicity in psychology.* https://www.apa.org/about/policy/guidelines-race-ethnicity.pdf

Anzaldúa, G. (1987). *Borderlands/la frontera: The new mestiza.* Spinsters/Aunt Lute.

Banks, M. E., & Lee, S. (2016). Womanism and spirituality/theology. In T. Bryant-Davis & L. Comas-Díaz (Eds.), *Womanist and* mujerista *psychologies: Voices of fire, acts of courage* (pp. 123–148). American Psychological Association. https://doi.org/10.1037/14937-006

Becker, D. (2005). *The myth of empowerment: Women and the therapeutic culture in America.* New York University Press.

Bowman, S. L., Rasheed, S., Ferris, J., Thompson, D., McRae, M., & Weitzman, L. (2001). Interface of feminism and multiculturalism: Where are the women of color? In J. G. Ponterotto, J. M. Casas, L. A. Suzuki, & C. M. Alexander (Eds.), *Handbook of multicultural counseling* (2nd ed., pp. 779–798). Sage.

Brown, L. S. (1990). The meaning of a multicultural perspective for theory-building in feminist therapy. *Women & Therapy, 9*(1–2), 1–22. https://doi.org/10.1300/J015v09n01_01

Brown, L. S. (2018). *Feminist therapy* (2nd ed.). American Psychological Association. https://doi.org/10.1037/0000092-000

Bryant-Davis, T. (Ed.). (2019). *Multicultural feminist therapy: Helping adolescent girls of color to thrive.* American Psychological Association. https://doi.org/10.1037/0000140-000

Bryant-Davis, T., & Adams, T. (2016). A psychocultural exploration of womanism, activism, and social justice. In T. Bryant-Davis & L. Comas-Díaz (Eds.), *Womanist and* mujerista *psychologies: Voices of fire, acts of courage* (pp. 219–236). American Psychological Association. https://doi.org/10.1037/14937-010

Bryant-Davis, T., & Comas-Díaz, L. (Eds.). (2016). *Womanist and* mujerista *psychologies: Voices of fire, acts of courage.* American Psychological Association. https://doi.org/10.1037/14937-000

Bryant-Davis, T., & Moore-Lobban, S. J. (2020). Black minds matter: Applying liberation psychology to Black Americans. In L. Comas-Díaz & E. Torres Rivera (Eds.), *Liberation psychology: Theory, method, practice, and social justice* (pp. 189–206). American Psychological Association. https://doi.org/10.1037/0000198-011

Bryant-Davis, T., & Rajan, I. (2019). Next steps: An integrated model for conducting multicultural feminist therapy. In T. Bryant-Davis (Ed.), *Multicultural feminist therapy: Helping adolescent girls of color to thrive* (pp. 189–207). American Psychological Association. https://doi.org/10.1037/0000140-007

Castañeda-Sound, C. L., Martinez, S., & Durán, J. E. (2016). *Mujeristas* and social justice: La lucha es la vida. In T. Bryant-Davis & L. Comas-Díaz (Eds.), *Womanist and* mujerista *psychologies: Voices of fire, acts of courage* (pp. 237–259). American Psychological Association. https://doi.org/10.1037/14937-011

Chesler, P. (1972). *Women and madness.* Doubleday.

Collins, P. H. (1986). Learning from the outsider within: The sociological significance of Black feminist thought. *Social Problems, 33*(6), S14–S32. https://doi.org/10.2307/800672

Collins, P. H. (2015). Intersectionality's definitional dilemmas. *Annual Review of Sociology, 41*(1), 1–20. https://doi.org/10.1146/annurev-soc-073014-112142

Comas-Díaz, L. (1994). An integrative approach. In L. Comas-Díaz & B. Greene (Eds.), *Women of color: Integrating ethnic and gender identities in psychotherapy* (pp. 287–318). Guilford Press.

Comas-Díaz, L. (2016). Mujerista psychospirituality. In T. Bryant-Davis & L. Comas-Díaz (Eds.), *Womanist and* mujerista *psychologies: Voices of fire, acts of courage* (pp. 149–169). American Psychological Association. https://doi.org/10.1037/14937-007

Comas-Díaz, L., & Bryant-Davis, T. (2016). Conclusion: Toward global womanist and mujerista psychologies. In T. Bryant-Davis & L. Comas-Díaz (Eds.), *Womanist and* mujerista *psychologies: Voices of fire, acts of courage* (pp. 277–289). American Psychological Association. https://doi.org/10.1037/14937-013

Comas-Díaz, L., & Torres Rivera, E. (Eds.). (2020). *Liberation psychology: Theory, method, practice, and social justice*. American Psychological Association. https://doi.org/10.1037/0000198-000

Combahee River Collective. (1983). The Combahee River Collective statement. *Home Girls: A Black Feminist Anthology, 1,* 264–274.

Crenshaw, K. (1989). Demarginalizing the intersection of race and sex: A Black feminist critique of antidiscrimination doctrine, feminist theory and antiracist politics. *University of Chicago Legal Forum, 1989*(1), 139–167.

Cruz, M. R., & Sonn, C. C. (2015). (De)colonizing culture in community psychology: Reflections from critical social science. In R. D. Goodman & P. C. Gorski (Eds.), *Decolonizing "multicultural" counseling through social justice* (pp. 127–146). Springer Science + Business Media. https://doi.org/10.1007/978-1-4939-1283-4_10

DiAngelo, R. (2018). *White fragility: Why it's so hard for White people to talk about racism*. Beacon Press.

Diemer, M. A., Rapa, L. J., Park, C. J., & Perry, J. C. (2017). Development and validation of the critical consciousness scale. *Youth & Society, 49*(4), 461–483. https://doi.org/10.1177/0044118X14538289

Enns, C. Z. (2004). *Feminist theories and feminist psychotherapies: Origins, themes, and diversity* (2nd ed.). Haworth Press.

Enns, C. Z., Díaz, L. C., & Bryant-Davis, T. (2021). Transnational feminist theory and practice: An introduction. *Women & Therapy, 44*(1–2), 11–26. https://doi.org/10.1080/02703149.2020.1774997

Escobar, A. (2007). Worlds and knowledges otherwise: The Latin American modernity/coloniality research program. *Cultural Studies, 21*(2–3), 179–210. https://doi.org/10.1080/09502380601162506

Freire, P. (1970). *Pedagogy of the oppressed*. Bloomsbury.

Freire, P. (1973). *Education for critical consciousness* (Vol. 1). Bloomsbury.

Gentles-Peart, K. (2020). "Fearfully and wonderfully made": Black Caribbean women and the decolonization of thick Black female bodies. *Feminism & Psychology, 30*(3), 306–323. https://doi.org/10.1177/0959353520912983

Gorski, P. C., & Goodman, R. D. (2015). Introduction: Toward a decolonized multicultural counseling and psychology. In R. D. Goodman & P. C. Gorski (Eds.), *Decolonizing "multicultural" counseling through social justice* (pp. 1–10). Springer. https://doi.org/10.1007/978-1-4939-1283-4_1

Gray, J. S., Isaacs, D. S., & Wheeler, M. J. (2019). Culture, resilience, and indigenist feminism to help Native American girls thrive. In T. Bryant-Davis (Ed.), *Multicultural feminist therapy: Helping adolescent girls of color to thrive* (pp. 43–77). American Psychological Association. https://doi.org/10.1037/0000140-003

hooks, b. (1989). *Talking back: Thinking feminist, thinking black* (Vol. 10). South End Press.

Hurtado, A. (1989). Relating to privilege: Seduction and rejection in the subordination of White women and women of color. *Signs: Journal of Women in Culture and Society, 14*(4), 833–855. https://doi.org/10.1086/494546

Joosub, N., & Ebrahim, S. (2020). Decolonizing the hijab: An interpretive exploration by two Muslim psychotherapists. *Feminism & Psychology, 30*(3), 363–380. https://doi.org/10.1177/0959353520912978

Kanu, I. A. (2021). Igwebuike philosophy and human rights violation in Africa. *AGORA-A Journal of Philosophical & Theological Studies, 2*(1).

Kirsh, B. (1974). Consciousness raising groups as therapy for women. In V. Franks & V. Burtle (Eds.), *Women in therapy: New psychotherapies for a changing society* (pp. 326–354). Brunner/Mazel.

Kurtiş, T., & Adams, G. (2015). Decolonizing liberation: Toward a transnational feminist psychology. *Journal of Social and Political Psychology, 3*(1), 388–413. https://doi.org/10.5964/jspp.v3i1.326

Kurtiş, T., Adams, G., & Estrada-Villalta, S. (2016). Decolonizing empowerment: Implications for sustainable well-being. *Analyses of Social Issues and Public Policy (ASAP), 16*(1), 387–391. https://doi.org/10.1111/asap.12120

Lara, I. (2008). Latina health activist-healers bridging body and spirit. *Women & Therapy, 31*(1), 21–40. https://doi.org/10.1300/02703140802145169

Lorde, A. (1984). *Sister outsider: Essays and speeches*. The Crossing Press.

Lykes, M. B., & Távara, G. (2020). Feminist participatory action research: Co-constructing liberation psychological praxis through dialogic relationality and critical reflexivity. In L. Comas-Díaz & E. Torres Rivera (Eds.), *Liberation psychology: Theory, method, practice, and social justice* (pp. 111–130). American Psychological Association. https://doi.org/10.1037/0000198-007

Macleod, C. I., Bhatia, S., & Liu, W. (2020). Feminisms and decolonising psychology: Possibilities and challenges. *Feminism & Psychology, 30*(3), 287–305.

Malone, N. J., & Hargons, C. N. (2021). Honoring the Ori: Mindfulness meditation at the intersection of Black women's spirituality and sexualities. *Journal of Psychology and Christianity, 40*(2), 120–127.

Marecek, J., & Kravetz, D. (1998). Power and agency in feminist therapy. In I. B. Seu & M. C. Heenan (Eds.), *Feminism and psychotherapy: Reflections on contemporary theories and practices* (pp. 13–29). Sage.

Matthews, N. A. (1994). *Confronting rape: The feminist anti-rape movement and the state*. Routledge. https://doi.org/10.4324/9780203993033

Noh, E. (2003). Problematics of transnational feminism for Asian American women. *CR: The New Centennial Review, 3*(3), 131–149. https://doi.org/10.1353/ncr.2004.0009

Norsworthy, K. L. (2017). Mindful activism: Embracing the complexities of international border crossings. *American Psychologist, 72*(9), 1035–1043. https://doi.org/10.1037/amp0000262

Norsworthy, K. L., & Khuankaew, O. (2020). Transnational feminist liberation psychology: Decolonizing border crossings. In L. Comas-Díaz & E. Torres Rivera (Eds.), *Liberation psychology: Theory, method, practice, and social justice* (pp. 225–243). American Psychological Association. https://doi.org/10.1037/0000198-013

Ratele, K., Cornell, J., Dlamini, S., Helman, R., Malherbe, N., & Titi, N. (2018). Some basic questions about (a) decolonizing Africa(n)-centred psychology considered.

South African Journal of Psychology. Suid-Afrikaanse Tydskrif vir Sielkunde, 48(3), 331–342. https://doi.org/10.1177/0081246318790444

Rawlings, E. I., & Carter, D. K. (1977). *Psychotherapy for women: Treatment toward equality*. Charles C. Thomas.

Shin, R. Q. (2015). The application of critical consciousness and intersectionality as tools for decolonizing racial/ethnic identity development models in the fields of counseling and psychology. In R. D. Goodman & P. C. Gorski (Eds.), *Decolonizing 'multicultural' counseling through social justice* (pp. 11–22). Springer Science + Business Media. https://doi.org/10.1007/978-1-4939-1283-4_2

Singh, A. A., Appling, B., & Trepal, H. (2020). Using the multicultural and social justice counseling competencies to decolonize counseling practice: The important roles of theory, power, and action. *Journal of Counseling and Development, 98*(3), 261–271. https://doi.org/10.1002/jcad.12321

Watts, R. J., Diemer, M. A., & Voight, A. M. (2011). Critical consciousness: Current status and future directions. *New Directions for Child and Adolescent Development, 2011*(134), 43–57. https://doi.org/10.1002/cd.310

Weatherall, R. (2020). Even when those struggles are not our own: Storytelling and solidarity in a feminist social justice organization. *Gender, Work and Organization, 27*(4), 471–486. https://doi.org/10.1111/gwao.12386

Wing, A. K. (2000). Polygamy from southern Africa to Black Britannia to Black America: Global critical race feminism as legal reform for the twenty-first century. *Journal of Contemporary Legal Issues, 11*(2), 811–880.

PART V QUEER FUTURES, SELF-CARE, AND COMMUNITY CARE

15 MOVING PSYCHOLOGY TOWARD ANTICOLONIAL QUEER FUTURES

DELLA V. MOSLEY, PEARIS L. JEAN, BRITTANY BRIDGES, MARIA SOBRINO, JEANNETTE MEJIA, SUNSHINE ADAM, GARRETT ROSS, AND ROBERTO ABREU

Prolific Black queer feminist writer Audre Lorde's poetry and prose takes up issues of identity, power, and wellness. Her poem "Who Said It Was Simple" (1997) invites us to consider the complexities of intersectional wellness and liberation. Her words encourage us to imagine an existence where those who face marginalization based on race, gender, and sexuality do not have to wonder about which identities will be liberated and survive. Queer psychology would benefit from visiting and revisiting Lorde's body of work, allowing her wisdom to help us move away from and eradicate the colonial ideas and practices that currently pervade our field and inhibit the liberation of queer people.

As currently constructed, the field of psychology, including queer psychology, is permeated by anti-Black, White supremacist, colonial, and violent theory and practices and restricts an uninhibited path to freedom for queer folx. For example, psychological research and theories are often focused on oppression and deficits rather than liberation and strengths (Valencia, 2010). The prevalent tendency is to focus on how communities experiencing harm can cope

Correspondence concerning this article should be addressed to Della V. Mosley at admin@wellshealing.org.

https://doi.org/10.1037/0000376-016

Decolonial Psychology: Toward Anticolonial Theories, Research, Training, and Practice,
L. Comas-Díaz, H. Y. Adames, and N. Y. Chavez-Dueñas (Editors)

or bounce back rather than on their resistance to harm and pathways toward holistic wellness (Buchanan & Wiklund, 2020; Somerfield & McCrae, 2000; Syed et al., 2018). This scholarship is generally not intersectional or inclusive (Burlew et al., 2019; Stevens et al., 2021). Additionally, the focus can be on promoting the personal advancement of White scholars and systems rather than the personal wellness of the public (Yakushko et al., 2016). Yakushko's findings highlight this point, having found the occurrence of epistemological violence inflicted on marginalized communities as collateral damage for hastily advanced research by White scholars who lacked regard for ethical concern. To truly work toward liberated, anticolonial queer futures, the norms and mores that have previously been the guiding principles of traditional psychology need to be recognized as antiquated; a fresh perspective needs to be offered.

The anticolonial queer futures outlined in this chapter necessitate decolonizing psychology. Instead of remaining complicit and enacting violence and harm-doing through propagating colonialism, psychologists need to adopt, cocreate and advance liberatory, anticolonial strategies. This chapter (a) delineates how colonialism has shaped queer psychology, (b) deepens understanding of decolonial and anticolonial approaches to queer psychology, and (c) provides recommendations, considerations, and resources for how to facilitate anticolonial queer futures through psychological practice.

QUEERNESS BEFORE COLONIZATION

The role of colonization on queerness, psychology, and queer psychology may be better understood in a historical context. Sexuality, gender identity, and kinship formations before colonization were vastly more expansive than they were during colonization. Provided that we were self-identifying and relating to one another in more expansive ways before colonization, it follows that the language we used to describe queerness, race, and gender and ultimately to understand identities was more expansive before the "history of oppression, exploitation, and abuse that our communities have experienced" as well (Adames & Chavez-Dueñas, 2021, p. 60). Indigenous cultures across the globe had sexuality, gender, and kinship customs, many of which are missing in today's literature and language. Despite this, we hope to share some accounts that convey what queerness looked like for some cultural groups before colonization.

Prior to colonization, gender was described many ways. Although cultural groups were diverse and may not have had a singular, universal definition for their identities, some terms and descriptions have been documented. For example, Two-Spirit describes certain Native Americans who embody masculine and feminine spirits and often hold spiritual leadership roles within their tribes (Sheppard & Mayo, 2013). Additionally, the *muxe* of Indigenous Mexico and the *hijras* of India are examples of nonbinary identities that existed before colonization (Adames & Chavez-Dueñas, 2021). This lack of endorsement of the binary gender system is also evidenced by the Diné people (Sheppard & Mayo, 2013), who lived on land now known as Colorado, New Mexico, and Arizona. The Diné historically viewed everything as constantly evolving and flowing processes, including gender (Sheppard & Mayo, 2013). Their language reflects their view of gender and gender roles as fluid and dynamic (Sheppard & Mayo, 2013). This dynamism is also reflected by Tallbear (2018), who described how Indigenous Americans have long had expansive ways of engaging in intimate relationships, forming kinship, or building families. However, although the diverse ways gender, sexuality, and kinship were lived, experienced, and practiced before colonization, queerness significantly shifted during colonization. Colonization would change, forever, how gender and sexuality would be explored and expressed.

QUEERNESS DURING COLONIZATION

Colonialism involves territorial expansions, exploitation of labor, and dispossession of resources "by powerful societies that then dominate other groups of people" (Gone, 2021, p. 260). The act of colonization maintains the hegemonic power of those in its metropole by actively claiming, absorbing, and exploiting the physical and emotional capital of those on the lower strata of its self-constructed power hierarchy. Some of the most common hierarchies advanced through colonization include, but are not limited to patriarchy, Christianity, and heterosexism. In "Black Atlantic, Queer Atlantic," for example, Tinsley (2008) documented the presence of queer relationships between recently captured Africans held in slave ships that crossed between West Africa and the Caribbean as "one way that fluid Black bodies refused to accept that the liquidation of their social selves—the colonization of oceanic and body waters" (p. 199). They write that the "emergence of intense shipmate relationships in the water-rocked, no-person's-land of slave holds created a Black Atlantic same-sex eroticism: a feeling of, feeling for the kidnapped that asserted the sentience of the bodies that slavers attempted to transform into brute matter" (p. 199). Colonialist thoughts and attitudes about gender and sexuality have impacted our contemporary attitudes and behaviors (Sewer, 2015). Morgensen (2010) argued that "colonization produced . . . 'settler sexuality:' a White national heteronormativity that regulates Indigenous sexuality and gender by supplanting them with the sexual modernity of settler subjects"

(p. 106). Individuals whose sexualities, gender, and relational formations fall outside settler subjectivity then face discrimination (e.g., isolation, violence) and may ultimately internalize the inferiority with which they are treated to survive (Fanon, 1963/2004).

The new gender norms were not enforced equally. Lugones's (2007) classic work on gender and heterosexism discusses how colonialism "imposed a new gender system that created very different arrangements for colonized males and females than for White bourgeois colonizers. Thus it introduced many genders and gender itself as a colonial concept and mode of organization" (p. 186). Put differently, this gender system was one under which colonizers were afforded a humanity, though fraught with patriarchal rule, and colonized beings were positioned as lacking gender and having a "sinful" and "bestial" hypersexuality overall (Lugones, 2007). This work aligns with Spillers's (1987) accounts of how kidnapped Africans were "unmade" or "ungendered" and located external to kinship and family units while traversing the Atlantic. Dignity and wellness were stripped away alongside the loss of land, familial ties, and ways of doing gender and sexuality for enslaved Africans. Colonization, then, is a double-edged sword that perpetuates the harmful systems in which we find ourselves and remains a continuing consequence. The harm this anti-Indigenous and eugenicist system enacts is, as Nancy Ordover (2003) wrote, "hydra-like in strategy and ideology" (p. 124). Colonization upholds the core value of Whiteness and utilizes predatory tentacles entwined with nationalism, liberalism, ableism, cis-heteronormativity,[1] racism, and homonegativity to keep those who uphold the colonial project and the wellness of the colonizers in power (Ordover, 2003). The confluence of these attitudes has infiltrated the dominant society and made it so that it is impossible to find a space free from these ideals—including the field of psychology.

PSYCHOLOGICAL THEORIES AND FRAMEWORKS AS PRODUCTS OF COLONIZATION

Dominant-culture ideologies and assumptions infiltrate psychological theory and practices. Psychology has and continues to serve as an active agent of the colonial empire, for example, the creation of "drapetomania" to facilitate the enslavement of Black people (Harrison, 2021). Those who coined the language and practices used in psychology today imposed their frameworks

---

[1] "A pervasive system of belief that centers and naturalizes heterosexuality and a binary system of assigned sex/gender" (Michigan State University, 2020).

and methodologies on society without viewing themselves as colonizers; they often saw themselves instead as catalysts of emancipatory good (Smith & Chambers, 2015). Nonetheless, these colonizers harmed Indigenous communities by ideologizing their actions as transgressive, pathologizing them, and ultimately pushing a framework onto them that would abandon Indigenous communities with the label of Other (Smith & Chambers, 2015).

The field of psychology is grounded in anti-Black, White supremacist, and colonial epistemology; current psychological practices are also rooted in harmful ideals of neoliberal economic subjectivity and neocolonial individualism (Kurtiş & Adams, 2015). Psychology models mental health and human wellness on these ideals of individual liberties, growth, and fulfillment of the self's desires and needs (Kurtiş & Adams, 2015). Moreover, the dominant psychological framework of being a "normal" human is rooted in colonial and neocolonial thought, and power (Fernando, 2017) that does not reflect or correspond to most people's lived experiences. This ideology is a cornerstone of the heterosexist, anti-Black, settler-colonial carceral state (Smith & Chambers, 2015). It is detrimental to marginalized groups because it enables and enacts the vicious cycles that reify and internalize colonialist thoughts even when professionals do not actively intend to cause harm (Smith & Chambers, 2015). This scholarship helps clarify how a psychologist may be acting within the established bounds of professionalism yet simultaneously upholding harmful, long held beliefs and practices rooted in White supremacy.

QUEER PSYCHOLOGY AND ITS WHITE ROOTS

Given the connection between colonialism and psychology, queer psychology requires us to practice psychology outside the frameworks of cisheteronormativity. Recognizing settler sexuality as one that naturalizes both gender and sexuality, queer psychology is a psychology concerned with sexualities beyond heteronormativity, gender beyond the binary, and—to a lesser extent—relationship styles beyond monogamy. This settler-colonial sexuality has shaped psychology such that a "queer psychology" even exists rather than a psychology that, without othering, recognizes various sexualities, genders, and relationship formations.

The American Psychiatric Association's decision to depathologize sexuality in 1973 has been noted for laying the groundwork for the development of queer psychology (APA, 2021). Queer psychology is vital to the development of psychology because it stresses that, in the long run, practices that propagate the heterosexist patriarchy in any form, including by reifying heteronormativity and the gender binary, only reproduce violence. Queer psychology aims to unravel the colonial roots of psychology that push us toward heteropatriarchy, nuclear families, and monogamy.

Despite its aims, much like psychological science broadly, queer psychology has historically expanded colonial, racist, patriarchal, and classist strategies and caused harm to queer and trans folks, particularly those who identify as Black, Indigenous, or People of Color (BIPOC). For example, Snorton (2017) argued that our institutions "perpetuate racialized gender as the norm and as the necessary and naturalized consequence of the current order of things" (p. ix). This has been the case within the subdiscipline of queer psychology. An overwhelming focus by White scholars in queer psychology has been on issues that maintain the colonial project, specifically White dominance, and capitalism (e.g., gay marriage). We can also recognize queer psychology as a consequence of colonization through the overwhelming focus on providing individual and short-term interventions for "coping" with violent oppressions at the expense of queer folx (Phillips et al., 2015). Today, psychological practices are often grounded in Western, educated, industrialized, rich, and democratic (or WEIRD) worlds (Henrich et al., 2010). As a result, full-fledged support to the queer community is lacking.

Even as its proponents have worked diligently to resist cis-heteronormativity, queer psychology is still White dominated and rooted in colonialism. Recent content analyses of psychology research and clinical practice spaces have helped underscore that queer psychology has not progressed beyond its colonial roots sustaining White supremacy, racial capitalism, anti-Blackness, and related oppressions. For example, in their content analysis of sexuality research, Hargons and colleagues (2017) uncovered that when the sexuality of BIPOC is covered in psychology, it is overwhelmingly from a deficit-oriented and sex-negative perspective. The authors found that sexuality researchers used predominantly White samples ten times more than predominantly BIPOC samples. When BIPOC samples were recruited intentionally, the focus was on "sex-negative, preventative discourses exclusively, with topics including sexual abuse, sexual objectification, HIV, and pregnancy prevention" (Hargons et al., 2017, p. 538). Similarly, in a content analysis of university counseling center websites, Mosley et al. (2021) illuminated that the group counseling offerings, counseling resources, and even the advertised specializations and interests noted by university counselors erased the needs and experiences of queer and transgender BIPOC. One example of the disparities found is in the group therapy offerings where 0.1% of the 1,693 groups advertised were for queer and transgender BIPOC students. Furthermore, 24.4% of staff indicated an interest in queer identities or issues in their biographies as opposed to the 13.7% reflecting an interest in BIPOC identities or issues (Mosley et al., 2021). The lack of visible support for BIPOC broadly and queer and transgender BIPOC reflects the ways the university and mental health system uphold the colonial project. We invite those who are in relation to the field of queer psychology to critically reflect on how they (we) benefited from "the erasure and assimilation of Indigenous peoples" broadly and of queer and gender expansive Indigenous people specifically (Tuck & Yang, 2012, p. 9). We contend that White supremacy and the cis-heteropatriarchy have advanced because of queer psychology's engagement in research, therapy, and training that, intentionally or not, serve the project of colonialism.

HOW QTBIPOC HAVE DISRUPTED, RESISTED, AND REIMAGINED QUEER PSYCHOLOGY

As queer scholars in psychology, we the authors (majority of queer-identified researchers) recognize that the verb *to queer* means to take an active part in deconstruction. It means living in the beast's belly and still squaring off with the forces of capitalism, racism, sexism, and ableism. Many queer and transgender BIPOC (QTBIPOC) psychologists and trainees have refused to bow in the face of the hegemony of queer psychology and instead opt for challenging normative knowledge, identities, behaviors, and spaces. For example, counseling psychologist Anneliese Singh's scholarship, advocacy, and leadership have centered on the resilience of transgender youth of color (Singh, 2013; Singh & McKleroy, 2011). Singh unapologetically called on the field to move from affirmation to liberation for the QTBIPOC community (Singh, 2016). Singh pushed us to "decolonize and re-Indigenize counseling psychology" (Singh, 2020, p. 1114). Despite colonization and White supremacy's continued attempts to destroy Indigenous ways of being and knowing, QTBIPOC folks like Singh have found ways to disrupt, resist, and reimagine queer psychology. Singh demonstrated these efforts by founding the Trans Resilience Project to translate their LGBTQ+ research findings into school and community-based change efforts, including NIH-funded work with trans and nonbinary people in Project AFFIRM.

Like Indigenous academic and writer Billy-Ray Belcourt, QTBIPOC psychologists and trainees have sought to uncover "the sort of possibilities, affective spheres, intimacies, modes of ethical life, paradoxes, and temporal and atmospheric disturbances" which Indigenous queerness elicits (Belcourt & Nixon, 2017). Evidence of this is seen in the work of the Immigration, Critical Race, and Cultural Equity (or IC-RACE) lab led by Hector Adames and Nayeli Chavez-Dueñas. From opening doors in psychology by mentoring numerous QTBIPOC psychology trainees to creating practical toolkits on QTBIPOC healing and sharing them on social media in a highly accessible manner (Adames et al., 2021), to the development and publication of a multidimensional model centered on QTBIPOC identity development (see Adames & Chavez-Dueñas, 2021) their work is a powerful exemplar of disrupting, resisting, and reimagining queer psychology.

The Trans Care Collaborative study, led by principal investigators Stephanie Budge and Elliott Tebbe, which is in data collection at the time of writing, stands out as a model for the disruption of the colonial, White supremacist, transnegative hegemony that pervades psychology research (see https://www.transcarecollabstudy.com). Through this study, QTBIPOC clinicians are working to uncover "what makes psychotherapy most effective and accessible to [BIPOC Two-Spirit, Transgender, and Nonbinary] folks" and, in the process providing access to 15 free psychotherapy sessions to participating members of this community. These efforts reflect the possibilities emerging when we envision and build pathways toward anticolonial queer futures.

ENVISIONING AND BUILDING AN ANTICOLONIAL QUEER PSYCHOLOGY

Many definitions of and approaches to decolonization and anticolonialism exist. As the terms grow in popularity, people with varying relationships to colonialism and Indigeneity use them differently based on people's positionality, needs, and contexts (Opara, 2021). For instance, Opara (2021) argued for "getting comfortable with [the] multiformity and fluidity" of decolonization because it has the potential to facilitate the successful end of colonialism in all its forms. The authors recognized the value in using multiple approaches to achieving anticolonial queer futures. This section synthesizes three pathways to anticolonial queer futures: consciousness-raising, research, and taking an anticolonial relational and political stance. We also share our recommendations for how anticolonial queer futures may be realized through each pathway.

Although these three approaches are relevant to psychological practice and may advance liberation, they should not be confused with what we view as the most critical and foundational definition of decolonization. At its core, decolonization means to give the land back to Indigenous people (Gone, 2021; Tuck & Yang, 2012) and to "un-colonize" the lands that have been colonized. Tuck and Yang's (2012) seminal article "Decolonization Is Not a Metaphor" explains the harm of using this term in ways that do not lead to the repatriation of all Indigenous land, making clear how using it as a synonym for liberation thwarts decolonization and solidifies settler futures. Much the same as an apology cannot replace the resource redistribution that reparations for the enslavement of those of African descent in the United States calls for, social change that does not repatriate land to Indigenous people across the globe can never replace true decolonization.

Anticolonial Queer Futures Through Consciousness-Raising

Frantz Fanon (1963/2004) was intentional in acknowledging land as "the most essential value" for colonized people (p. 44), but he and many others in the mental health fields recognize consciousness-raising as a key component and first step of decolonization (Fanon, 1963/2004; Tuck & Yang, 2012). Achieving decolonization (noun) requires a decolonizing (verb) of people's minds. Fanon (1963/2004) posited that this growth process was both cognitive (e.g., increased sociopolitical awareness, learning histories) as well as psychological (e.g., having hope, gaining self-efficacy, valuing collectivism). In psychology, critical consciousness development requires gaining a social awareness, developing a sense of sociopolitical efficacy, and taking actions focused on systems of power and oppression (Adames et al., 2022; French et al., 2020; Mosley et al., 2021). For psychology to reach its potential in contributing to anticolonial queer futures, consciousness-raising must be an integral component of practice. Moreover, critical consciousness—which always includes action—will need to be prioritized and consistently practiced by psychologists and trainees. Decolonizing one's mind through critical consciousness development enables critical questioning of how the current practice of psychology perpetrates cis-heteronormativity. For example, consider why diverse genders, sexualities, and relationship styles are addressed as afterthoughts. Why are all of my colleagues cisgender or heterosexual? Smith (2015) argued that decolonizing starts with counselors and psychologists taking ownership of integrating systems of oppression into their work. Adames et al. (2018) found that it is not enough to merely be able to identify these systems of oppression in the outside world. Counselors need to consistently and readily reflect on internalized heterosexism and cissexism within themselves to create an empowering therapeutic space where clients can trust that their counselor does not recreate the colonial norms forced upon them in their daily lives. Smith (2015) described this process as "moving away from affirming counseling" and "moving toward anti-heteronormative counseling" (pp. 34–36). Consciousness-raising work may help clinicians understand that the very act of affirming a client's queer or trans identity perpetuates the power a straight counselor has as the dominant identity by whom the oppressed identity should strive to be accepted. The anticolonial future of psychological practice with queer and trans people could require approaching our work from a different relational starting point rather than simply altering the work already being done. Imagine the following: what if we only entered into research, clinical, or teaching relationships with those we have already established trusting relationships? What if our ethical principle of doing no harm required mutual respect, boundary setting, and good communication with members of this community?

Psychologists striving to facilitate anticolonial queer futures may benefit from critically exploring non-Westernized avenues to elicit change with clients. For example, Zepeda (2014) described how Queer Latina and Xicana Indígenas "enact forms of remembering through their art to regain cultural and ancestral memory and story" (p. 120). This example is not simply art therapy but an entirely new frame of clinical work, allowing the client to bring their wellness traditions into the therapeutic space. Other research has shown spiritual practices to provide healing to BIPOC populations, which could also be incorporated more into counseling work if clients desire (Comas-Díaz, 2021). By creating space for client-driven techniques and collaborating with queer and trans people in counseling, clinicians can affirm the traditions of these populations. This work could help clients feel understood by their counselor, strengthening trust in the therapeutic relationship. Integrating these techniques may also validate clients' identities by subverting the colonial health care system that primarily uses interventions created by hegemonic, White society.

Consciousness-raising may also move psychologists to legitimate non-professional therapeutic practices in our communities. Gone (2021) recommended identifying providers within the community who already have established relationships with community members and creating a space to include them in traditional clinical work. Further, they stated that "a decolonization approach to practice that emphasizes accompaniment will collaborate with community experts and leaders toward local innovations in counseling and therapeutic services based on tailored responses to community needs" (p. 267). A few community initiatives doing therapeutic work that has been delegitimized through colonialism and are inclusive of queer and trans populations include Harriet's Apothecary and the Radical Healing Collaborative. Harriet's Apothecary is an intergenerational, healing collective led by BIPOC and QTBIPOC healers, artists, health professionals, magicians, activists, and ancestors who provide diverse healing interventions to BIPOC communities. Radical Healing is a healing campus where diverse healers—bodyworkers, artists, social workers, physicians, musicians, energy workers, clinical and counseling psychologists, activists, caregivers, peacemakers, movement guides, yogis, workers, scholars—work individually and collectively to promote wellness for BIPOC, queer, trans and other people marginalized in society. This type of decolonial therapeutic work disrupts the myth that only licensed counselors and psychologists can provide healing practices to queer and trans people or focus on queer and trans concerns. Such notions perpetuates the colonial dominance of Western therapeutic practices when it is widely understood that countless organizations within the community do healing work and, in many cases, garner greater trust from queer and trans people than traditional clinicians.

As counselors working with this population, we need to be conscientious that all groups and cultures have ways of care and wellness. When we forget this notion, we devalue those populations and erode any trust we may have with them (Goodman, 2015). We also devalue the strengths of communities, eroding trust further. Goodman and colleagues (2015) explained that it is not enough only to acknowledge that communities have their own established wellness practices. To truly decolonize clinical work, we need to privilege delegitimized Indigenous practices (including queer and trans practices) as the primary or dominant ways these populations find healing.

Anticolonial Queer Futures Through Research

Historically, psychological research has been used as a colonial tool to further oppressive hierarchies of race and ethnicity and to pathologize queerness. Therefore, decolonization has also been posited as a social justice-oriented approach to engaging in psychological research and described as "an innovative and generative framework for conducting research that encompasses diverse qualitative methodologies and methods" (Gone, 2021, p. 260). This approach is not novel, given that Indigenous communities have long used qualitative methods such as oral storytelling, writings, and artistic expression to archive and explore their histories, stories, and experiences. However, these approaches have not been meaningfully and respectfully incorporated or documented in most U.S. psychological research. Decolonizing as an approach to research requires that researchers interrogate and reject the "expert" status bestowed on them to move toward pursuing research led by and in equitable collaboration with historically marginalized communities (such as queer, Indigenous communities).

Decolonial and anticolonial research with queer populations will require a comprehensive reimagining of what it means to do psychological research. Pillay (2017) wrote that "our research agendas must be cracked to challenge the relevance of our research topics, methods, assumptions, analyses, and dissemination methods" (p. 139). The primary recommendation here is that, by nature, research cannot be done on queer and trans populations but must be done with them. The following recommendations are paramount to the notion of being in relationship with queer and trans people throughout the research process. To accomplish this, the authors proposed adopting liberation-based methodologies, such as the healing methodologies of Lee and colleagues (2023) and the critical bifocality of Weis and Fine (2012). The framework presented for healing-centered research methods involves six components: maintaining social justice ethics, adopting liberation methodologies, implementing healing methods, embracing interdisciplinary approaches, catalyzing action, and promoting community accessibility (Lee et al., 2023). Critical bifocality calls for research designs that evaluate how history and systems shape the topics we study today (Fine, 2016).

Additionally, Chavez-Dueñas and colleagues (2019) provided a framework for healing that can work together with these methods to reshape the ways we approach research with queer and trans people by encouraging counselors and psychologists to adopt practices that venture deeply into the communities we are studying. Evaluating systems and structures will also require us to collaborate with those who "have stronger frameworks for studying structural processes (e.g., sociology, social work, ethnic studies)" (Syed & McLean, 2021, p.1). Other fields were doing work related to social identities and worldviews long before the field of psychology developed. To be in relationship with those who have more expertise and can consult to improve our work is to begin to decolonize the field of psychology.

One pathway to decolonizing research is participatory action research (PAR). PAR subverts traditional processes of science by reframing the relationship between the researcher and the researched (Brydon-Miller, 1997). Gone (2021) stated that through PAR, we can "exchange the familiar expert–client relationship for participatory action in which trusted researchers are invited by these communities to provide facilitation, support, and resources for efforts whereby formerly colonized people solve their own problems on their own terms" (p. 267). PAR presents a research method that allows colonized queer and trans people to advocate for themselves for the research they genuinely need, and to develop transformative new knowledge. This frame will further anticolonial queer futures as it intentionally seeks to position agency within the communities that colonization took it from. Research for anticolonial queer futures will reflect the belief that queer and trans people are the most equipped to answer the questions of their existence.

Anticolonial Queer Futures Through Relationship Building, Training, Education

We posit that anticolonial queer futures may also be achieved by taking an anticolonial relational and political stance. Benaway (2017), in an article focused on queer and Two-spirited Indigenous artists, explored how they are reenvisioning and embracing the concept of decolonial love, which they defined as learning to "hold and navigate each other's traumas experienced through generations of colonization" and "the resurgence of the Indigeneity of oneself" (para. 8). To love a person or a group of people, one must also learn about them. Decolonial love deepens and builds on the work of critical consciousness. This process involves working to understand the impact of colonization on our communities and learning, in community with others, to love the aspects of ourselves and our communities that colonialism has pathologized, condemned, and isolated. Decolonial love necessitates finding our way back to the beauty, value, and strength the colonizers have attempted to hide and destroy. Interrogating how we have internalized cis-heterosexism, transnegativity, anti-Blackness, ableism, and related oppressions is an important action to take in this process. Decolonial love also needs to look to create new love that has yet to exist, that which exists beyond what we know and have had stolen from us (Harrison, 2021).

Decolonization as a relational and political approach is the foundation for an anticolonial future. To create this future, we must examine the role of power embedded in ideas, culture, knowledge, politics, and resistance (Foucault, 1980; Moore, 1997). Dei and Asgharzadeh (2001) described how an anticolonial approach challenges the human tendency to create systems of oppression and subjugation. Anticolonialism would suggest that it is not enough to decolonize ourselves and psychology but that we also need to take an approach that does not recreate the colonial world we live in today. An anticolonial relational and political approach moves beyond liberation and is focused on sustaining our liberation from colonialism with the opportunity to queer our future. We desire a queer psychology that strives toward such anticolonialism.

Training and education are important to explore from a relational and political perspective if we are to achieve anticolonial queer futures. As scholars and educators, we need to ensure that our courses and curriculum use decolonial, anticolonial, antiracist, antipatriarchal, antisexist, anticapitalistic, and otherwise inclusive frameworks (Goodman et al., 2015). This means going beyond addressing social identities in multicultural psychology courses to weave the topics and issues most relevant to the lives of queer and trans people into every course throughout training, thereby shifting the epistemology and ontology that undergirds traditional psychology training (Pillay, 2017). These curricula need to not only address queer and trans topics, but also decolonize how we conceptualize training and its purpose. As Pillay (2017) states, "the curriculum must be cracked, and the contents and processes laid bare" (p. 139). Pillay's (2017) scholarship urged us to ask several questions:

- What is being taught?
- Why is it being taught?

- How is it being taught?
- Who is teaching it?
- What is the purpose of teaching it?
- How is competence being examined?
- Is there a hidden curriculum? (p. 139).

The answers to these questions will often uphold colonial narratives that continue to exclude the most marginalized from teachings and conversations. However, by continuous reflection, reshaping, and reimagining, we can begin to center instead the voices that have been stifled for so long and shatter the systems that have silenced them.

Psychology programs should begin by reimagining and rebuilding the selection process for students admitted into psychology programs. Presently, colonial and oppressive university systems continue to exclude Indigenous, queer, trans, and other marginalized students from psychology spaces and conversations altogether through their reliance on racist, classist, and elitist selection processes. Pillay (2017) stressed that "selection processes must be cracked to determine whether the selection of students into psychology courses—especially the key Honours and master's degrees—and the hiring of psychologists in all settings is fair and equitable" (p. 139). Psychologists need to be in constant conversation and relationship with each other, administration, trainees, and applicants' communities in their programs. Transparency in the selection process and dismantling the oppressive barriers (e.g., reliance on biased assessment and grading schemes, stereotypes held by faculty members) that discriminate against queer and trans applicants will be necessary for this process.

Consequently, psychologists must actively participate in creating anticolonial systems that value Indigenous, queer, and trans populations in the ways they deserve. It is not enough to passively wait for change to occur and believe that what we currently do as a field to be inclusive of these populations is enough. This belief is colonial and makes us complicit in the continued harm to these communities. We must act as accomplices in the liberation of Indigenous, queer, and trans communities in and beyond psychology.

The following recommendation asks psychologists to critically examine how they understand and express love. "Decolonial love . . . breaks down hundreds of years of oppression in how we love one another" (Benaway, 2017, para 8). Stewart's (2017) poem "In My Decolonized Black Queer Love Story" describes decolonial love as full of contradiction, negotiation, care, growth, and relational and familial possibility. Building such a decolonized relationship with others and ourselves is political. Queering White settler colonialism and colonial gender and sexual identity deconstruct and challenge what is considered normal (Hunt & Holmes, 2015). As researchers and colonized beings on the continuous journey of decolonization, we recognize the importance of uplifting the voices of Black, Indigenous, and other queer artists and activists of color. We encourage readers to listen to Stewart's (2017) poem on YouTube and to read the descriptions of decolonized love offered by Indigenous artists in Benaway's (2017) article. For example, Kiley May, a Mohawk trans, Two-spirit woman from Six Nations of the Grand River in Ontario, Canada, who is a community ambassador and artist, describes decolonial love as "[The world] fully embrace[ing] my past, present and future, including my culture and spirituality." Furthermore, Lindsay Nixon, a Nehiyaw-Saulteaux-Métis curator, editor, writer, and art history graduate student, shared their view of decolonial love as

> [A] pathway . . . to resisting scarcity-driven cruelty within our relationships . . . I need decolonial love to heal myself, even from my own community, to envisage an Indigenous world, Indigenous possibility, that is gentler, kinder. I need decolonial love to quite literally love my body back to life. (Benaway, 2017, para 14)

As these statements underscore, decolonial love is a way of being in relationship with self, others, and the world that is unapologetically communal and healing, breaking boundaries associated with time, place, and the entire project of colonization.

The artists mentioned have shared their journey to decolonial love, which first requires them to reflect on their relationship with colonialism and desire to return to Indigeneity. We invite psychologists to consider the meaning of decolonial love in their personal and professional lives. We can learn from this vulnerable process that it is through deep reflection on our relationship to decolonized love that we can begin to embrace a decolonial queer politic in our work and coconstruct an anticolonial future for all of us.

CONCLUSION

This chapter highlights an agenda for doing anticolonial and decolonial queer psychology work in a way that acts against current frameworks of queerness that operate, thrive, and accommodate White supremacist, capitalist, sexist, ableist, and Christian hegemony. In this way, we "revive the sense of possibility for those who still believe in lost causes, including redistribution, recognition, and radical transformation" (Fine, 2016, p. 362). Because practices of domination and subjugation guide the narrative in queer psychology, we sought to provide recommendations for facilitating anticolonial queer futures. Could queer psychology exist outside colonial mentality, White supremacy, and capitalism? We dream that queerness will not need to be (re)defined and deconstructed because queerness will be synonymous with thriving and not merely existing. However, for this to become actualized, we would need both to acknowledge and address coloniality (including internalized coloniality) and anti-Blackness as the root of the psychopathological frameworks for understanding queerness and to engage in the described psychological practices that have promise for facilitating anticolonial queer futures.

RESOURCES

BBC World Service. (2020, July 30). *Gender identity: How colonialism killed my culture's gender fluidity* [Video]. YouTube. https://www.youtube.com/watch?v=AqEgsHGiK-s

brown, a. m. (2019). *Pleasure activism*. AK Press.

Project 562. (n.d.). *Decolonizing sexuality at the largest Two-Spirit pow wow in the nation* [Blog]. https://www.project562.com/blog/decolonizing-sexuality-at-the-largest-two-spirit-pow-wow-in-the-nation

Snorton, C. R. (2021, April 15). *Black Freedom Lectures Q&A* [Video]. YouTube. https://www.youtube.com/watch?v=5OP_YCx284c

REFERENCES

Adames, H., & Chavez-Dueñas, N. Y. (2021). Reclaiming all of me: The racial queer identity framework. In K. L. Nadal & M. Scharron-del Río (Eds.), *Queer psychology: Intersectional perspectives* (pp. 59–79). Springer. https://doi.org/10.1007/978-3-030-74146-4_4

Adames, H. Y., Chavez-Dueñas, N. Y., Cruz, X., & Mchabcheb, R. (2021). *Our collective healing: A toolkit for queer and trans people of color (QTPOC)*. https://www.icrace.org

Adames, H. Y., Chavez-Dueñas, N. Y., Lewis, J. A., Neville, H. A., French, B. H., Chen, G. A., & Mosley, D. V. (2022). Radical healing in psychotherapy: Addressing the wounds of racism-related stress and trauma. *Psychotherapy*, *60*(1), 39–50. https://doi.org/10.1037/pst0000435

Adames, H. Y., Chavez-Dueñas, N. Y., Sharma, S., & La Roche, M. J. (2018). Intersectionality in psychotherapy: The experiences of an AfroLatinx queer immigrant. *Psychotherapy*, *55*(1), 73–79. https://doi.org/10.1037/pst0000152

American Psychological Association (APA). (2021). *Speaking of psychology: The history of LGBTQ psychology from Stonewall to now, with Peter Hegarty, PhD* [Video]. https://www.apa.org/research/action/speaking-of-psychology/stonewall

Belcourt, B., & Nixon, L. (2017). What do we mean by queer Indigenous ethics? *Canadianart*. https://canadianart.ca/features/what-do-we-mean-by-queerindigenousethics/

Benaway, G. (2017, July 4). *Decolonial love: These Indigenous artists are taking back the self-love that colonialism stole*. Canadian Broadcasting Corporation. https://www.cbc.ca/arts/decolonial-love-these-indigenous-artists-are-taking-back-the-self-love-that-colonialism-stole-1.4189785

Brydon-Miller, M. (1997). Participatory action research: Psychology and social change. *Journal of Social Issues, 53*(4), 657–666. https://doi.org/10.1111/j.1540-4560. 1997.tb02454.x

Buchanan, N. T., & Wiklund, L. (2020). Why clinical science must change or die: Integrating intersectionality and social justice. *Women & Therapy, 43*(3–4), 309–329. https://doi.org/10.1080/02703149.2020.1729470

Burlew, A. K., Peteet, B. J., McCuistian, C., & Miller-Roenigk, B. D. (2019). Best practices for researching diverse groups. *American Journal of Orthopsychiatry, 89*(3), 354. https://doi.org/10.1037/ort0000350

Chavez-Dueñas, N. Y., Adames, H. Y., Perez-Chavez, J. G., & Salas, S. P. (2019). Healing ethno-racial trauma in Latinx immigrant communities: Cultivating hope, resistance, and action. *American Psychologist, 74*(1), 49–62. https://doi.org/10.1037/amp0000289

Comas-Díaz, L. (2021). Afro-Latinxs: Decolonization, healing, and liberation. *Journal of Latina/o Psychology, 9*(1), 65–75. https://doi.org/10.1037/lat0000164

Dei, G. J. S., & Asgharzadeh, A. (2001). The power of social theory: The anti-colonial discursive framework. *The Journal of Educational Thought (JET)/Revue De La Pensée Éducative*, 297–323. https://doi.org/10.11575/jet.v35i3.52749

Fanon, F. (2004). *The wretched of the earth* (Richard Philcox, Trans.). Grove. (Original work published 1963)

Fernando, S. (2017). *Institutional racism in psychiatry and clinical psychology.* Palgrave Macmillan. https://doi.org/10.1007/978-3-319-62728-1

Fine, M. (2016). Just methods in revolting times. *Qualitative Research in Psychology, 13*(4), 347–365. https://doi.org/10.1080/14780887.2016.1219800

Foucault, M. (1980). *Power/knowledge: Selected interviews and other writings.* Vintage. https://doi.org/10.1007/BF00142984

French, B. H., Lewis, J. A., Mosley, D. V., Adames, H. Y., Chavez-Dueñas, N. Y., Chen, G. A., & Neville, H. A. (2020). Toward a psychological framework of radical healing in communities of color. *The Counseling Psychologist, 48*(1), 14–46. https://doi.org/10.1177/0011000019843506

Gone, J. P. (2021). Decolonization as methodological innovation in counseling psychology: Method, power, and process in reclaiming American Indian therapeutic traditions. *Journal of Counseling Psychology, 68*(3), 259–270. https://doi.org/10.1037/cou0000500

Goodman, R. D. (2015). A liberatory approach to trauma counseling: Decolonizing our trauma-informed practices. In R. Goodman & P. Gorski (Eds.), *Decolonizing "multicultural" counseling through social justice* (pp. 55–72). Springer. https://doi.org/10.1007/978-1-4939-1283-4_5

Goodman, R. D., Williams, J. M., Chung, R. C. Y., Talleyrand, R. M., Douglass, A. M., McMahon, H. G., & Bemak, F. (2015). Decolonizing traditional pedagogies and practices in counseling and psychology education: A move towards social justice and action. In R. Goodman & P. Gorski (Eds.), *Decolonizing "multicultural" counseling through social justice* (pp. 147–164). Springer. https://doi.org/10.1007/978-1-4939-1283-4_11

Hargons, C., Mosley, D. V., & Stevens-Watkins, D. (2017). Studying sex: A content analysis of sexuality research in counseling psychology. *The Counseling Psychologist, 45*(4), 528–546. https://doi.org/10.1177/0011000017713756

Harrison, L. D. (2021). *Belly of the beast: The politics of anti-fatness as anti-Blackness.* North Atlantic Books. https://doi.org/10.1080/21604851.2021.2010334

Henrich, J., Heine, S. J., & Norenzayan, A. (2010). The weirdest people in the world? *Behavioral and Brain Sciences, 33*(2–3), 61–83. https://doi.org/10.1017/S0140525X0999152X

Hunt, S., & Holmes, C. (2015). Everyday decolonization: Living a decolonizing queer politics. *Journal of Lesbian Studies, 19*(2), 154–172. https://doi.org/10.1080/10894160.2015.970975

Kurtiş, T., & Adams, G. E. (2015). Decolonizing liberation: Toward a transnational feminist psychology. *Journal of Social and Political Psychology, 3*(1), 388–413. https://doi.org/10.5964/jspp.v3i1.326

Lee, B. A., Ogunfemi, N., Neville, H. A., & Tettegah, S. (2023). Resistance and restoration: Healing research methodologies for the global majority. *Cultural Diversity & Ethnic Minority Psychology, 29*(1), 6–14. https://doi.org/10.1037/cdp0000394

Lorde, A. (1997). *The collected poems of Audre Lorde.* W. W. Norton.

Lugones, M. (2007). Heterosexualism and the colonial/modern gender system. *Hypatia, 22*(1), 186–209. https://doi.org/10.1111/j.1527-2001.2007.tb01156.x

Michigan State University. (2020). Glossary. *The Gender and Sexuality Campus Center.* https://gscc.msu.edu/education/glossary.html

Moore, D. L. (1997). Rough knowledge and radical understanding: Sacred silence in American Indian literatures. *American Indian Quarterly, 21*(4), 633–662. https://doi.org/10.2307/1185717

Morgensen, S. L. (2010). Settler homonationalism: Theorizing settler colonialism within queer modernities. *GLQ, 16*(1–2), 105–131. https://doi.org/10.1215/10642684-2009-015

Mosley, D. V., Gonzalez, K. A., Abreu, R. L., & Kaivan, N. C. (2019). Unseen and underserved: A content analysis of wellness support services for bi+ People of Color and Indigenous people on US campuses. *Journal of Bisexuality, 19*(2), 276–304. https://doi.org/10.1080/15299716.2019.1617552

Mosley, D. V., Hargons, C. N., Meiller, C., Angyal, B., Wheeler, P., Davis, C., & Stevens-Watkins, D. (2021). Critical consciousness of anti-Black racism: A practical model to prevent and resist racial trauma. *Journal of Counseling Psychology, 68*(1), 1–16. https://doi.org/10.1037/cou0000430

Opara, I. N. (2021, July 29). It's time to decolonize the decolonization movement. *Speaking of Medicine and Health.* PLOS Blog. https://speakingofmedicine.plos.org/2021/07/29/its-time-to-decolonize-the-decolonization-movement/

Ordover, N. (2003). *American eugenics: Race, queer anatomy, and the science of nationalism.* University of Minnesota Press. https://doi.org/10.1086/433039

Phillips, N. L., Adams, G., & Salter, P. S. (2015). Beyond adaptation: Decolonizing approaches to coping with oppression. *Journal of Social and Political Psychology, 3*(1), 365–387. https://doi.org/10.5964/jspp.v3i1.310

Pillay, S. R. (2017). Cracking the fortress: Can we really decolonize psychology? *South African Journal of Psychology [Suid-Afrikaanse Tydskrif vir Sielkunde], 47*(2), 135–140. https://doi.org/10.1177/0081246317698059

Sewer, H. (2015, July 7). *We must talk about race and American colonialism* [Video]. YouTube. https://www.youtube.com/watch?v=BD1Pk_9hcsg

Sheppard, M., & Mayo, J. B., Jr. (2013). The social construction of gender and sexuality: Learning from two spirit traditions. *Social Studies, 104*(6), 259–270. https://doi.org/10.1080/00377996.2013.788472

Singh, A. A. (2013). Transgender youth of color and resilience: Negotiating oppression and finding support. *Sex Roles, 68*(11–12), 690–702. https://doi.org/10.1007/s11199-012-0149-z

Singh, A. A. (2016). Moving from affirmation to liberation in psychological practice with transgender and gender nonconforming clients. *American Psychologist, 71*(8), 755–762. https://doi.org/10.1037/amp0000106

Singh, A. A. (2020). Building a counseling psychology of liberation: The path behind us, under us, and before us. *The Counseling Psychologist, 48*(8), 1109–1130. https://doi.org/10.1177/0011000020959007

Singh, A. A., & McKleroy, V. S. (2011). "Just getting out of bed is a revolutionary act": The resilience of transgender people of color who have survived traumatic life events. *Traumatology, 17*(2), 34–44. https://doi.org/10.1177/1534765610369261

Smith, L., & Chambers, C. (2015). Decolonizing psychological practice in the context of poverty. In R. D. Goodman & P. C. Gorski (Eds.), *Decolonizing "multicultural" counseling through social justice* (pp. 73–84). Springer. https://doi.org/10.1007/978-1-4939-1283-4_6

Smith, L. C. (2015). Queering multicultural competence in counseling. In R. D. Goodman & P. C. Gorski (Eds.), *Decolonizing "multicultural" counseling through social justice* (pp. 23–39). Springer. https://doi.org/10.1007/978-1-4939-1283-4_3

Snorton, C. R. (2017). *Black on both sides: A racial history of trans identity*. University of Minnesota Press. https://doi.org/10.5749/minnesota/9781517901721.001.0001

Somerfield, M. R., & McCrae, R. R. (2000). Stress and coping research. Methodological challenges, theoretical advances, and clinical applications. *American Psychologist, 55*(6), 620–625. https://doi.org/10.1037/0003-066X.55.6.620

Spillers, H. J. (1987). Mama's baby, papa's maybe: An American grammar book. *Diacritics, 17*(2), 64–81. https://doi.org/10.2307/464747

Stevens, K. R., Masters, K. S., Imoukhuede, P. I., Haynes, K. A., Setton, L. A., Cosgriff-Hernandez, E., Lediju Bell, M. A., Rangamani, P., Sakiyama-Elbert, S. E., Finley, S. D., Willits, R. K., Koppes, A. N., Chesler, N. C., Christman, K. L., Allen, J. B., Wong, J. Y., El-Samad, H., Desai, T. A., & Eniola-Adefeso, O. (2021). Fund Black scientists. *Cell, 184*(3), 561–565. https://doi.org/10.1016/j.cell.2021.01.011

Stewart, I. F. (2017, November 18). *In my decolonized Black queer love story* [Video]. YouTube. https://www.youtube.com/watch?v=AUSSh8XLiTM

Syed, M., & McLean, K. C. (2021). Who gets to live the good life? Master narratives, identity, and well-being within a marginalizing society. *Cultural Diversity and Ethnic Minority Psychology, 29*(1), 53–63. https://doi.org/10.1037/cdp0000470

Syed, M., Santos, C., Yoo, H. C., & Juang, L. P. (2018). Invisibility of racial/ethnic minorities in developmental science: Implications for research and institutional practices. *American Psychologist, 73*(6), 812–826. https://doi.org/10.1037/amp0000294

TallBear, K. (2018). Making love and relations beyond settler sex and family. In A. E. Clarke & D. Haraway (Eds.), *Making kin not population* (pp. 145–164). Prickly Paradigm Press.

Tinsley, O. E. N. (2008). Black Atlantic, queer Atlantic: Queer imaginings of the middle passage. *GLQ, 14*(2–3), 191–215. https://doi.org/10.1215/10642684-2007-030

Tuck, E., & Yang, K. W. (2012). Decolonization is not a metaphor. *Decolonization: Indigeneity, Education & Society, 1*(1), 1–40.

Valencia, R. R. (2010). *Dismantling contemporary deficit thinking: Educational thought and practice*. Routledge. https://doi.org/10.4324/9780203853214

Weis, L., & Fine, M. (2012). Critical bifocality and circuits of privilege: Expanding critical ethnographic theory and design. *Harvard Educational Review, 82*(2), 173–201. https://doi.org/10.17763/haer.82.2.v1jx34n441532242

Yakushko, O., Morgan Consoli, M. L., Hoffman, L., & Lee, G. (2016). On methods, methodologies, and continued colonization of knowledge in the study of "ethnic minorities": Comment on Hall et al. (2016). *American Psychologist, 71*(9), 890–891. https://doi.org/10.1037/amp0000060

Zepeda, S. J. (2014). Queer Xicana Indígena cultural production: Remembering through oral and visual storytelling. *Decolonization: Indigeneity, Education & Society, 3*(1), 119–141.

16 YOUR SELF-CARE IS MADE OF CAPITALISM

A Decolonial Approach to Self and Community Care

ARIANNE E. MILLER AND NELLIE TRAN

I had to examine, in my dreams as well as in my immune-function tests, the devastating effects of overextension. Overextending myself is not stretching myself. I had to accept how difficult it is to monitor the difference. Necessary as cutting down on sugar. Crucial. Physically. Psychically. Caring for myself is not self-indulgence, it is self-preservation, and that is an act of political warfare.

—Audre Lorde, 1988, p. 130

Capital is dead labor, which, vampire-like, lives only by sucking living labor, and lives the more, the more labor it sucks.

—Karl Marx, 1867/1967, p. 342

"Caring for myself is not self-indulgence, it is self-preservation, and that is an act of political warfare" (Lorde, 1988, p. 130) is possibly one of the most cited quotes about self-care on the internet. Noticeably absent from it is what

https://doi.org/10.1037/0000376-017
Decolonial Psychology: Toward Anticolonial Theories, Research, Training, and Practice,
L. Comas-Díaz, H. Y. Adames, and N. Y. Chavez-Dueñas (Editors)

comes before it: an examination of overextension that produces ill health and an intensified need to care for oneself. One reading of this is that individuals should or can stop overextending themselves. Another is that it has become difficult to monitor the difference between stretching and overextension, because it has become an expectation that we should or can extend ourselves to produce more. The word *overextension* is perhaps a uniquely concise term that describes an essential impact of capitalism and essential focus of self-care. Capitalism extracts as much labor as humanly possible because production is always required (Marx, 1867/1967). Audre Lorde wrote these words in the context of managing liver cancer, being an academic, continuing her social justice work, and needing to make intentional choices with her time and actions. As we write this chapter, we are at a notable moment in history: the push is renewed for a more radical self-care as an antiracist and anticapitalist endeavor, at least implicitly. Yet, because of the current state of labor and our capitalist system that has created a multibillion-dollar self-care industry (IRi, 2018), the push for self-care also works in favor of capitalism. Workers require self-care to survive and keep their jobs, and, more recently, some businesses have begun to invest in worker self-care to maintain and increase production (Thrive Global, n.d.).

The goal of this chapter is to critically interrogate the concept, discourse, and practice of self-care through the lens of decoloniality and propose a path toward a more liberatory understanding and practice of self-care. The chapter explores how self-care is rooted in connected colonial systems of capitalism and White supremacy such that efforts to make self-care an accessible, useful tool for the health and well-being of society ultimately fail. We discuss the possibility that self- and community care are not two ends of a single spectrum, argue that the dominant understanding and practice of self-care functions as a tool of coloniality, and explore how we can begin to decolonize it. We describe the ways in which self-care functions as a vague concept that presumes the existence of economic resources (money, time, childcare), an ability or inclination to prioritize the self as opposed to the community, as well as its intermingling with indulgence. Finally, we suggest that this conceptualization of self-care focuses on what "the self" can do to feel better in the world as we know it and delineate how the practice of self-care relies on colonized versions of ancient and traditional cultural and religious practices (e.g., yoga, meditation) that make invisible the cultural, spiritual, and religious histories from which these practices originate. In summary, this chapter offers a decolonial critique of traditional public and evidence-based notions of self-care as well as a proposal for how we might approach building decolonial community care.

WHY THE NEED FOR A NEW APPROACH TO SELF-CARE?

It can seem that self-care and activism stand in opposition to one another. In undertaking self-care, the individual may be seen as selfish and unwilling to sacrifice for the good of the community. In undertaking activism, the individual sacrifices the self (sometimes literally) in service of the community. Given the current interlocking socioeconomic conditions and systems of oppression, it may seem that a person needs to choose between self and community given the time, energy, and resources required for basic survival. This situation is facilitated by a dominant discourse of self-care and Western individualism in which the self is positioned as separate from family and community. Even when the dominant self-care discourse directs us to reconnect with people, it is to maintain the self, not the community. Moreover, it ignores the fact that people cannot be extracted from their collective and individual racial, ethnic, and cultural position. This dominant formulation alienates the majority of those who are non-White and view family, community, and cultural identity as central to their existence from self-care. Any version of self-care that seeks to meaningfully improve well-being within a White supremacist and capitalist system of interlocking oppressions needs to attend to the broader social context.

DECOLONIAL CONCEPTS AND TERMINOLOGY

The discussion of self-care presented here incorporates several concepts from decolonial and liberation psychology scholars. We agree with the perspective and use the term coloniality to refer to the long-standing effects and transformed continuation of U.S. colonization that has defined all aspects of society, knowledge production, labor, and the like (Maldonado-Torres, 2007). We understand that colonialism describes a relationship in which a nation extracts and steals resources, land, or people to become dominant, and that this relationship leaves impressions on every aspect of our lives (Jackson, 2018) including how we relate to, experience, and express ourselves (Maldonado-Torres, 2007), how domination and exploitation continue to operate beyond colonization (Quijano, 2000), as well as what we believe is true and how we understand the world to have been defined by colonialism (Martín-Baró, 1994). We turn to the concept of coloniality to reconsider self-care because it reminds us that if we use only concepts grounded in the perspective of the dominant group, we will reproduce that dominance even when we do not intend to do so (Mignolo, 2002). Moreover, the power of the colonial legacy suggests that it can lead us to believe that our current reality is the only one possible (Martín-Baró, 1994).

Self-care, like all other things, is shaped and informed by coloniality. It has been deracinated and depoliticized such that a dominant discourse of self-care is defined and limited by its relationship to White supremacy and capitalism. Thus we take a decolonial perspective and approach that seeks to "delink" or "detach" (Mignolo, 2007, 2017) self-care from White supremacist and capitalist structures of power and knowledge that define and control our relationship to, and understanding of, self-care. We offer an alternate view of self-care that creates the potential for other versions of self-care in which community and societal well-being become possible.

"FIND WHAT FEELS GOOD": U.S. CONCEPTUALIZATIONS OF SELF-CARE

In the public domain, the definition of self-care is often broad, oversimplified, and misleading. It is generally defined as doing "an activity that's good for your physical or mental well-being" (Cabotaje, 2020), coping with daily stressors (Lawler, 2021), preventing illness, and doing anything from exercise and meditation to shopping and watching television (Scott, 2021). Yet "its essence is so diverse, that any action which ends in oneself feeling happier and more positive can be attributed to it" (Taylor, 2020). This is in part how we have 57.6 million #selfcare Instagram posts as of January 2022 that share vastly different images of self-care and a self-care industry that earns an estimated $10 billion; and if you include technology like wearable devices such as health watches, self-care audio books, and apps, the estimates jump to hundreds of billions of dollars (IRi, 2018). In the context of consumerism, which seeks to anesthetize people with goods, food, and media, self-care easily becomes aligned with doing something that feels good, and thus indulgent. Additionally, the notion that self-care is akin to indulgence is ubiquitous. This is evident in articles, memes, and images related to self-care that depict bubble baths, manicures, alcohol, shopping for unnecessary goods, and watching television (Lawler, 2021). The number of online articles and blogs imploring people to understand the difference between self-care and self-indulgence (Forman, 2017; Lissy, 2019; Noonan, 2018) is in and of itself evidence that the message of self-care has been co-opted and depoliticized.

The dominant self-care discourse has also been deracinated. The image most associated with this depoliticized dominant narrative of self-care is of a White, cisgender, presumably heterosexual woman in yoga pants overlaid in a meme about taking time for herself. This portrayal of self-care reinscribes the idea that self-care is not for People of Color, queer, or disabled people and requires economic resources. In its association with White, heterosexual women, self-care is further sold as a form of indulgence; if it is only for White women, it must be indulgent. This racialized portrayal of self-care is then exported to People of Color, insisting that People of Color should have equal access to White women's form of self-care. When the message is adapted for People of Color, particularly for Black women, the message is that it is radical for Black women to engage in self-care, like Audre Lorde, because Black women experience so many forms of over overlapping structural oppression (e.g., racism, sexism, classism, homophobia) that any attempt to care for the Black body is radical (Lorde, 1988). Although it is true that Black self-care is a radical individual act, the Black radical tradition of self-care does not end with the individual (Lorde, 1988; Newman-Bremang, 2021). If it ends at caring only for the self, it remains focused on survival and does little to change the conditions that oppress Black women and Black people more generally. It is also unsurprising that even the renewed use of the term *radical self-care* has been co-opted to apply to all people in need of authentic self-care (cf. Degges-White, 2020). This once again reinscribes self-care as a deracialized and depoliticized practice and most notably is authored by a psychologist.

A popular example of this is *Yoga With Adriene*, a free yoga YouTube channel that has been operating since 2012. It has been credited with making yoga more accessible by offering yoga for free, in shorter doses, and tailored to specific populations (e.g., "Yoga for Manual Labor") or problems (e.g., yoga for foot pain) that do not usually receive the attention they deserve. On the one hand, Yoga With Adriene is an exemplary model of what making self-care resources free and widely available can do. Mishler's audience was extensive prepandemic, but exploded to 11 million YouTube subscribers and more than 1.1 billion views (Yoga With Adriene, 2012) during the pandemic. On the other hand, in an effort to welcome Americans to self-care, this version of yoga is completely disconnected from its religious, ethnic, and cultural origins, such that she is engaging in a lucrative business selling, and offering for free, a sanitized and deracinated version of yoga for financial gain.

In addition, the channel and the creator, Adriene Mishler, is known for the trademarked phrase "Find What Feels Good" (Yoga With Adriene, 2012). "Find What Feels Good" or FWFG, as seen on t-shirts, is an invitation to experience pleasure in yoga and to avoid injury by being aware of pain for the novice practitioner. As applied to yoga, the strategy is helpful and encouraging for beginners to maintain a yoga practice and feel invited. However, the phrase is also highly representative of the current state of self-care in the United States. "Find What Feels Good" is very much the perspective and even goal of many self-care seekers who are following the described, overly broad definitions of self-care. Yet what feels good is deeply entwined in a capitalist system and, as a guide, does not inherently direct people to good health or well-being.

The discourse of self-care also presumes the existence of economic resources, such as money, time, and childcare (El-Ghoroury et al., 2012; Restorick Roberts, 2017; Zeb et al., 2021). The most insidious aspect to practicing self-care is how difficult it has become. Neoliberal politics and policies (Duggan, 2014) have replaced easy and free public access to recreation centers, parks, libraries, and food co-ops with private health clubs, expensive organic markets, Little Free Libraries, book stores, and home food delivery. It has become more expensive to engage in any kind of self-care. For example, in the context of the global COVID-19 pandemic, ordering groceries online became a form of self-care that only wealthy people could access; it created an increase in working-class people and People of Color risking their health to provide for themselves and their families, all in the name of self-care and protection. Buddhist temples continue to provide free meditation and mindfulness practices. Public libraries provide access to books, computers, and internet. However, these public goods have been co-opted by individuals seeking personal credit for their offering. For example, the Little Free Library (https://littlefreelibrary.org) movement allows homeowners to install a small library on their property to give away books. In addition, that self-care is equated with indulgence and economic resources means that self-care has real monetary costs; spending more money is likely to signify greater indulgence and potentially produce greater self-care. Combined with the message that the individual ought to prioritize the self before family and community, the result is a public discourse of self-care that may be perceived as taking resources intended to be shared with family and community and redirecting them to the individual.

Current Evidence Base Supports Capitalistic Self-Care

Despite more than 75 similar and overlapping definitions of self-care in the scholarly literature (Godfrey et al., 2011), no singular definition has been agreed upon across the allied fields of psychology, counseling, and social work (Dorociak et al., 2017; Lee & Miller, 2013). In the psychology and medical research literature, the definition of self-care is similar to the public definition. Self-care is generally understood as engaging in behaviors that maintain a person's health and well-being and prevents burnout and illness (Lee & Miller, 2013); "ongoing practice of self-awareness and self-regulation for the purpose of balancing the physical, psychological and spiritual needs of the individual" (Carter & Barnett, 2014, p. 112); a person's efforts and capacity to promote their optimal health and well-being, prevent illness and manage chronic conditions (Woods et al., 1989); and engaging in behaviors that maintain and promote physical, emotional, cognitive, and spiritual well-being (Reese &

Meyers, 2012). The World Health Organization (WHO) defines self-care as "the ability of individuals, families and communities to promote health, prevent disease, maintain health, and to cope with illness and disability with or without the support of a health care provider" (WHO, n.d., para. 1).

One notable difference between the medical and psychological literature is that medical self-care emanates from the field of nursing and therefore focuses on building patient capacity for independence after an illness, surgery, or procedure as well as how to independently manage a chronic disease (Orem, 1985). Practically, this means a focus on physically caring for the body (e.g., taking medicine, eating what the body needs, seeing the doctor, tending to wounds). In psychology, the focus is on maintaining cognitive, emotional, relational, and spiritual well-being and functioning of practitioners in the context of trauma, burnout, stress, and overwork. Medical self-care is focused on patients, the broader population of society, whereas psychological self-care arises from trauma therapy and the need to specifically take care of clinicians, not the broader population. Thus psychological self-care has always been focused on how clinicians remain well in the face of bearing their client's trauma. It is also grounded in the notion that the aim of self-care is to help clinicians continue working. Although maintaining well-being in the face of trauma is a helpful professional goal given the amount of violence, trauma, economic hardship, and limited social safety networks, this kind of maintenance unintentionally encourages the belief that workers should be able to sustain themselves no matter the conditions, and thus encourages maintenance of the status quo. The public self-care discourse that discusses self-care among the general population is more aligned with this psychological framing that aims to help people maintain their wellness to keep working in the face of hardship, whereas the medical framing does not. Arguably, the public would be better served by a definition of self-care that emphasizes the medical framing's independent functioning over coping, because independence allows for self-determination and collective action rather than coping or maintenance that leads to surviving and managing the status quo.

The discourse of self-care often positions the self as separate from the community, that is, self-care is a time to focus on oneself and not others. Similar to how the practice of coloniality has sanitized and removed the religious and cultural meaning of specific ancient practices in service of the status quo, so has self-care been stripped of its political roots (Spicer, 2019). Professional psychology training, which focuses the most on self-care out of all psychology subspecialties, implicitly and explicitly suggests that self-care is an individual imperative and responsibility of the student (Callahan & Watkins, 2018; Miller, 2022; Pakenham, 2015). Despite cultural expectations that psychologists take good care of themselves for the ethical protection of the public, as well as specific self-care training benchmarks, self-care is still treated as an individual responsibility. This is exemplified by the minimal efforts within the field to provide self-care training to psychology graduate students because it is deemed their personal responsibility (Bamonti et al., 2014; Callahan & Watkins, 2018; Zahniser et al., 2017).

Even when the self-care discourse directs us to reconnect with people, it is for maintaining the self, not maintaining the community or building collective resistance and power. In this way, it has functioned as a professional survival mechanism. In the public, we are directed to reconnect with others because it brings us joy, decreases isolation, reminds us of who we are, and can make us feel more connected to our communities (Carlton-Smith et al., 2021). All of this is accurate, yet it still centers and focuses on benefits for the individual, leaving those who value their family and community as central to their existence remain alienated from the project of improving well-being that self-care is supposed to help achieve.

Taken together, we have a public working definition of self-care that says we should do healthy things, but we are encouraged and lured into doing individualized, indulgent, sometimes unhelpful activities. This understanding has developed in the gap between the idea of a health focused self-care and our actual capacity to practice self-care in our current racialized socioeconomic system. In the context of a racial capitalism (Gilmore, 2017) that requires people, particularly People of Color and working-class people, to work multiple jobs for long hours in unsafe working conditions for decreasing amounts of money, it becomes more likely and relatable that people will do what feels good with their remaining time, energy, and pay.

More troubling is that because of our capitalistic ideals and requirements that we should always be working and producing, even when we are exhibiting adaptive self-care behaviors, it feels indulgent. This is true for multiple reasons. First, related to capitalist requirements for constant production and our commercialization of self-care, we have lost sight of the line between stretching and overextension; overextension and good health are incompatible expectations that we are trying to adapt to. When we try to make time for good health, we feel indulgent. When we fail to achieve good health while overworking, we feel guilty. Second, the idea that we should take good care of ourselves to be in good health has morphed into an expectation that we should just be in good health without needing to the necessary steps to create good health. Finally, the cost of self-care and good health more generally has increased as an impact of neoliberal politics and policies (Duggan, 2014) that have removed public access into private entities, such as privatized medical and mental health care, private health clubs and gyms, and specialty health food.

The Business of Self-Care and the Self-Care Business

Self-care is sold as a way to prevent illness and burnout and avoid going to the doctor (IRi, 2018) so that the individual can perform and remain employed. Thus, without adequate self-care, the individual may spend large amounts of money on hospitals, may not remain employed, and may ultimately fall lower in the stratified economic system. The self-care industry is controlled by and supports neoliberal economic policy (Duggan, 2014) that emphasizes privatization and the withdrawal of state funded resources from public works (e.g., parks, pools, libraries), health care, and education. Individuals are asked to engage in better self-care, rather than demand better health insurance, more paid leave, and free childcare. The dominant discourse of self-care calls individuals to adapt to ruthless White supremacist, capitalist systems rather than challenge them, which ultimately strengthens the infrastructure of the oppressive system. Thus self-care comes to function as a method for helping individuals adapt to a neoliberal world in which increasing inequity, declining pay, and declining labor conditions have become the norm.

Self-care has also become critical to employers, to the functioning of the overall economic system, and in particular to the emergence of the gig or hustle economy. Employers want to push people beyond 40 hours a week and a 9-to-5 day by maintaining more part-time positions (Zundl et al., 2022) to avoid providing paid time off or health insurance—and have them continue to show up. Companies function with the understanding that turnover will be constant and plan for constantly training new people to address the situation. For companies that do not want turnover, they need employees to use their benefits (i.e., health insurance) and engage in self-care. In this context, self-care has become a necessary tool of capitalism and neoliberal economic policy.

For example, *Thrive Global* is a company that helps other companies such as Walmart, Verizon, and Microsoft, "end stress and burnout . . . and increase well-being and resilience." Their website tagline reads, "Employee well-being is no longer a benefit. It's a strategy" (Thrive Global, n.d.). They advertise "A Continuous, Real-time Behavior Change Ecosystem" that aims to improve well-being, resilience, and productivity. They provide examples of helping a Walmart Distribution Center associate who has learned to set "small goals, take baby steps . . . to finally feel that he is making progress, appreciating [his] small wins and heading in the right direction" (Thrive Global, n.d.). It is a strategy for company longevity to have "healthy" and "happy" employees through individualism and private initiatives to get each individual employee to take care of themselves, rather than provide additional benefits. Walmart is notorious for low wages, poor labor practices, inadequate health insurance (Layne & Carvale, 2014), and lawsuits. Unsurprisingly, Thrive Global's well-being and social justice section does not promote strategies for changing workplace labor practices, negotiating higher salaries, starting unions, or advocating for universal health insurance or childcare—actions that facilitate improved health and happiness.

In many ways, capitalism pathologizes employees by blaming their feelings of suffering on personal attributes that can be fixed by using wellness practices that the workplace has co-opted from other cultures, such as Buddhism (cf. Dawson, 2021). This is one way corporations help reduce the turnover in their toxic workplaces where profit is put ahead of employee wellness. For example, corporations and mental health professionals offer secular mindfulness (cf. Dawson, 2021) workshops in hopes of helping employees find peace in their otherwise toxic workplace. In this system, employees are taught to remain calm and complicit in an oppressive and toxic workplace.

The dominant discourse and practice of self-care reflect "an ensemble of ideological practices that help legitimize a world of growing inequality and shrinking possibilities by promoting and embodying a configuration of self compatible with that world" (Aschoff, 2015, May 9). Originally written to describe the role of Oprah Winfrey's enterprise in promoting the U.S. "neoliberal focus on the self," this statement is an equally accurate description of how self-care functions in the United States today. The self-care industry promotes self-care ideologies, practices, and even spirituality (e.g., Oprah's Super Soul Sunday), to help the individual adapt and feel better in a dehumanizing oppressive socioeconomic system that is unlikely to change, rather than promoting resistance and the desire to change the oppressive systems that cause ill health and unhappiness. Like the American dream, self-care is advertised as something that anyone can do, yet at the same time it is out of reach. It is technically true that anyone can engage in acts of self-care, take five minutes to breathe (quick), or go to church or temple or mosque (free). In practice, five minutes of breathing and regular attendance at church may help you to survive, but it will not change a White supremacist, capitalist system working to maintain the status quo where People of Color especially are often considered replaceable.

ERASING THE HISTORY OF SELF-CARE

Another aspect of the mainstream business and practice of self-care is that it significantly relies on, or looks to, ancient or traditional cultural and religious practices (e.g., yoga, meditation) with minimal recognition or education about the cultural and religious histories from which these practices originate. The coloniality of self-care is that it continues to extract, translate, and transform aspects of these practices as it promotes, studies, and approves of them with their self-imposed authority for use as a self-care method. These certified practices are then sold to the public, which of course includes the very people whose religious and cultural practices were co-opted. By omitting or even minimally referring to information about the histories of these practices, individuals and organizations promote themselves as a creator, trustworthy translator, and teacher of traditional cultural and religious practices and knowledge, all the while gentrifying them.

Elite universities tout their embrace of meditation and offer validation via the scientific method followed by commodification. "Although the practices of mindfulness and meditation are thousands of years old, research on their health benefits is relatively new, but promising" (Harvard University, n.d.). These institutes promise their stamp of evidence-based authority over practices that are admittedly "thousands of years old" but whose benefits need to be verified by a Western scientific method. These institutions become the experts who validate and "prove" that meditation, for example, works and can thus justify selling it. When the public wants to advance their practice and knowledge, they are directed to institutes of mindfulness (e.g., UCSD Center for Mindfulness, Mindfulness Based Stress Reduction Training) and certified yoga training offered by the very people and organizations who have extracted and commodified these ancient practices. Rarely do they refer the "buyer" to the "source." For example, Buddhist monasteries around the world offer mediation training for visitors. Mindfulness practitioners can visit one of Thich Nhat Hanh's many monasteries and learn directly from his disciples at no cost (e.g., Deer Park, Plum Village) rather than buying books written about him and his mindfulness work. Even better, people can visit any of the lesser-known Buddhist monasteries in the world, such as the Phap Vuong Monastery in Escondido, California, which runs free mindfulness retreats for families.

The translation, validation, and transmission of religious practices for profit is at once particularly egregious and consistent with colonial practice. Meditation and yoga, two of the most widely recommended activities, are ancient religious practices that are available at no cost. However, when offered by those outside the cultural and religious practice, they are rarely offered for nothing. Instead, free yoga or mindfulness classes are often taught by new practitioners as a method of furthering their individual training and careers and to sell other services or practices. Beyond these outlets, both practices, which usually do require instruction and practice, are all offered at ever-increasing prices. In addition, in the United States, consumers of meditation and yoga are overwhelmingly White and middle to upper class, such that teachers and practitioners of color have created POC-only spaces to reach and welcome People of Color who have largely been left out of the now well-documented health benefits of meditation and yoga. These include mobile apps specifically for People of Color, such as Insight Timer offering yoga, and Liberate Meditation offering meditation practices. In-person offerings also exist, such as Yoga for People of Color Sangha in Albuquerque, New Mexico.

WE NEED A NEW STARTING POINT: SELF-ACTUALIZATION WILL NOT LEAD TO LIBERATION

Maslow's (1943) hierarchy of needs is one of psychology's most cited models of human motivation and sets the stage for the development of our current conceptualization of self-care, which focuses on the individual to care first for their basic needs, then relational needs, and only then the ultimate purpose of personal enlightenment (self-actualization). As individuals begin to meet their basic needs, they gain the motivation to work toward achieving relational and other higher needs (Maslow, 1987). By placing a personal goal at the top of the hierarchy, Maslow presumes that all human interactions, even relational ones, are intended to further the individual's goal for the self. Emanating from this model of development, self-care is a tool for individual enlightenment and development.

Maslow developed his hierarchy after being inspired by learnings from Blackfoot Nation (Blackstock, 2011; Blackstock, 2014, as cited in Lincoln Michel, 2014; Jacobs, 2022). First Nation beliefs hold self-actualization as a first step and innate quality leading to community actualization and ultimately to cultural perpetuity. Individual goals thus also continue the historical and cultural history and legacy of the group (Wadsworth, 2008, as cited in Blackstock, 2011). As is common among White Western colonizers, Maslow took generously from Blackfoot beliefs to rewrite it and claim it as his own (Blackstock, 2011). Furthermore, he used this presumed inspiration to understand how individual humans might be motivated to function without understanding the human motivation of community. His ignorance of community and relational life presumably led him to drop those features he could not relate to. This pattern has been repeated time and time again with many Indigenous and cultural practices around the world.

Self-care is often discussed as a supporting mechanism to survive, thrive, and achieve greater life goals. Reframing the Blackfoot belief system in full allows us to consider an Indigenous model of self-care. Caring for the self then serves a purpose far beyond the individual. Self-care becomes a necessary first step to allow individuals to have healthy and effective family and community relationships. These relationships in turn serve to maintain and cultivate cultural preservation, not personal preservation.

Similarly, French and colleagues (2020) recently proposed a model of radical healing that also promotes collectivism and cultural preservation. Their vision and framework for authentic healing for People of Color asserts that seeking liberation and social justice are required for healing and well-being, as are critical consciousness and the capacity to collectively resist oppression and its resulting trauma, such that a sense of shared struggle prevents or minimizes misattribution and pathologizing the individual. In the description of radical healing, the authors note that People of Color and Indigenous people (POCI) also need self-care to cope with symptoms of racial trauma. In this model, self-care is needed as a tool and among other tools to achieve radical healing. Yet self-care that aligns with the current dominant discourse will not likely facilitate radical healing.

Self-care is not well understood as something distinct from healing, much less radical healing. Self-care is a tool; it is not an end unto itself. The dominant self-care discourse offers methods for coping that can distract from healing or, worse still, reinscribe the conditions that POCI are trying to heal from. Similar to radical healing, a decolonial approach to self-care requires critical consciousness (Prilleltensky, 2003) to be able to critically reflect on the relationship between self-care and White supremacy, capitalism, and coloniality. We suggest that a decolonial approach to self-care will help facilitate radical healing that centers the relationship between the self and community, attempts to detach and delink from the dominant discourse and practice of self-care, and is restorative.

A DECOLONIAL APPROACH TO SELF AND COMMUNITY CARE

In his work mentoring future psychology leaders, Alvin Alvarez (personal communication, 2018) often shares his description of community care in the context of leadership work using the image of geese flying in the V-formation. Geese fly in the V-formation to conserve energy and to assist in communication and coordination (Library of Congress, n.d.). The leader of the group flies in front and each pair of birds flies behind and slightly higher than the bird in front of it. When the leader gets tired, it moves back and inside the formation to be protected by the group and to recuperate. It then rejoins the formation at the back and moves forward as other geese take their turn leading the group. Under this model, leadership and service become an act that every group member takes on, as are the tasks of caring and protecting other group members. This is in stark contrast to Western versions of teams and leadership as modeled by the competitive cycling community, in which team members expend all their energy to burn out solely to propel a single rider to the top of the podium at the expense of all the others.

We propose that a decolonial approach requires delinking (Mignolo, 2007) self-care from the expectation of maintaining production or being more productive, as well as not limiting it to a survival response to exploitation and overextension. Self-care should move beyond a list of sanitized and authorized actions to an internal and community-based awareness of and attunement to personal needs, values, and culture that can guide individuals and communities toward health, wellness, and radical healing (French et al., 2020). The trap remains, however, that even when we are working for communities we can still overextend and be so rooted in the coloniality of production that we do not feel we can stop and share the burden and responsibility. We feel guilt, desperation, want power or control, and so we work no matter the consequence.

Instead, when individuals and communities contend with exploitation, feeling burned out, isolated, unwell, and so on, they can return to their needs, values, and culture to determine the most useful coping strategies that will provide relief and lead to a healthier way forward.

They can question situations they find themselves in to become grounded in a critical understanding of how colonial and capitalist systems created or contributed to their experience of being unwell, isolated, burned out, or exploited. This can be a process we engage in frequently and iteratively. It can also become a practice of telling a more truthful story about the conditions we live in that can lead to more systemic solutions and less individualization and personalization (guilt, shame, and the like) of why we feel unwell.

Thus a decolonial approach uses self-care to develop a "conscious and sober assessment of everyday reality" so that imagining and working toward better alternate realities become possible (Martín-Baró, 1994; Phillips et al., 2015). This approach includes a critical awareness and understanding that self-care is often used in service of capitalism, current socioeconomic conditions make self-care a necessary tool of capitalism, and current conceptions of self-care are directly responding to, coping with, and maintaining a system of racial capitalism.

We can begin a decolonial process of self-care by asking critically conscious questions about self-care (Table 16.1). These questions can return us to the purpose of our self-care and force difficult but meaningful questions about self- and community care. They can help us not fall into the trap of overextension, guilt, self-blame, equating our worth with work, and engaging in

TABLE 16.1. A Decolonial Approach to Self-Care: Questions to Reorient Your Self-Care

Domain	Questions
Beginning self-care	Who and what is my self-care for?
	What does my self-care allow me to do beyond my survival?
Developing a critically conscious self-care	What do I want to do with a healthy body, mind, and spirit?
	Why does doing self-care feel so difficult?
	Why do I feel guilt when caring for myself?
	Where did the idea that I should have to choose between myself and my community come from?
	Who does this choice benefit and who does it harm?
	How is my self-care shaped and influenced by my community?
	How is my self-care connected to the self-care of others and my ability to be in, with, and for my community?
	How does my self-care help and sustain my community?
	How might my self-care reinforce capitalist and colonial values of work and exploitation?

Note. Adapted from "When Your Graduation Gift Is Cancer: The Making of a Psychotherapist," by A. E. Miller, 2019, *Journal of Psychotherapy Integration, 29*(2), pp. 175–187 (https://doi.org/10.1037/int0000141). Copyright 2019 by the American Psychological Association.

indulgence and self-protection rather than resistance and self-determination. Interrogating and being intentional about self-care forces us to acknowledge that something is making us ill and stressed that we must survive, leading us to take a closer look at what is oppressing us. These questions also seek to reconnect and expose the entwined nature of all self-care. This is the critical consciousness that self-care should cultivate.

A decolonial approach to self-care includes being open to moving beyond normative methods of self-care (e.g., yoga, mindfulness) that are Western-ized and sanitized versions of ancestral, culturally, and spiritually grounded methods of self- and community care. Current day mainstream practices of yoga and mindfulness in particular have removed the cultural and religious traditions from their practice, exploring and reengaging in methods orig-inally described and practiced by cultures of origin and ancestors has the potential to lead to increased connection and healing, in community and for the self (Ayuk, 2020).

For example, a person of Burmese, Buddhist ancestry might reengage in mindfulness within the traditions of Buddhist temples and explore the historical adaptations that Burmese monks such as Ledi Sayadaw made to mindfulness practices to survive and attempt to end British occupation and colonization of Burma (Braun, 2013). As in the case of the authors of this chapter, one might choose to not try to "return to how things were" after a serious medical illness with respect to work (see Miller, 2019, for personal narrative), or might manage their despair about family separations at the border by helping organize individuals, communities, and systems that could best aid in and manage the overwhelming influx of migrants being abandoned by the state. In each of these cases, the critical aspect is being attuned to the needs, values, and culture that facilitate the kind of self-care that the person or community need in that moment. The choices we question are those that attempt to care for self through surface-level fixes and those that reinforce capitalistic demands. Although these self-care choices are helpful some of the time, they do not work toward a sustainable and liberated collective future. There is no one way to decolonize self-care, thus the questions we propose are meant to help guide rather than to instruct.

CONCLUSION

> I tell my students, when you get these jobs that you have been so brilliantly trained for, just remember that your real job is that if you are free, you need to free somebody else. If you have some power, then your job is to empower somebody else. This is not just a grab-bag candy game. (Toni Morrison as quoted in Houston, 2003, p. 212)

Although Morrison is specifically talking about students, her message applies. Self-care should not be a "grab-bag candy game" that we use to benefit only ourselves.

Current U.S. mainstream formulations and practices of self-care help people adapt to rather than change oppressive systems. They rely on extracted pieces of ancient cultural practices that are sold without permission or benefit to the cultures they are stolen from. It shames anyone who does not practice self-care. Benefits are also disproportionately conferred on those who are White and wealthy. The current culture of self-care is infused with coloniality and requires delinking and rethinking how, who, and what self-care is serving. Self-care should be a force for resistance and liberation from dehumanizing social, political, and economic conditions, rather than a tool to manage, accept, and perpetuate oppressive conditions. Yet coloniality means that the line between these two realities is constantly blurred and shifting. Therefore, it must be critically recontextualized as existing in and responding to a White supremacist, capitalist system. Claiming and deploying a more honest understanding of self-care means acknowledging the limits of the dominant discourse and putting into practice a self-care the goal of which is not merely individual survival, but also collective freedom.

RESOURCES

Achbar, S. B., & Abbott, J. (Directors). (2005). *The corporation* [Film]. Zeitgeist Films.

Ayuk, M. E. (2020, June 4). Decolonizing wellness: An ancestral approach to self-care. What would our ancestors do? [Blog]. *An Injustice!* https://aninjusticemag.com/decolonizing-wellness-an-ancestral-approach-to-self-care-b34664999fb

Francis, M., & Pugh, M. (Directors). (2017). *Walk with me* [Film]. Speakit Films. https://walkwithmefilm.com/

Heath, T. (2019, October 4). *Self-care to communities of care* [Video]. TedxMSU Denver. YouTube. https://www.youtube.com/watch?v=beOWvqBFK3I

Jacobs, D. T. (2022, March). Unsettling coloniality in the psychological sciences by restoring our kinship worldview. *Transcend Media Service.* https://www.transcend.org/tms/2022/03/unsettling-coloniality-in-the-psychological-sciences-by-restoring-our-kinship-worldview/

Lorde, A. (1988). *A burst of light and other essays.* Ixia Press.

REFERENCES

Aschoff, N. (2015, May 9). Oprah Winfrey: One of the world's best neoliberal capitalist thinkers. *The Guardian.* https://www.theguardian.com/tv-and-radio/2015/may/09/oprah-winfrey-neoliberal-capitalist-thinkers

Ayuk, M. E. (2020, June 4). Decolonizing wellness: An ancestral approach to self-care. *An Injustice!* https://aninjusticemag.com/decolonizing-wellness-an-ancestral-approach-to-self-care-b34664999fb

Bamonti, P. M., Keelan, C. M., Larson, N., Mentrikoski, J. M., Randall, C. L., Sly, S. K., Travers, R. M., & McNeil, D. W. (2014). Promoting ethical behavior by cultivating a culture of self-care during graduate training: A call to action. *Training and Education in Professional Psychology, 8*(4), 253–260. https://doi.org/10.1037/tep0000056

Blackstock, C. (2011). The emergence of the breath of life theory. *Journal of Social Work Values and Ethics, 8*(1), 1–16. https://indigenouslanguagelearning.ca/wp-content/uploads/2017/11/Blackstock-C_2011_The-emergence-of-breath-of-life-theory.pdf

Blackstock, C. (2014). *When everything matters: What happens to children when they are brought into care?* [Conference session]. National Indian Child Welfare conference, Fort Lauderdale, FL, United States.

Braun, E. (2013). *The birth of insight: Meditation, morning Buddhism, and the Burmese monk Ledi Sayadaw.* University of Chicago Press. https://doi.org/10.7208/chicago/9780226000947.001.0001

Cabotaje, A. (2020, December 30). What does self-care mean—And why is it important? *Right as Rain.* https://rightasrain.uwmedicine.org/mind/mental-health/self-care-meaning

Callahan, J. L., & Watkins, C. E., Jr. (2018). The science of training III: Supervision, competency, and internship training. *Training and Education in Professional Psychology, 12*(4), 245. https://doi.org/10.1037/tep0000208

Carlton-Smith, A., Whelan, D., & Mackenzie, M. (2021, February 17). Why social support is the most overlooked self-care routine. CampusWell. https://www.campuswell.com/social-support-for-self-care/

Carter, L. A., & Barnett, J. E. (2014). *Self-care for clinicians in train: A guide to psychological wellness for graduate psychology students*. Oxford University Press.

Dawson, G. (2021). Zen and the mindfulness industry. *The Humanistic Psychologist, 49*(1), 133–146. https://doi.org/10.1037/hum0000171

Degges-White, S. (2020, October 20). Radical self-care to protect your overall well-being. *Psychology Today Blog*. https://www.psychologytoday.com/us/blog/lifetime-connections/202010/radical-self-care-protect-your-overall-well-being

Dorociak, K. E., Rupert, P. A., Bryant, F. B., & Zahniser, E. (2017). Development of the professional self-care scale. *Journal of Counseling Psychology, 64*(3), 325–334. https://doi.org/10.1037/cou0000206

Duggan, L. (2014). Neoliberalism. In B. Burgett & G. Hendler (Eds.), *Keywords for American cultural studies* (2nd ed., pp. 181–183). New York University Press.

El-Ghoroury, N., Galper, D. I., Sawaqdeh, A., & Bufka, L. F. (2012). Stress, coping, and barriers to wellness among psychology graduate students. *Training and Education in Professional Psychology, 6*(2), 122–134. https://doi.org/10.1037/a0028768

Forman, T. (2017, December 3). Self-care is not an indulgence. It's a discipline. *Forbes*. https://www.forbes.com/sites/tamiforman/2017/12/13/self-care-is-not-an-indulgence-its-a-discipline/

French, B. H., Lewis, J. A., Mosley, D. V., Adames, H. Y., Chavez-Dueñas, N. Y., Chen, G. A., & Neville, H. A. (2020). Toward a psychological framework of radical healing in communities of color. *The Counseling Psychologist, 48*(1), 14–46. https://doi.org/10.1177/0011000019843506

Gilmore, R. S. (2017). Abolition geography and the problem of innocence. In G. T. Johnson & A. Lubin (Eds.), *Futures of Black radicalism* (pp. 225–240). Verso.

Godfrey, C. M., Harrison, M. B., Lysaght, R., Lamb, M., Graham, I. D., & Oakley, P. (2011). Care of self—care by other—care of other: The meaning of self-care from research, practice, policy and industry perspectives. *International Journal of Evidence-Based Healthcare, 9*(1), 3–24. https://doi.org/10.1111/j.1744-1609.2010.00196.x

Harvard University. (n.d.). *In Focus: Mindfulness and meditation*. https://www.harvard.edu/in-focus/mindfulness-meditation/

Heath, T. (2019). Self-care to communities of care [Video]. TedxMSU Denver. YouTube. https://www.youtube.com/watch?v=be0WvqBFK3I

Houston, P. (2003, November). The truest eye: The legendary Toni Morrison sits down with Pam Houston to discuss the beginning (Ohio), the middle (her revolutionary first novels), and her latest (the magisterial Love). *O, The Oprah Magazine, 4*(11), 212. https://link.gale.com/apps/doc/A111146315/ITOF

IRi. (2018, November). *Taking charge: Consumers grabbing hold of their health and wellness drives $450-billion opportunity*. https://www.iriworldwide.com/en-us/insights/publications/self-care-trends

Jackson, S. N. (2018). Colonialism. In E. R. Edwards, R. A. Ferguson, & J. O. Ogbar (Eds.), *Keywords for African American studies*. New York University Press.

Jacobs, D. T. (2022, March 28). Unsettling coloniality in the psychological sciences by restoring our kinship worldview. Transcend Media Service. https://www.transcend.org/tms/2022/03/unsettling-coloniality-in-the-psychological-sciences-by-restoring-our-kinship-worldview/

Lawler, M. (2021, May 19). What is self-care and why is it so important for your health? *EveryDay Health*. https://www.everydayhealth.com/self-care/

Layne, N., & Carvale, S. (2014, October 7). Wal-Mart raises healthcare costs, cuts benefits for some part-timers. *Reuters.* https://www.reuters.com/article/us-walmart-healthcare/wal-mart-raises-healthcare-costs-cuts-benefits-for-some-part-timers-idUSKCN0HW1G220141007

Lee, J. J., & Miller, S. E. (2013). A self-care framework for social workers: Building a strong foundation for practice. *Families in Society, 94*(2), 96–103. https://doi.org/10.1606/1044-3894.4289

Library of Congress. (n.d.). Why do geese fly in a V? https://www.loc.gov/everyday-mysteries/zoology/item/why-do-geese-fly-in-a-v/

Lincoln Michel, K. (2014, April 19). Maslow's hierarchy connected to Blackfoot beliefs. https://lincolnmichel.wordpress.com/2014/04/19/maslows-hierarchy-connected-to-blackfoot-beliefs/

Lissy, K. (2019, Oct. 15). The fine line between self-care and self-indulgence. *Ascent Publication.* https://medium.com/the-ascent/the-fine-line-between-self-care-and-self-indulgence-6a643f0765ac

Lorde, A. (1988). *A burst of light and other essays.* Ixia Press.

Maldonado-Torres, N. (2007). On the coloniality of being. *Cultural Studies, 21*(2–3), 240–270. https://doi.org/10.1080/09502380601162548

Martín-Baró, I. (1994). Writings for a liberation psychology (A. Aron & S. Corne, Eds.). Harvard University Press.

Marx, K. (1967). *Capital: A critique of political economy* (Vol. 1, B. Fowkes, Trans.). Penguin Books. (Original work published 1867)

Maslow, A. H. (1943). A theory of human motivation. *Psychological Review, 50*(4), 370–396. https://doi.org/10.1037/h0054346

Maslow, A. H. (1987). *Motivation and personality* (3rd ed.). Pearson Education.

Mignolo, W. D. (2002). The geopolitics of knowledge and the colonial difference. *The South Atlantic Quarterly, 101*(1), 57–96. https://doi.org/10.1215/00382876-101-1-57

Mignolo, W. D. (2007). DELINKING: The rhetoric of modernity, the logic of coloniality and the grammar of de-coloniality. *Cultural Studies, 21*(2–3), 449–514. https://doi.org/10.1080/09502380601162647

Mignolo, W. D. (2017, January 21). Interview – Walter Mignolo/Part 2: Key concepts. *E-International Relations.* https://www.e-ir.info/2017/01/21/interview-walter-mignolopart-2-key-concepts/

Miller, A. E. (2019). When your graduation gift is cancer: The making of a psychotherapist. *Journal of Psychotherapy Integration, 29*(2), 175–187. https://doi.org/10.1037/int0000141

Miller, A. E. (2022). Self-care as a competency benchmark: Creating a culture of shared responsibility. *Training and Education in Professional Psychology, 16*(4), 333–340. https://doi.org/10.1037/tep0000386

Newman-Bremang, K. (2021, May 28). Reclaiming Audre Lorde's radical self-care. Refinery29. https://www.refinery29.com/en-us/2021/05/10493153/reclaiming-self-care-audre-lorde-black-women-community-care

Noonan, S. J. (2018, March 2). Self-care is not self-indulgent. Why taking care of yourself is important to your emotional health. *Psychology Today.* https://www.psychologytoday.com/us/blog/view-the-mist/201803/self-care-is-not-self-indulgent

Orem, D. E. (1985). A concept of self-care for the rehabilitation client. *Rehabilitation Nursing, 10*(3), 33–36. https://doi.org/10.1002/j.2048-7940.1985.tb00428.x

Pakenham, K. I. (2015). Effects of acceptance and commitment therapy (ACT) training on clinical psychology trainee stress, therapist skills and attributes, and ACT processes. *Clinical Psychology & Psychotherapy, 22*(6), 647–655. https://doi.org/10.1002/cpp.1924

Phillips, N. L., Adams, G., & Salter, P. S. (2015). Beyond adaptation: Decolonizing approaches to coping with oppression. *Journal of Social and Political Psychology, 3*(1), 365–387. https://doi.org/10.5964/jspp.v3i1.310

Prilleltensky, I. (2003). Understanding, resisting, and overcoming oppression: Toward psychopolitical validity. *American Journal of Community Psychology, 31*(1–2), 195–201. https://doi.org/10.1023/A:1023043108210

Quijano, A. (2000). Coloniality of power and eurocentrism in Latin America. *International Sociology, 15*(2), 215–232. https://doi.org/10.1177/0268580900015002005

Reese, R. F., & Myers, J. E. (2012). EcoWellness: The missing factor in holistic wellness models. *Journal of Counseling & Development, 90*(4), 400–406. https://doi.org/10.1002/j.1556-6676.2012.00050.x

Restorick Roberts, A., Betts Adams, K., & Beckette Warner, C. (2017). Effects of chronic illness on daily life and barriers to self-care for older women: A mixed-methods exploration. *Journal of Women & Aging, 29*(2), 126–136. https://doi.org/10.1080/08952841.2015.1080539

Scott, E. (2021, December 9). *5 self-care practices for every area of your life.* VeryWellMind. https://www.verywellmind.com/self-care-strategies-overall-stress-reduction-3144729

Spicer, A. (2019). 'Self-care': How a radical feminist idea was stripped of politics for the mass market. *The Guardian.* https://www.theguardian.com/commentisfree/2019/aug/21/self-care-radical-feminist-idea-mass-market

Taylor, S. (2020, July 13). Self-care, Audre Lorde and Black radical activism. *Dissolving Margins Blog.* https://www.dissolvingmargins.co/post/self-care-audre-lorde-and-black-radical-activism

Thrive Global. (n.d.). *About.* https://thriveglobal.com/solutions/

Wadsworth, B. (2008). *Personal conversation with Billy.* Wadsworth, Blood First Nation.

Woods, N. F., Yates, B. C., & Primomo, J. (1989). Supporting families during chronic illness. *The Journal of Nursing Scholarship, 21*(1), 46–50. https://doi.org/10.1111/j.1547-5069.1989.tb00098.x

World Health Organization. (n.d.). *Self-care interventions for health.* https://www.who.int/health-topics/self-care#tab=tab_1

Yoga With Adriene. (2012). *Yoga With Adriene* [Video]. YouTube. https://www.youtube.com/c/yogawithadriene

Zahniser, E., Rupert, P. A., & Dorociak, K. E. (2017). Self-care in clinical psychology graduate training. *Training and Education in Professional Psychology, 11*(4), 283–289. https://doi.org/10.1037/tep0000172

Zeb, H., Younas, A., Ahmed, I., & Ali, A. (2021). Self-care experiences of Pakistani patients with COPD and the role of family in self-care: A phenomenological inquiry. *Health & Social Care in the Community, 29*(5), e174–e183. https://doi.org/10.1111/hsc.13264

Zundl, E., Schneider, D., Harknett, K., & Bellew, E. (2022). *Still unstable: The persistence of schedule uncertainty during the pandemic.* Shift Project Research Brief. https://shift.hks.harvard.edu/still-unstable

Index

A

Abandonment of racism phase, 259
Accapadi, M. M., 351
Accountability, 285
Accreditation status, 232
Acculturation, 22–23
Acompañamiento, 53, 54, 230–231, 306
Active concentration, 281
Activism
    education as decolonial, 50–52
    by Impacto Juventud, 49
    related to climate change, 189–190
    and self-care, 391
    social justice, 304
    spiritual, 298, 310
Adames, Hector, 3–4, 275, 375–377
ADDRESSING framework, 28
Advice, 312
Affirmative action, 209
Africa, 69
African American Buddhist teachers, 273
African Americans
    and gun violence, 111–112
    soul wounds among, 301
African psychology, 183–184
Africans
    kidnapped, 372
    in slave ships, 371
Afşin, B., 250
Aiello, M., 286
Aliento program, 221, 223–229, 234
"All lives matter," 340
Alvarez, A., 401
American Dream, 330
American Indians, 359

American Psychiatric Association, 308, 373
American Psychological Association (APA)
    accreditation by, 232
    APA Guidelines for Psychological Practice With Girls and Women, 355–358
    APA Guidelines on Race and Ethnicity in Psychology, 355–359
    APA Task Force on The Warrior's Path, 311
    Apology to People of Color, 263
    on coloniality, 4
    decolonization as deconstructing, 224
    Ethical Principles of Psychologists and Code of Conduct, 222, 271–272, 285, 309
    first black president of, 301
    guidelines of, 345
    Task Force on The Warrior's Path, 311
Ancestrality, 297
Anti-Blackness, 326–328
Anticolonial curriculum, 210
Anticolonial future, 262–263
Anticolonialism
    as contemporary and historical movement, 123–124
    as critical lens, 124–125
Anticolonial methodologies, 119–137
    case example of, 129–135
    enacting, in psychology, 135–137
    foundations of, 123–128
    and role of settler colonialism, 121–122
    shortcomings of decolonial research, 122–123

Anticolonial psychology, 6
Antioppression, 308
Antioppressive education, 214
Antiracism, 221, 308
Anti-Semitism, 328, 329
Anxiety symptoms, 24
Anzaldúa, Gloria, 152, 153, 162, 178, 189,
    219, 229, 241, 298–299, 310, 352
APA. *See* American Psychological
    Association
Apache people, 129–135
APA Ethics Code Task Force (ECTF), 272
*APA Guidelines for Psychological Practice
    With Girls and Women*, 355–358
*APA Guidelines on Race and Ethnicity in
    Psychology*, 355–359
Apartheid system, 175, 182, 192
APA Task Force on The Warrior's Path, 311
Apology to People of Color (APA), 263
Appropriate attention, 281
Archives, 73–76
Arendt, Hannah, 191
Artivism, 310
Asgharzadeh, A., 381
Asian American feminism, 352–353
Asian Indians
    colonial mentality expressed by, 19, 20
    mental health and colonial mentality in,
        33
Association of Black Psychologists, 222
Atallah, D. G., 157–158
Attention, 281
Attneave, Carolyn, 125
Aula en la Montaña (School in the
    Mountain), 50–52
Autoethnography, 148–149
Awe, 276
Aymara, 298

B

Bailey, T.-K. M., 19
Baldwin, James, 180
Banking system of education, 226–227
Baños, 312
Barad, Karen, 177
Bargero, M., 154, 155
Becker, D., 349
Belcourt, B., 375
Bell, D., 158
Benaway, G., 380–381, 383
Beshara, R. K., 325

Bhatia, S., 79
Bicultural conflict, 212–213
Bierer, L. M., 303
Bifocality, critical, 380
Big Other, 327
Bilingual speakers, in *Aliento* program,
    226, 228
Black, Indigenous, and other People of
    Color (BIPOC), 374
    colonization's mental health effects for,
        235
    consequences of White supremacy
        culture on, 247
    critical psychological approaches
        developed by and for, 263
    cultural resilience among, 304
    dehumanized, under coloniality, 5
    and Eurocentric values, 296
    internalized racism expressed by, 19
    marginalization of perspectives on
        illness/healing of, 250
    psychological theories/interventions
        with limited applicability for, 221
    racial identity development for, 259
    rationalization of harm done to, 222
    research by, and structural equity, 110
    research experience with, 225
    resistance among, 304
    resistance to pathologizing, 146
    sexuality of, 374–375
    supporting businesses owned and
        operated by, 262
Black, Indigenous, and other People of
    Color (BIPOC) mentees
    conscientization for, 256
    de-ideologization and denaturalization
        for, 255
    honoring strengths of, 254–255
    praxis for, 257
    problematization for, 256
    recovering of historical memory by,
        253–254
Black, Indigenous, and other People of
    Color (BIPOC) psychologists, 285–286
"Black Atlantic, Queer Atlantic" (Tinsley),
    371
Black feminism, 352
Blackfoot Nation, 400
Black Lives Matter movement, 255
Black people
    enslavement of, 371, 372
    impact of segregation on, 327
    sleep and health for, 284

Black psychology, 252
Black woman feminism, 306
Black women, 354
Blanket Exercises, 34
Blood memory, 301
Blood Memory: A Story of Removal and Return (documentary), 301
Blume, Art, xix
Bodhisattva, path of, 273, 282–283
Body language, 333
Body-positive views, 358
Boggs, Grace Lee, 353
Bomba, 50
Boonzaier, F., 89, 90
Borderlands, 152, 162, 241
Bottom-up approaches, 105, 106
Brain health, 303
Britain, 64–65
Brodkin, Karen, 175
brown, a. m., 287
Brown, D., 225
Bryant-Davis, T., 6, 308, 353–354
Buddhism, 273, 280–283, 398, 399, 403
Budge, Stephanie, 376
Buen vivir, 298
Bulhan, H. A., 91, 109, 110
Bull Lodge, 92, 104
Burnout, 402
Butler, Judith, 191
Byrd, Desiree, 193

C

Cabotaje, A., 392
Campón, R. R., 19
Canada, 76
Canadian Museum for Human Rights, 184
Capielo Rosario, C., 19, 23, 25
Capitalism, self-care and, 390–392, 396–398, 402
Caribbean women, 358
Carjuzaa, J., 94
Carlson, Teah Anna Lee, 178
Carolissen, Ronelle, 161
Carter, R. T., 19
Casswell, M., 73
Causadias, J. M., 97–98
CBPR. *See* Community-based participatory research
Celebrating Life program, 129–135

Center for American Indian Health, 137
Center for Latinx Communities, 225.
    See also Aliento (breath) program
Cermeño, I. E., 154–155
Chavez-Dueñas, N., 3–4, 257, 275, 375–376, 380
C-HeARTS (Community Healing and Resistance Through Storytelling), 111–112
Cheng, P., 284
Chicago, Ill., 52–55
Chicana/Latina feminism, 352
Chicano affirmative psychology, 356
Chilisa, B., 33
Chin, Jean Lau, xix
Choctow, 136, 137
Choque, 189
Christian syndrome (tolerance), 209
Churchill, Winston, 64–65
Çiftçi, A., 19
Circle, joining the, 305–307
Circular model of learning, 236–237
Civil rights movements, 346
Clark, K. B., 301
Classism, 222
Cleansings, spiritual, 312
Climate change
    effect of, on children, 51
    and Indigenous worldviews, 181
    youth activism related to, 189–190
Clinical approaches, colonial mentality in, 26–27
Clinical training requirements, 219
CM. *See* Colonial mentality
CM-IAT, 21–22
CMS (Colonial Mentality Scale), 18, 20
Cocreation, in supervision process, 237
Cognitive-behavioral therapy, 26–27
Collaboration
    between academia and communities, 172
    ethical principle of, 276
    between mental health professionals and communities, 51–52
    in participatory action research, 161
Collectivism, 401
Collins, P. H., 352
Colonial debt, 18–20
Colonial differences, 43
Colonial discourse, deconstruction of, 206
Colonialism, phases of, 16–17

Coloniality
    addressing effects of, 296
    defining, 63–64
    enduring nature of, 4
    interrupting, in daily interactions, 262
    and modernity, 67
    and self-care, 391–392
    as term, 391
    and White supremacy culture, 247
Coloniality positionality–decoloniality
    praxis, 6–8
Colonial mentality (CM), 15–35
    addressing, in clinical context, 26–27
    automaticity of, 20–22
    decolonial clinical approaches, 27–29
    decolonial community efforts to
        address, 29–32
    decolonial interventions, 34–35
    decolonizing research, 32–34
    manifestations of, 18–20
    pervasiveness of, 16–18
    psychological implications of, 22–25
Colonial Mentality Scale (CMS), 18, 20
Colonial resilience, 32
Colonial trauma, 301
Colonization
    no universal experiences of, 136
    in psychology, 228
    stages of, 208–209
Colonizing (term), 348
Colonizing viewpoints and practices,
    219–220
Color-blind racial ideologies, 250, 260
Comas-Díaz, L., 27, 52, 230, 251, 309,
    311, 339, 346–347, 352
Combahee River Collective, 346
Common core curriculum and
    accreditation standards, 208
Communities
    collaboration with, 194
    efforts to address colonial mentality in,
        29–32
    engaging in local, 190
    intervention strategies for, 193
    learning with and from, 105
Community-based healing, 238–239
Community-based historical research, 76
Community-based participatory research
    (CBPR)
    and anticolonial methodologies,
        125–128, 136–137
    used by WMAT-JHU partnership, 129, 131

Community-based research, 33–34
Community Healing and Resistance
    Through Storytelling (C-HeARTS),
        111–112
Community knowledge, 44–45
Community programs, 29
Community psychology, 252. See also
        Decolonial community psychology
        praxis
    developed in Majority World, 144
    history of, in U.S., 145–148
    in Puerto Rico, 47
Community relationships, 98–99, 103–104
Community storytelling efforts, 106
Compartmentalism, 277
Competence, 283
Concentration, active vs. selective, 281
Concientización, 54, 96
Connectedness, 98, 178
Connection, ethical principle of, 276
Conocimiento, 306
Conscientização, 147
Conscientization, 253, 256–257
Conscientization stage, in decolonization
    of curriculum, 213–214
Consciousness raising, 54, 377–379
Consejos, 312
Consumerism, 392
Contact zones, 177, 189
Corazón, teaching with, 229–233
Council of International Schools, 213
Covi, Ratu, 297–298
COVID-19 pandemic
    graduate training during, 233
    initiatives in response to, 50, 53
    isolation and community during, 191
    self-care during, 394
Create empowering teaching-learning sites
        (DPS framework), 101, 106–108
Creativity, colonialism and loss of, 225
Crenshaw, K., 350
Critical bifocality, 380
Critical collaboration inquiry, 213
Critical consciousness
    and anticolonial queer futures, 377
    for decolonization of curriculum, 213
    definition of, 347
    ethical, 100, 104–105
    and feminist therapy, 356–357
    in graduate education and training,
        221–223
    intertwined knowledge as, 153–155

local populations' need fort, 284
in mentorship, 256–257
Critical fabulation, 74
Critical feedback, on *Aliento* program, 224
Critical race theory, 229
Critical reflexivity, 150–153
Critical thinking, in decolonization of
curriculum, 206, 207, 211, 213
Cross-cultural psychology, 67–68
Critical race theory, 206
Cuentos, 212–213
Cultural appropriation
of Indigenous healing practices, 227
and stages of colonization, 209
Culturally responsive research practices,
103
Cultural research system, 98
Cultural wealth, 304
Cultural wisdom, 274–277
Culture
attending to, in decolonial mentoring,
250
colonizer's reconstruction of, 208
as contribution of oppressed
communities, 44
eradication of, 208
maintaining, as Indigenous resistance,
131
teaching, with language, 129–130
Curanderismo, 296
Curry Rodríguez, J., 220
Cusicanqui, Silvia Rivera, 153
Cwik, M., 129–134, 136–137
Cycles of life and development, 276

D

Danziger, Kurt, 80
David, Angela, 352
David, E. J. R., 18, 20–21, 23, 31
Davis, Angela, 156
Decision-priming tasks, 21
Declarations of the Rights of the Child
(United Nations), 48
Decolonial action, 235
Decolonial action stage, in decolonization
of curriculum, 212–213
Decolonial clinical approaches, 27–29
Decolonial community psychology praxis,
143–163
autoethnography, 148–149
definition of, 295

embodied critical reflexivity, 150–153
history of U.S. community psychology,
145–148
intertwined knowledge in action,
153–155
radical relationality, 156–159
transdisciplinarity, 159–162
Decolonial feminism, 169–194
epistemic justice, 187–194
pedagogical spaces, 180–187
Decolonial interventions, 34–35
Decolonialism, postcolonialism vs., 42–43
Decoloniality, 5–6
Decolonializing Methodologies (Smith), 91
Decolonial love, 380–382
Decolonial mentoring, defined, 248
Decolonial mentoring framework (DMF),
247–265
defined, 247
in everyday practice, 263–265
racial identity social interaction model
in, 261–262
rebuilding for an anticolonial future,
262–263
recognizing racial identity and power,
258–261
reorienting to a decolonial psychology,
251–258
resisting psycolonization, 250–251
Decolonial mentors, characteristics of, 264
Decolonial practice, 251
Decolonial psychology, 252
Buddhist contributions to, 280–283
competence in, 283
ethics for, 283–285
external saviors in, 280
multiculturalism in, 284–285
as paradigm shift to liberation, 5–6
Puerto Rican, 46–55
reorienting to a, 251–258
Decolonial psychotherapy, 295–313
coloniality addressed by, 296
epigenetics in, 302–303
guiding concepts of, 297–300
healing circles, 305–307
intergenerational resilience and
resistance, 304–305
naming the Wound in, 300–302
as racial trauma-informed therapy,
307–309
therapeutic relationship in, 309–312
Decolonial research, 122–123

Decolonial turn, 63–68
  to historical praxis, 71–76
  to history of psychology, 68–71
  to psychologies, 77–81
  in U.S. community psychology, 147–148
Decolonization
  challenges with, 122
  conceptualization of, 205–206, 220
  efforts in, 43–46
  epistemological, 65–66
  in framework of settler-colonialism, 63
  of graduate education and training,
    220–221, 232–233
  intellectual, 71
  of methodologies, 91–92
  of oneself, 286
  operationalizing, 251
  pluralism/complexity of, 205
  positionality and, 64–65
"Decolonization is Not a Metaphor"
  (Tuck & Yang), 376
Decolonization literacy, developing,
  352–353
Decolonization movement, 206
Decolonizing, 330–331, 379
Decolonizing interventions, 239–240
Decolonizing psychological sciences (DPS)
  framework, 89–113
  in action, 111–112
  create empowering teaching-learning
    sites, 101, 106–108
  facilitate human and community
    relationships, 98–99, 103–104
  foundations of, 93–97
  generate reciprocal knowledge and
    translation, 101, 105–106
  increase structural equity, 102, 108–111
  promote critical ethical consciousness,
    100, 104–105
  and psychologies for liberation, 92–93
Decolonizing Psychology course, 193
DeGruy, J., 301–302
Dei, G. J. S., 381
De-ideologization, 253, 255
De-ideologization stage, in decolonization
  of curriculum, 211–212
Deinistitutionalization movement, 146
Del Castillo, R., 295
Delinking, 402
Denaturalization, 253, 255
Denial and withdrawal stage of
  colonization, 208

Denigration, belittlement, and insulting
  stage of colonization, 208–209
Depression symptoms, 24–25
De Sahagún, Fray Bernardino, 272
Desenvolvimiento, 298, 310–312
Destruction and eradication stage of
  colonization, 208
Diab, M., 108
Diagnoses, 356
*Diagnostic and Statistical Manual of Mental
  Disorders*, 223, 227
Diaz, Junot, 8
Dichos, 312
Difficult Dialogues, 287
Diné people, 371
Disciplinary reflexivity, 348
Discrimination, with-in group, 18, 19
Diversity, absence of, 4–5
Diversity of standpoints paper, 232
DMF. *See* Decolonial mentoring framework
DNA, 302
Domestic violence crisis centers, 349
Domestic Violence Survivors Justice Act
  (DVSJA), 185–186
"Do no harm" principle, 221–222, 283
DPS framework. *See* Decolonizing
  psychological sciences framework
Drapetomania, 372
Dunford, R., 286
Duran, E., 104, 296, 297
Dussel, E., 279
Dutta, U., 149, 156–158
DVSJA (Domestic Violence Survivors
  Justice Act), 185–186

E

Ecologically attuned graduate curriculum,
  220
ECTF (APA Ethics Code Task Force), 272
Education. *See also* Graduate education
  and training; High school and
  undergraduate curriculum
  about oppression, 29–30
  banking system of, 226–227
  as decolonial activism, 50–52
Educational settings, 206
Eightfold Path, 280–281
El Centro, 150–152
Elements of Decolonial Healing Justice
  (Nixon), 312
Elimination, as colonial strategy, 121

Ellison, R., 327
Embarrassment, 18, 20
Embodied awareness, 150
Embodied critical reflexivity, 150–153
Embodying decoloniality, 220
Emotional labor, 238
Emotions
    as healing mechanism, 96
    theory connected to, 152
Empathy, radical, 310
Empowering teaching, 107
Empowerment, 349
Enculturation, 23–25
Energy work, 236
English language
    instruction in, 206
    translation of Náhuatl texts in, 273
Enriquez, V. G., 208
Entanglements, 177
Epigenetics, 302–303
Epistemes, 122
Epistemic justice, 187–194
Epistemic violence, 5, 121–122, 156
Epistemological decolonization, 65–66
Erased history
    in colonization, 208
    reflecting on, 211–212
    searching for, 210–211
ERI (ethnic or racial identity), 23–24
Espiritismo, 296, 308
Ethical consciousness, in DPS framework,
    100, 104–105
Ethical decolonial behavior, 274
Ethical Principles of Psychologists and Code
    of Conduct (APA), 222, 271–273,
    275–277, 285
Ethics, 271–287
    in Buddhism, 280–283
    in cultural wisdom and historical
        memory, 274–277
    for decolonial psychology, 283–285
    existing ethics guidelines, 271–274
    Indigenous African approaches to, 178
    in pre-Columbian Náhuatl beliefs,
        277–280
    reflection and continued growth in,
        285–287
Ethics codes, 223
Ethics in Psychotherapy and Counseling
    (6th ed., Pope et al.), 283
Ethnic or racial identity (ERI), 23–24
Ethnopolitical psychology, 252

Ethnoracial trauma, 300
Eugenics, 76
Eurocentric ideals
    dismantling, within psychology, 286
    and feminism, 350
    upholding, in psychology, 4
Eurocentric psychology
    constructed on narrow social basis, 80
    critiques of, 65–66
    decolonizing methodologies of, 91–92
    epistemological concerns about, 92
    ontological concerns about, 91
    oppression maintained in, 89–90
    and psycolonization, 122
    taught, in India, 64–65
    U.S. community psychology as,
        145–146
Eurocentric values, 248, 296
European-based psychology, 274–275
European Enlightenment, 324
Evangelical Christianity, 209
Even the Rat Was White (Guthrie), 263
Everyday experience, 255
Evolution, 303
Experiences
    embodied, 150
    everyday, 255
    knowledge produced through, 153
Experiential knowledge, 155
Expert knowledge
    prioritizing, over community
        knowledge, 44–45
    refusing, in favor of Indigenous
        knowledge, 134
External saviors, decolonial psychologists
    as, 280

F

Faaleava, F., 32
Facilitate human and community
    relationships (DPS framework),
    98–99, 103–104
la facultad, 298, 304, 312
Fallist protests, 69
Fallon, Thomas, 150–151
Fals-Borda, Orlando, 109, 187
Family statement (community statement),
    227
Fanon, Frantz, 9, 15–17, 22, 26, 35,
    92–93, 147, 175, 179, 322, 323, 326,
    327, 335, 336, 377

Feedback, in supervision, 237
#FeesMustFall movement, 183
Feliciano-Graniela, F., 323–324
Fellner, K. D., 220
Feminism. *See also* Decolonial feminism
  Asian American, 352–353
  Black, 352
  Black woman, 306
  Chicana/Latina, 352
  transnational, 347
  White, 350
Feminist methodology
  autoethnography as, 148–149
  and embodied critical reflexivity,
    152–153
Feminist therapy, 345–360
  and existing decolonization practices,
    352–355
  existing guidelines in, 355–359
  future directions for, 359–360
  issues and challenges in, 348–350
  and privilege, 351–352
Feminist therapy collectives, 349
Fenichel, O., 326, 329, 332
Fenimore-Smith, J. K., 94
Ferenczi, S., 326
Fernández, J. S., 154–155
Figueroa, Maria, 229
Filipino Americans
  colonial mentality expressed by, 17–20
  mental health and colonial mentality in,
    24–25, 33
  psychological decolonization
    frameworks for, 30–31
  research on colonial mentality with,
    20–22, 32
"Find What Feels Good" (FWFG), 393
Fine, M., 179, 380, 383
Firehammer, J., 104
First Nations, 400
First Peoples, 301
Fish, Jillian, 104
Flexibility, in supervision, 237
Flowering, 304
Floyd, George, 233
4Rs of decolonial mentoring framework,
    248–249
Four Noble Truths, 280
Free association, 333
Freedom's Journal, 172
Freire, Paolo, 17, 96, 147, 211, 213,
    226–227, 229, 256, 340, 347

French, B. H., 401
Freud, S., 322, 325, 326, 331, 339, 340
Fuentes, M. J., 74–75
Fuentes, Marisa, 72
FWFG ("Find What Feels Good"), 393

G

Gandhi, Mohandas, 124
García, C., 323–324
García, M. A., 273, 275–277
Garrett, J. T., 299
Garrett, M. W., 299
Gautama, Siddhartha (the Buddha), 280
Gaztambide, D. J., 322, 333
Gender, before colonization, 370–372
Generate reciprocal knowledge and
    translation (DPS framework), 101,
    105–106
Gespe'gewa'gi Mi'gmawei Mawiomi, 80
Ghaddar, J. J., 73
Ghanaians
  colonial mentality expressed by, 18–19
  mental health and colonial mentality
    in, 25, 33
Gherovici, P., 308
Gig economy, 397
Global Majority, 90
  community psychology developed in,
    144
  cultivating authentic partnerships with,
    98
  including, in psychology, 110
  increasing structural equity for, 109
Global North, 295, 347
Global South
  cultural healing practices of, 310
  decolonization efforts in, 68–69
  and epistemic decolonization, 66
  epistemologies from, 295
  and feminism, 347
  influence of, in Puerto Rican psychology,
    47
  knowledge from, as undervalued, 4–5,
    188, 324
  psychoanalysis from, 339
  psychoanalysis of, 321
  psychotherapy concepts from, 297
  talk therapy from, 296
Gone, J. P., 92, 104, 371, 378–380
Good health, 396
Goodman, R. D., 44, 228, 379

Gorski, P. C., 44, 228
Gqola, Pumla, 184
Graduate Center, 193
Graduate education and training, 219–242
  challenges of decolonizing, 232–233
  colonizing viewpoints and practices in, 219–220
  creating space for student voices in, 223–229
  critical consciousness and social justice ethic in, 221–223
  decolonization of, 220–221
  decolonizing courses in, 193
  deconstructing Western Euro-settler perspectives in, 223
  increasing structural equity in, 110
  supervision norms, perspectives, and process in, 233–241
  teaching with spirit and *corazón* (heart) in, 229–233
Graeber, D., 325
Great Puerto Rican migration, 47
Greene, Maxine, 194
Group counseling, 374
Group supervision, 238
Group therapy, 374
Guiding Principles for Engaging in Research With Native American Communities (Straits et al.), 273, 275
Gun violence, 111–112
Guthrie, R., 263

H

Halagao, P. E., 31
Hanh, Thich Nhât, 280–281, 399
Hargons, C., 374
Harriet's Apothecary, 378
Hartman, Saidiya, 73, 74
Hartman, W. E., 124–125, 131, 135
Harvard University, 399
Hatuey (Taino hero), 340
Healing, radical, 401, 402
Healing circles, 305–307
Healing practices, holistic, 357–358
Healing research methodologies framework, 95–97
Health
  good, 396
  Western/European vs. Indigenous view of, 277
Health intervention efforts, 135

The Heart of the Buddha's Teaching (Hanh), 280–281
Hegarty, P., 79–80
Heine, H., 328
Helms, J. E., 5, 24, 248, 258, 259
Help-seeking, 25
Here and Now (podcast), 284
Hernández-Wolfe, P., 241
Hersey, Tricia, 237, 284
Heteronormativity, 222
Heterosexism, 371–372
Hierarchy of needs, 400
High school and undergraduate curriculum, 205–215
  approaches to decolonizing, 209–214
  increasing structural equity in, 110
  stages of colonization, 208–209
Hijras, 371
Hinojosa, Maria, 225
Historical memory, 109, 253–254, 274–277
Historical praxis, 71–76
Historical trauma, 301
Holistic healing practices, in feminist therapy, 357–358
Honoring, ethical principle of, 276
hooks, bell, 107, 211, 229, 346, 350, 352
Ho'oponopono, 296
Horney, K., 326
Human rights, 223
Humility, 241
Hurricane Maria, 332
Hurtado, A., 346, 352
Hustle economy, 397

I

IAT (Implicit Association Test), 21–22
Identity
  context for, 277
  ethnic or racial identity, 23–24
  ontological markers of, 69, 70
IK. *See* Indigenous Knowledges
Ill health, 389–390
Image teaching, 280
Imagination, colonialism and loss of, 225
Impacto Juventud (Youth Impact), 48–50
Implicit Association Test (IAT), 21–22
Inappropriate attention, 281
Inclusive curriculum, 210
Increase structural equity (DPS framework), 102, 108–111

India, 64–65, 371
Indigenous ancestral wisdom, 236
Indigenous cultures, 273, 370
Indigenous healing practices, 227
Indigenous Knowledges (IK)
    and anticolonial methodologies, 126
    elimination of, in colonization, 121
    learning to listen to, 181–182
    recovery, reclamation, or revitalization
        of, 120, 127–128, 132–134
Indigenous languages, access to, 129–130,
    235
Indigenous people
    best-practices for engaging research
        with. *See Guiding Principles for
        Engaging in Research With Native
        American Communities* (Straits
        et al.)
    and conscious mind, 324–325
    and feminism, 350
    histories of, 77–78
    Latin American colonization from
        perspective of, 213
    leading the way, in research, 127–128,
        133
    respecting and valuing, 263
Indigenous research methodologies,
    33–34, 91–92
Indigenous resistance, 126–127, 130–132
Indigenous science, 250
Indigenous ways of knowing, 206, 220,
    251
Individualism, 296, 324, 391, 395–396
Inferiority, 18–20
"In My Decolonized Black Queer Love
    Story" (Stewart), 382
Insight Timer (app), 400
Insomnia, racial discrimination and, 284
Instagram, 392
Integrative awareness stage, of racial
    identity development, 259
Intellectual decolonization, 71
Interdependence, 98
Interdisciplinary approaches
    in community psychology, 159–162
    in healing research methodologies, 96
    increasing structural equity with, 109
    in story science, 105
Intergenerational transfer, 300
Intergenerational trauma, 311
Intergeneration aspects, of decolonial
    psychotherapy, 304–305

Internalization stage, of racial identity
    development, 259
Internalized racism, 18, 19, 26
Intersectionality, 95, 96, 287, 355
Intertwined knowledge in action, 153–155
Intuition, 240, 276
Intuthuko embroidery collective, 184–185
Iroquois people, 324

J

Jacobsen, F., 302, 309
Jean-Louis, Girardin, 284
Jews and Judaism, 175, 322, 326, 329
Johns Hopkins University (JHU), 129–135,
    137
Jones, S. H., 149
Jordan, M., 306
Jouissance, 327, 328–331, 336, 337
Jung, C. G., 297
Justice
    epistemic, 187–194
    injustice as focus of liberation
        psychology, 93
    social justice, 236, 340, 358
    social justice action, 228–229
    social justice activism, 304
    as tenet of community psychology, 144
    transformative justice, 287

K

Kanesatake Resistance, 124, 132
Keating, A., 219
Kessi, S., 89, 90, 190
Kidsbridge Tolerance Center, 211
Kiguwa, Peace, 64
Kluckhorn, C., 309
Knowledge. *See also* Indigenous
        Knowledges
    alternative histories as, 77–78
    community, 44–45
    creating, in educational programs, 50
    in epistemological decolonization, 65–66
    experiential, 155
    Indigenous approaches to, 92
    intertwined, in action, 153–155
    local, place-based, and situated, 62, 79
    pluriversal, 68
    as process and outcome of relationships,
        158
    reciprocal, 101, 105–106

recognizing multiple systems of, 188
shared, 154–155
Knowledge production
acknowledging different sources and
types of, 44–45
as domain of academia, 172
with embodied critical reflexivity, 152
research as, 120
and rival ways of knowing, 70
through experiences, 153
Kochiyama, Yuri, 353
Korean War, 308
Kornfield, J., 282

L

Lacan, J., 327, 332
Laenui, P., 30, 208
Land acknowledgment, 377
Latin America, 68–69
Latin American cultures, 212–213
LatiNegra, 7
Latinx communities, 225–226
Latinx people
ancestral healing and wisdom of, 312
Queer, 378
sleep and health for, 284
Latinx psychology, 44
Latinx women, 354
Law, John, 79
Lebeloane, L. D. M., 207, 209
Lee, B. A., 380
Lee, Martin, 286
Lee, Rich, 286
León-Portilla, M., 277, 278
Lessons, events as, 276
Letters of accountability, 171–172
Lewis, T., 221
Liberate Medication (app), 400
Liberation
decolonial action for, 212–213
self-care and, 400–401
Liberation Now podcast, 263
Liberation praxis, 52, 147, 170
Liberation psychology, 321, 326
and *Aliento* program, 226
and community psychology, 147
and DPS framework, 92–93
essential elements of, 252
in graduate education, 230
and model to decolonize curriculum,
211–213

reorienting with principles of, 252–258
supervision rooted in, 235–236
transmodernity vs., 279–280
Liberation psychotherapy, 27–28
Liebert, Rachel, 178
Limpias, 312
Linklater, R., 308
Little Free Libraries, 394
Local knowledge, 79
Lorde, A., 237, 346, 350, 352, 369, 389,
390, 393
Love, decolonial, 380–382
Lugones, M., 179, 321, 330, 331, 372
Luiggi-Hernandez, J., 323
Lumadi, M. W., 210

M

Madres Emprendedoras, 154–155
Madyaningrum, Monica, 161
Mal de palea, 308
Maldonado-Torres, N., 63, 160, 251, 279,
322
Mannoni, O., 327
Māori Language Act of 1987, 124
Māori people
anticolonial activism by, 124
Ormand's experience as, 174–175
research with Indigenous research
methodologies, 91–92
Tipuna Project with, 178
worldview of, 180–182
Māori protest movement, 124
Marcos, S., 3, 265
Marginalization, 356
Marginalized people
in healing research methodologies, 96
primary sources from and about, 74
resistance to pathologizing, 146
Martín-Baró, Ignacio, 34, 93, 147, 210–212,
229, 252, 297, 325–326
Marx, K., 389, 390
Maslow, A. H., 400
Matrix of power, 214
May, Kiley, 383
Mbembe, A., 70
Mbiti, John, 178
McGowan, T., 327
McLean, K. C., 380
McWhirter, Ellen, 242
Medical self-care, 395
Medicine Wheel, 299

Medina, L., 233
Medina Escobar, E. V., 323
Meditation, 281–282, 398–399
Mehl-Madrona, L., 298
Memmi, Albert, 17
Menakem, R., 301
Mental health, 24–25, 32–33
Mental health services, 51–52
Mentorship
    Eurocentric values upheld in, 248
    resisting psycolonization through,
        250–251
    RISIM model for analyzing, 261–262
Mentorship relationship, 255
Merchant Marine Act (Jones Act) of 1917,
    46
Mestizaje de saberes, 153–154
Mexico, 371
Microsoft, 397
Mignolo, W. D., 45, 63, 174, 298
Mi hogar, mi lugar (My home, My place)
    collective poem, 242
Miles, Tiya, 74, 75–76
Miller, A. E., 404
Million, Dian, 74
Mindfulness, 280–282, 399
Mindfulness Based Stress Reduction
    Training, 399
Miracles, 276
Mishler, Adriene, 393
Mitchell, T., 301
Miya communities, 158
Mkhize, N., 177–178
Moane, G., 207
Modernity, 67, 79
Mohawk Nation, 124, 132, 383
Moore-Lobban, S. J., 353–354
Moraga, C., 152
Morgensen, S. L., 371
Morphic resonance, 311
Morrison, T., 404
Morrison, Toni, 108–109
Morse, Gayle Skawen:nio, xix
Mosley, D. V., 308, 374
Moura, James Ferreira, 161
Mujerista psychology, 230, 236, 353–355
Multiculturalism, 284–285
Multicultural principles, in ethics codes,
    223
Multiple consciousness, 352–353
Multiple knowledge systems, 188
Murray, H. A., 309

Muwekman Ohlone communities, 151
Muxe, 371
Mystery, 276
Myth of Empowerment (Becker), 349

N

Nadal, K. L., 23
Náhuatl culture, 272–273, 277–280
Náhuatl language, 235
Naknanuk, E. K., 61
Nandy, Ashis, 79
Nap Ministry, 237, 284
Nash, R. J., 228
National Association of Black Studies,
    106
National Council of Teachers of English
    (NCTE), 212
National Latinx Psychological Association,
    242
National Latinx Psychological Association
    (NLPA), 222
Native Americans, 298, 304, 306, 370–371
Native culture
    appropriation of, 209
    eradication of, 208
Native Hawaiians, 30
Native Land Digital, 263
Native ways of knowing, 206
NCTE (National Council of Teachers of
    English), 212
Ndlovu-Gatsheni, S. J., 66
"Nea Onnim No Sua a, Ohu" (the one who
    does not know) symbol, 249
Neoliberalism, 394, 397
Nepantla, 241
Neville, H. A., 103
Nichols, L., 154–155
Nikalje, A., 19
Nixon, A., 312
Nixon, L., 375
Nixon, Lindsay, 383
NLPA (National Latinx Psychological
    Association), 222
Noble Eightfold Path, 273, 280–281
Nonmaleficence, moving beyond, 104
Nonracist identity development phase, 259
Non-Western interventions, 240
Norms, questioning, 233
North America, 273
Nos-otras, 178, 188
"Not-knowing" stance, 332

Nta'tugwaqanminene: Our Story, Evolution of the Gespe'gewa'gi Mi'gmaq (Gespe'gewa'gi Mi'gmawei Mawiomi), 80

O

Objects
  as archives, 75–76
  sharing findings through, 106
  in visual methodologies, 184
Ocampo, C., 308
Ohlone communities, 151
Oka Crisis, 124
Okazaki, S., 18, 20–21, 23
One World World, 79
Online grocery ordering, 394
Opara, I. N., 376
Ordover, N., 372
Original Peoples of the Abya Yala, 279–280
OrigiNatives, 104–105
Orloff, J., 311
Orozco, A. R., 154–155
Ortega, N., 332–333
Overextension, 389–390, 396

P

Palestinian communities, 158
Parallel dyads, 260
Paranjpe, A. C., 77
PAR Entre-mundos, 172–173
Participatory action research (PAR), 160, 178, 184–185, 380
Participatory contact zones, 177, 189
Participatory history, 76
Participatory research, 33–34
Patriarchy
  and feminism, 351, 353
  and psychotherapy relationship, 346
Pavón-Cuéllar, D., 332
PBS in the Classroom, 212
PBS Teachers' Lounge, 212
PCSD (postcolonial stress disorder), 301
Peace Prayer, 311
Pedagogy
  decolonial feminism in, 180–187
  empowering and healing, 107–108
Pedagogy of the Oppressed (Freire), 226
People of Color
  and feminism, 350, 351
  and self-care, 393, 399–400

People of Color and Indigenous people (POCI), 401
Pepperdine University, 225
Pérez Ortega, R., 284
Perspectives, inviting divergent, 188–189
Peterson, Bhekizizwe, 191
Phap Vuong Monastery, 399
Pickren, W. E., 71
Pillay, S. R., 379, 381–382
Pillay, Suntosh, 173
Pláticas, 236
Platt, Jason, 231
Pluriversality, 70, 78, 286
Pluriversal knowledge, 68
POCI (People of Color and Indigenous people), 401
"Poetry as data, data as poetry" workshop, 242
Political action, 338
Political mentalization, 338
Pope, K. S., 274, 283
Positionality, 64–65, 231–232
Postcolonialism
  decolonialism vs., 42–43
  focus of scholarship on, 63–64
Postcolonial psychology, 46–55
Postcolonial stress disorder (PCSD), 301
Posttraumatic slave syndrome (PTSS), 301–302
Posttraumatic stress disorder (PTSD), 303
Power dynamics
  being mindful of, 28–29
  in the global academy, 70
  racial identity and relational, 260–261
  reproducing colonial, 41
#PowerUp, 111–112
PPLTM (Public Psychology for Liberation Training Model), 94–95, 98
Pratt, M. L., 177
Pratto, F., 79–80
Praxis. *See also specific praxes*
  in rebuilding for an anticolonial future, 262–263
  for reorienting to a decolonial psychology, 253, 257–258
PRIA (Puerto Rican Influence Area), 53
Prilleltensky, I., 225
Primary sources, 73–76
Primitive, 79
Privatization, 397
Privilege, 351
Problematization, 253, 256

Professionalism, 233–234
Progressive dyads, 261, 264
Project AFFIRM, 375
Promote critical ethical consciousness
    (DPS framework), 100, 104–105
Protection, 241
Protective factors, 130
Proverbs, 312
Psychoanalysis, 321–340
    in broader historical context, 324–326
    clinical illustrations of, 333–338
    decolonizing approach to clinical and
        community work, 331–333
    Fanon's views on race, 329–330
    Freud's views on race, 328–329
    history of, 326–327
    practice recommendations for, 338
    theoretical implications of decolonizing,
        330–331
Psychological coloniality, 41–55
    and decoloniality efforts, 43–46
    in decolonialization efforts, 44–45
    necessity of Puerto Rican postcolonial
        and decolonial psychology, 46–55
    terminology, 42–43
Psychological decolonization frameworks,
    30–31
Psychological self-care, 395
Psychologists
    expanding roles of, 34–35
    filling multiple roles, 54
    prioritization of expert knowledge by,
        44–45
    tlamatinime as, 277–279
Psychology (field). See also specific fields
    changing, for ethical decolonial
        psychology, 283–285
    colonization in, 228
    decolonial turn to, 77–81
    enacting anticolonial methodologies in,
        135–137
    to history of, 68–71
    types of knowledge valued by, 121
Psychology programs, 382
Psychosocial accompaniment, 159
Psychotherapists, 219
PsycInfo, 16
Psycolonization
    epistemic violence through, 121–122
    refusing the terms of, 134
    resisting, 250–251, 265

PTSD, 307–308
PTSD (posttraumatic stress disorder), 303
PTSS (posttraumatic slave syndrome),
    301–302
Public Psychology for Liberation Training
    Model (PPLTM), 94–95, 98
Public Science Project, 185, 193–194
PubMed, 302
Puerto Rican Influence Area (PRIA), 53
Puerto Ricans
    acculturation and stress in, 23
    colonial mentality expressed by, 19
    mental health and colonial mentality
        in, 25
    postcolonial and decolonial psychology
        for, 46–55
    postimmigration status as Others, 47
Puerto Rican syndrome, 308
Puerto Rico, 46–55, 332, 336–338
Putnam, James Jackson, 75

Q

Queer and transgender BIPOC (QTBIPOC),
    375–376
Queer people, 326
Queer psychology, 369–384
    creating an anticolonial, 376–383
    QTBIPOC and disruption/reimagining
        of, 375–376
    and queerness before colonization,
        370–371
    and queerness during colonization,
        371–372
    and theories/frameworks as products of
        colonization, 372–373
    White roots of, 373–375
¿Quién eres, quienes somos? (Who are
    you, who are we?) collective poem,
    242
Quijano, A., 214, 279

R

Race
    attending to, in decolonial mentoring,
        250
    as contribution of oppressed
        communities, 44
    Fanon's views on, 329–330
    and feminism, 350

Freud's views on, 328–329
  silencing of, 335–336
Racial capitalism, 111, 325, 330, 396
Racial differences, 43–44
Racial discrimination, insomnia and, 284
Racial equity, for decolonialization, 251
Racial Equity Action Plan, xx
Racial identity
  recognizing, 259–260
  and relational power dynamics,
    260–261
Racial identity social interaction model
    (RISIM), 258–262
Racial identity theory, 259
Racial silencing, 335–336
Racial socialization, 258
Racial trauma, 300, 307
Racism, 307
  and coloniality, 247
  confronting modern day, 254
  and mental health, 111
  systemic, 222, 254
Radical empathy, 310
Radical healing, 252, 263, 401, 402
Radical Healing Collaborative, 378
Radical honesty, 173
Radical humanity, 230–231
Radical listening, 284
Radical relationality, 156–159
Radical self-care, 393
Rape crisis centers, 349
Ratele, K., 90
Ratts, M. J., 28
Readsura Decolonial Editorial Collective, 5
Rebuilding for an anticolonial future
    (pillar 4), 262–263
Reciprocal knowledge, 101, 105–106
Recognizing racial identity and power
    dynamics (pillar 3), 258–261
Recombinant narratives, 74
Red path, 312
Red Power movement, 125
Reed, T., 301
Reflexivity, 96, 150–153, 155, 348,
    355–357
Reflexivity rituals, 336–338
Reframing discussion stage, in
    decolonization of curriculum,
    210–211
Regressive dyads, 260–261
Reich, W., 332

Reiki, 236
Relational power, 260–261
Relevance, of psychology, 68
Relevant healing, 276
Religiosity, 354
Reorienting to a decolonial psychology
    (pillar 2), 251–258
  with conscientization, 256–257
  with de-ideologization and
    denaturalization of everyday
    experience, 255
  by honoring people's strengths,
    254–255
  praxis for, 257–258
  with principles of liberation psychology,
    252–258
  with problematization, 256
  by recovering historical memory,
    253–254
Repatriation, of land, 122–123
Resilience
  in Celebrating Life curriculum, 129–135
  recognizing, 356
Resisting psycolonization (pillar 1),
    250–251
Respect, 276
Respectability politics, 234
Responsibility, for self-care, 395–396
Rest, 237–238
Rest, liberation and, 284
Reyes, K., 220
Reyes Cruz, M., 160
#RhodesMustFall movement, 183
Richter, Agnes, 75
Right Action, 281, 287
Right Concentration, 281
Right Diligence, 281
Right Effort, 281
Right Livelihood, 281, 287
Right Mindfulness, 280–281
Right Speech, 281, 284
Right Thinking, 280
Right View, 280
RISIM (racial identity social interaction
    model), 258–262
Rituales de reflexividad, 332–333
Rizal, Jose, 17
Roach, M., 247
Robinson, C. J., 325
Rodriguez, P., 154–155
Rojas-Arauz, Brian, 242
Roman Catholicism, 296

Roots and Routes of Decoloniality in Community Psychology (RRD-CP) Project, 161
RRD-CP (Roots and Routes of Decoloniality in Community Psychology) Project, 161
Rutherford, A., 70, 78

S

Saberes compartidos, 154
Saberes entrelazados, 153–155
Sacredness, 276, 286
Said, E., 322
Saint Francis Prayer, 311
Salomon, M., 330
San José, California, 150–152
Santería, 296
Santos, B. S., 65, 80
Sartre, J.-P., 329
"Savior" mentalities, 352
Sayadaw, L., 403
Schemas, racial identity, 258
Scientific method, 399
SC-PAR (Sociopolitical Citizenship Participatory Action Research) Project, 157
Segalo, Puleng, 64, 179, 192
Segundo Ruiz Belvis Cultural Center (SRBCC), 52–55
Sekhem, 325
Selective concentration, 281
Self-care, 389–404
  and activism, 391
  business of, 397–398
  decolonial approach to, 401–404
  and decolonial concepts/terminology, 391–392
  definitions of, 394–395
  erasing the history of, 398–400
  and liberation, 400–401
  medical, 395
  need for new approach to, 391
  psychological, 395
  radical, 393
  for therapists, 237–238
  U.S. conceptualizations of, 392–398
Self-determination, 131
Self-esteem, 24
Self-reflection, 110
Self-report measures, 20
Sentipensando, 178

Serrano-García, I., 159, 160
Settler colonialism
  and anticolonial methodologies, 121–122
  confronting and resisting, in research, 120
  decolonization in framework of, 63
  Indigenous resistance to, 130
Sexism, 222
Sexual orientation, 336–338
Shakur, Assata, 31
Shame, 18–20
Shared knowledge, 154–155
Sheldrake, R., 311
Siempre Vivas Metro, 324
Silencing of race, 335–336
Simpson, A., 132
Simpson, Leanne, 119
Singh, A. A., 348, 375
Six Nations of the Grand River, 383
SJP (Survivors Justice Project), 185–187
Slavery, 329, 372
Slavery, narrative of, 72
Slave ships, 371
Smith, L. C., 377
Smith, Shardé, 111
Snorton, C. R., 374
Social change, advancing, 358
Social cognition studies, 26
Socialization, attending to, 250
Social justice, 236, 340, 358
Social justice action, 228–229
Social justice activism, 304
Social Justice Counseling Model, 28
Social justice ethic, 221–223
Social justice mentoring, 103
Social media, 49
Social sciences, 45
Social support, 25
Society of Indian Psychologists, 125, 274–277
Society of Indian Psychologists Commentary on the American Psychological Association's Ethical Principles of Psychologists and Code of Conduct (García & Tehee), 273, 275–277
Sociopolitical Citizenship Participatory Action Research (SC-PAR) Project, 157
Sociopolitical context
  addressing, in conceptualizations, 27
  ignored, in Eurocentric psychology, 5

therapists' awareness of, 34
of U.S. community psychology, 146
Somatic interventions, 236
Sonn, C. C., 106
Sonn, Christopher, 161
Soul, 325
Soul wounds, 301
South Africa, 175, 182–183
South African Freedom Park, 193
South Africans, 359
Space, for student voices, 223–229
Spanish language, 234–235
Spillers, H. J., 372
Spirit, teaching with, 229–233
Spirita, 354
Spiritual activism, 298, 310
Spiritual cleansings, 312
Spirituality, 297–298, 354
Spiritual pedagogy, 229
SRBCC (Segundo Ruiz Belvis Cultural
    Center), 52–55
Standing Rock resistance, 124
Status quo, resisting reinforcement of,
    263
Stevens, Garth, 161
Stewart, I. F., 382, 383
Story science, 104–105
Storytelling, 176
Straits, K. J. E., 273, 275
Strengths, recognizing, 356
Strengths-based approach
    in anticolonial methodologies,
        130–131
    to decolonial action, 212
    to decolonized psychology, 274
    for reorienting to decolonial psychology,
        253–255
Stress reduction, meditation and, 282
Strobel, L. M., 30–31
Structural equity, 102, 108–111
Substance teaching, 280
Suicide prevention programs, 129–135
Sullivan, H. S., 326–327
Super Soul Sunday, 398
Supervision
    in graduate education and training,
        228, 233–241
    RISIM in mentorship vs., 261
Survivance, 177, 304
Survivors Justice Project (SJP), 185–187
Sustainability, ethical principle of, 276
Swampscott Conference, 144

Syed, M., 380
Synchretistic healing, 295
Systemic-level interventions, 34–35
Systemic oppression, 300
Systemic racism, 222, 254
Systemic transformation, advancing, 358

T

Taino people, 340
Tait, Lawson, 75
Talk therapy, 296
TallBear, K., 371
Tate, C., 329
Tate, K. A., 210
Tatum, Becky, 16
Taylor, S., 392
Teaching, with spirit and corazón,
    229–233
Teaching-learning sites, 101, 106–108
Tebbe, Elliott, 376
Tehee, M., 273, 275–277
Tejeda. C., 210
Tension, in transdisciplinarity, 162
Teo, T., 250
Tepehuán Revolt, 124
Testimonio, 155, 305–306, 308, 310, 312
Testimonio method, 220, 232, 234
Texas Board of Education, 207
Theatre of the Oppressed, 231
Therapeutic relationship, 309–312
Thrive Global, 397–398
Tibetan Buddhist Bodhisattva vow, 282
Ticktin, Miriam, 191
Tinsley, O. E. N., 371
Tipuna Project, 178
Tlamatinime (wise ones), 273, 278–280
Tokenism, 208
Tolerance (Christian syndrome), 209
Torres-Kortright, Omar, 53
Torres Rivera, E., 52, 254, 256
Trail of Tears, rewalking, 136, 137
TransCare Collaborative study, 376
Transdisciplinarity, 159–162
Transformation and exploitation stage of
    colonization, 209
Transformative justice, 287
Transgenerational trauma, 303
Transmodernity, 279–280
Transnational feminism, 347
Transnational feminist commons, 191–192
Trauma, 332

Trauma-informed lens, 236
Tribal nationalism, 125
Tribal Nation of the Year Award, 129
Tuck, E., 76, 123, 251, 376
Tuhiwai Smith, Linda, 62, 77–78, 91–92, 176, 179
Tummala-Narra, P., 339
Two Eye Seeing perspective, 295–296
Two-Spirit, 370–371

U

UCSD Center for Mindfulness, 399
United Nations, 48
Universal Declaration of Ethical Principles for Psychologists, 221–222
Universal dialogue principles, 210
Universal theories, push for, 91
University of Puerto Rico, 324
University of Puerto Rico Mayaguez (UPRM), 48
University of Waterloo, 211
U.S. community psychology, 144–148
Utsey, S. O., 18–19, 25

V

Verizon, 397
V-formation, 401
Villanueva, E., 251
Vincularidad, 298, 306–307, 309–310, 312
Violence
    domestic violence, 185–187
    epistemic violence, 5, 121–122, 156
    gun violence, 111–112
Viray, S., 228
Vizenor, G., 177

W

Walker, M., 310
Walmart, 397
Walters, K. L., 136, 137
Warrior's Path, 312
Warrior's Path Report (WPR), xix–xxi
Warrior's Path Task Force, 283
Watkins, M., 53
Webb, Kinari, 284
Weil, Marie C., xix
WEIRD. *See* Western, educated, industrialized, rich, and democratic
Weis, L., 380

Wendat people, 324
Wendt, D. C., 222
Wengrow, D., 325
Wertham, F., 327
West, Cornell, 224
Western, educated, industrialized, rich, and democratic (WEIRD), 77, 205–207, 374
Western Eurocentrism, 250
Western Euro-settler perspectives, 223
Western (European) view of health, 277
White, heterosexual men with power and privilege (WHMP), 5
White dominance, 374
White feminism, 350, 354
White mentees
    conscientization for, 256
    de-ideologization and denaturalization for, 255
    honoring of people's strengths by, 255
    praxis for, 257
    problematization for, 256
    recovering of historical memory by, 254
White Mountain Apache Tribe (WMAT), 129–135
Whiteness, 327, 330, 372
White people, 259
White Supremacy, 192, 350, 373, 375, 390–392, 397
White supremacy culture
    and coloniality, 247
    psycolonization and propagation of, 250, 265
    and racial identity development, 251, 259
White Western psychology, 43–44
WHMP (White, heterosexual men with power and privilege), 5
WHO (World Health Organization), 395
"Who Said It Was Simple" (Lorde), 369
Williams, Bianca, 173
Wilson, Shawn, 188
Winfrey, Oprah, 398
Wiradjuri land warfare, 124
Wise Face and Firm Heart, of *tlamatini*, 278–279
With-in group discrimination, 18, 19
Wiyot people, 123
WMAT (White Mountain Apache Tribe), 129–135

Womanism, 306
  in graduate education, 230
  supervision rooted in, 236
Womanista model, 263
Womanist psychology, 353–355
Women of Color
  and embodied critical reflexivity, 150
  and feminism, 350, 354–355
  and feminist therapy, 346
  and spirituality, 354
Wonder, 276
Word-completion tasks, 20–21
World Health Organization (WHO), 395
World War II, 326
Wound, healing the, 300–302, 305
WPR (Warrior's Path Report), xix–xxi
Wretched of the Earth (Fanon), 92
Wright, R., 327

Y

Yakushko, O., 370
Yang, K. W., 123, 251, 376
Yappali: Choctaw Road to Health (Walters), 136
Yerbas, 312
Yoga, 393, 398–400
Yoga for People of Color Sangha, 400
Yoga With Adriene, 393
Youth
  and Imapcto Juventud, 48–50
  Māori, 181–182
YouTube, 383, 393

Z

Zepeda, S. J., 378
Zinn Education project, 211

About the Editors

Lillian Comas-Díaz, PhD, is a clinical psychologist in private practice and a clinical professor at George Washington University Department of Psychiatry. She directed the Yale Hispanic Clinic as a past faculty member at Yale University's Psychiatry Department. She is a former director of the Office of Ethnic Minority Affairs at the American Psychological Association (APA). Dr. Comas-Díaz is the author or senior editor of over 170 scholarly publications, including *Liberation Psychology: Theory, Method, Practice, and Social Justice* (coedited with Edil Torres Rivera; 2020); *Latina Psychologists: Thriving in the Cultural Borderlands* (coedited with Carmen Inoa Vazquez; 2018); *Womanista and* Mujerista *Psychologies: Voices of Fire, Acts of Courage* (coedited with Thema Bryant-Davis; 2016); *Psychological Health of Women of Color: Intersections, Challenges, and Opportunities* (coedited with Beverly Greene; 2013); and *Multicultural Care: A Clinician's Guide to Cultural Competence* (2012). A former president of Psychologists in Independent Practice (APA Division 42), Dr. Comas-Díaz is the recipient of the American Psychological Foundation and APA 2019 Gold Medal for Life Achievement in the Practice of Psychology.

Hector Y. Adames, PsyD, received his doctorate in clinical psychology from the APA-accredited program at Wright State University in Ohio and completed his APA predoctoral internship at the Boston University School of Medicine's Center for Multicultural Training in Psychology. Currently, he is a licensed psychologist and a professor at The Chicago School of Professional Psychology and the codirector of the IC-RACE Lab. Dr. Adames has coauthored or coedited several books including *Speaking the Unspoken: Breaking the*

Silence, Myths, and Taboos That Hurt Therapists and Patients (with Kenneth S. Pope, Nayeli Y. Chavez-Dueñas, Janet L. Sonne, and Beverly Greene; 2023); *Succeeding as a Therapist: How to Create a Thriving Practice in a Changing World* (with Nayeli Y. Chavez-Dueñas, Melba J. T. Vasquez, and Kenneth S. Pope; 2023); the sixth edition of *Ethics in Psychotherapy and Counseling: A Practical Guide* (with Kenneth S. Pope, Melba J. T. Vasquez, and Nayeli Y. Chavez-Dueñas; 2021); *Caring for Latinxs With Dementia in a Globalized World: Behavioral and Psychosocial Treatments* (with Yvette N. Tazeau; 2020); and *Cultural Foundations and Interventions in Latino/a Mental Health: History, Theory, and Within Group Differences* (with Nayeli Y. Chavez-Dueñas; 2016). He has earned several awards, including the 2018 Distinguished Emerging Professional Research Award from the Society for the Psychological Study of Culture, Ethnicity and Race (APA Division 45). Visit https://icrace.org/ to learn more about his lab.

Nayeli Y. Chavez-Dueñas, PhD, received her doctorate in clinical psychology from the APA-accredited program at Southern Illinois University at Carbondale. She is a professor at The Chicago School of Professional Psychology, where she serves as the faculty coordinator for the concentration in Latinx mental health in the Counseling Psychology Department. She also is the codirector of the IC-RACE Lab (Immigration, Critical Race, and Cultural Equity Lab). Dr. Chavez-Dueñas has coauthored four books: *Speaking the Unspoken: Breaking the Silence, Myths, and Taboos That Hurt Therapists and Patients* (with Kenneth S. Pope, Hector Y. Adames, Janet L. Sonne, and Beverly Greene, 2023); *Succeeding as a Therapist: How to Create a Thriving Practice in a Changing World* (with Hector Y. Adames, Melba J. T. Vasquez, and Kenneth S. Pope, 2023); the sixth edition of *Ethics in Psychotherapy and Counseling: A Practical Guide* (with Kenneth S. Pope, Melba J. T. Vasquez, and Hector Y. Adames; 2021) and *Cultural Foundations and Interventions in Latino/a Mental Health: History, Theory, and Within Group Differences* (with Hector Y. Adames; 2016). Her research focuses on colorism, skin-color differences, parenting styles, immigration, unaccompanied minors, multiculturalism, and race relations. She has earned a number of awards, including the 2018 APA Distinguished Citizen Psychologist Award. Visit https://icrace.org/ for more information about her lab.